ADVANCE PRAISE FOR *YOUR BODY CAN TALK*, Second Edition

I have conducted wellness seminars for thousands of health professionals over the years, and no one surpasses speaker Dr. Susan Levy in the ability to mesmerize audiences with the powerful message of how the body communicates with us to let us know what it needs. That same gift translates to her writing, and in her newly revised book, *Your Body Can Talk*, 2nd edition, Dr. Levy once again transcends the mystery of what's happening in our bodies and simplifies the steps to learn its language, allowing us to hear its story firsthand. The new additions for leaky gut, candida, children's health, etc., are fresh, captivating, and not to be missed. Version 1 taught us to listen to the body's message; version 2 is like giving the body a smartphone to increase speed and efficiency.

> **—Dr. Lynn Toohey, Ph.D., nutrition.**
> Wellness consultant, and organizer of nutrition-related and wellness seminars; author of numerous articles in peer-reviewed journals.

Dr. Levy's book is easy to read and understand. The information presented is clear and insightful, empowering the reader to exercise their health freedom rights. I feel it offers a path to success in shifting illness to wellness.

> **—Theresa I. Dale, Ph.D., C.C.N., N.P., N.D.**
> Pres & CEO: Wellness Center for Research & Education, Inc., Dean and Founder: California College of Natural Medicine, Inc. http://www.wellnesscenter.net ; http://www.cconm.com

Dr. Levy presents a great amount of valuable information in a user-friendly manner. Apply her insights and work with a professional applied or clinical kinesiologist to help in restoring and maintaining your health.

> **—Robert M. Blaich, D.C.**
> Author, *Your Inner Pharmacy*.

This is a valuable read for parents, prospective parents and professionals who have heard about or already understand the importance of holistic principles in caring for our and our family's health, and how these principles translate into do-able self care and making wise choices for using health care professionals. Dr. Levy's perspective is both broad and deep.

> **—Suzanne Arms**
> Author, health advocate, Director of Birthing The Future®;
> www.BirthingTheFuture.org

ACKNOWLEDGEMENTS FROM THE FIRST EDITION

These simple testing procedures…can be followed easily by anyone. Gives hope and enlightenment on what can be done for the mysterious symptoms that have "no pathological basis," according to orthodox approaches. I recommend it to anyone who isn't feeling optimum health.

> **—John F. Thie, D.C.**
> Author and founder, *Touch for Health*; International College of Applied Kinesiology, founding chairman.

Muscle Testing provides instant access to the knowledge which the body and mind are offering us… Integrates knowledge about the body and the way to stay well. An excellent book.

> **—Daniel R. Condron**, D.M., D.D., M.S.
> Chancellor, College of Metaphysics; author, *Permanent Healing*.

Without question, a classic…destined to become one of healing's greatest reference books of modern times. I highly recommend it.

> **—John A. Amaro, D.C., F.I.A.C.A.**
> Dipl. Ac.: International Academy of Clinical Acupuncture, President.

One of the finest texts on Clinical Kinesiology. A must have.

> **—Christopher Beardall, B.S., D.C.**

Your Body Can Talk

Second Edition

How to Use Simple Muscle Testing for Health and Well-Being

The Art and Application of Clinical Kinesiology

Susan L. Levy, D.C.

Kalindi Press
Chino Valley, Arizona

COPYRIGHT © 2014 Peaceful Valley Retreat

All rights reserved. No part of this book may be reproduced in any manner for public or private use without the written permission of the publisher, except in cases of quotes embodied in critical articles or reviews.

Design and Layout: Becky Fulker, Kubera Book Design, Prescott, Arizona
Cover: Adi Zuccarello

Library of Congress Cataloging-in-Publication Data

Levy, Susan, 1952-
  Your body can talk : how to use simple muscle testing for health and well-being : the art and application of clinical kinesiology / Susan L. Levy, D.C. -- Second edition.
      pages cm
  First published: Prescott, AZ : Hohm Press, 1996.
  Includes bibliographical references and index.
  ISBN 978-1-935826-36-1 (trade pbk. : alk. paper)
 1. Applied kinesiology--Popular works. 2. Muscle strength--Training. I. Title.
  RZ251.A65L48 2014
  613.7--dc23
                            2014026309

Kalindi Press
PO Box 4410
Chino Valley, Arizona 86323
www.kalindipress.com

Disclaimer: Any information in this book is not intended to be a replacement for medical advice. Any person with a condition requiring medical attention should consult a qualified health professional.

This book was printed in the U.S.A. on recycled paper using soy ink.

A Moment of Silence

In honor of the following individuals who have passed from this life, I express my deep and confident belief that they have indeed entered the realm of ultimate healing, wisdom, and peace.

Family
Dr. Burt Espy – passed from this life 11/19/1999
I miss you, and will always love you, my darling.

Justin Houghton – 1985-2005
Your entire family loves and misses you, we honor your memory.

Kay Lynn Willis Rogers – 1951-2014
My cousin, my childhood playmate, I miss you.

Colleagues, Mentors, Friends and Health Seekers
Dr. Alan Beardall – 1938-1987
Dr. George Goodheart – 1918-2008
Dr. John Thie – 1933-2005
Dr. Paul White – 1939-2009
Dr. Linus Pauling – 1901-1994
Dr. William Crook – 1917-2002
Anne Wigmore – 1909-1993

Dr. Otto Warburg – 1883-1970
Dr. Bernard Jensen – 1908-2001
Dr. Guy Abraham – deceased 2013
Dr. Hazel Parcells – 1889-1996
Thomas Beardall – 1973-1989
Annette Ross – 1960-2011
Dottie – 1917-2007
Debbie – 1952-2012
Arlene – 1954-2013

World Community Members
Let us acknowledge the thousands of people lost due to wars and conflicts, greed and terrorism, drug failures, addictions and overdoses; as well as those taken in natural disasters such as earthquakes, tsunamis, tornadoes, fires, floods and other such tragic events.

Our thoughts are with you, and we are thankful for our brief time together.
Your presence has made the world a better place. Farewell.

Dedication

This book is dedicated to our children and grandchildren, and their children and grandchildren. Our future is in your hands and hearts. The Great Law of the Iroquois Confederacy states that **"In our every deliberation, we must consider the impact of our decisions on the next seven generations."**

Dr. Burt Espy's children:
   Tony
   David

Dr. Burt Espy's grandchildren; sons of David:
   Cameron Anthony
   Theodore Burtis

Dr. Susan Levy's nieces:
   Chelsea and son James
   Lorrin and sons Trevin and Kingston

Dr. Susan Levy's nephews:
   Max
   John
   Sam

Dr. Alan G. Beardall's children:
   Christopher and children Amanda, Caitlin, Elena, Emily, Christina, and Christopher
   Timothy and son Teegan
   Michael
   Matthew

Dr. Paul White's Children and Grandchildren:
   Paul A. White II (Tony) and sons Anthony, Andrew and Austin
   Michele White Ediss and children Jordan, Taylor, and Megan Lisco Forgey - Great Grandchild – Mallory Jean Forgey
   Tiffany White Moore and son Cooper Moore

Dr. Linus Paulings' four children, fifteen grandchildren, and nineteen great-grandchildren

Carol Lehr's grandchildren:
   Jasmine
   Natasha

Annette Ross' children:
   Trillo and children Elisha, Nathaniel, Asher, and Jubilee
   Michael and son Cowen
   Roze and son Locke

Acknowledgements

This book could not have been possible without the contributions of so many people. I am indebted to the pioneering doctors who invested years of research into the new sciences which now bring great benefit to numerous patients. I am grateful that they have shared their expertise by teaching their colleagues, such as myself. Unfortunately, three of these pioneers have passed from this life. I was blessed to have had my life touched by each of them. Thank you Dr. Alan G. Beardall, the founder of Clinical Kinesiology. Applied Kinesiology was researched and developed by the late Dr. George Goodheart. Touch for Health, an outgrowth of Applied Kinesiology, was developed and taught to many by the late Dr. John Thie.

My enduring thanks go to Dr. John Amaro, who has digested volumes of acupuncture information and teaches his colleagues in a succinct and logical fashion. Again, my thanks to Dr. John Amaro for graciously allowing me to reproduce the excellent acupuncture meridian illustrations.

I especially want to acknowledge my late husband, Dr. Burt Espy, my primary consultant during the first edition of *Your Body Can Talk* on procedural facts, for his contribution to the field of Clinical Kinesiology. Though you are no longer here with me in the physical realm, my love for you doesn't cease. I think of you often and I love you always.

For helping me navigate the tangled and daunting World Wide Web and for all of her help and patience, I thank my niece, Chelsea. Without her the 2nd edition, would not have been possible in this decade. You need special recognition for mastering the task of reading my handwriting! Thank you for countless hours at the keyboard, at all hours of the day and night. I so appreciate your logical and systematic approach, and your uncanny ability to track down references and citations to which I barely allude. You deserve acknowledgement for reading the first edition and noting discrepancies, and out of date information. Every very right-brained person needs an extremely left-brained counterpart. Thank you, Chelsea for bringing balance.

My deep appreciation to the professional staff at Kalindi Press for their unending support and faith in this book, especially my editor, Regina Sara Ryan, for her gentle guidance and for the trust she has placed in me. Regina, I see you as a mentor, and I appreciate you. I so much appreciate the support of Dasya Zuccarello, Publisher, of Hohm Press and Kalindi Press. Thank you for bringing my work to several new audiences in Eurasia. I thank you for encouraging me to move forward to our next proposed projects.

My enduring thanks to Dr. Christopher Beardall for providing editorial contributions and valuable insights on the life of his father, Dr. Alan Beardall. My gratitude also to the late Dr. William Crook and Dr. Guy Abraham who directly counseled me during their lives. Though they have passed on from this life, their work is still significant. Thanks to Dr. Theresa Dale for graciously sharing her information and research. Special thanks to Jim Butler and Ken Lesser for their outstanding contribution on EMFs.

Thanks also to my graphic designers, Tom Mares and Edward Adamic, for their creation of the majority of the graphics in this book. To Regis University reference librarian Judy Anders for her valuable research assistance, and of course to Carol Lehr, who worked tirelessly on the first edition.

My thanks to the numerous people that worked behind the scenes on the first edition, without you this second, expanded, and revised edition would not have been possible.

During the years it took to write the first and second editions of this book, many wonderful friends stood by with encouragement, love, support and many various contributions. They are Maggie Ohmert, Glenn Ohmert, Constance Richardson, Susan Stark, Ken Lesser, Cheri Chairo, Suzanne Fox, Glenda Hanover, Trillio and Danielle Ross to name only a few.

A very special thanks to Dr. Barbra Walters for mentoring me from graduation on, and bringing many new and outside-the-box treatments and technologies to my attention. Thank you as well for your artistic contributions.

Thank you to Jody Gardner for long discussions about critically important topics, and for your thumbs of steel, when my trigger points needed goading.

Also, to my family who provided daily unconditional support and devotion, especially my mother, Allorah Jo, who remains one of my biggest supports and inspirations. I love you, Momma. Thanks to my sister Lori for lightening my load in many ways. Thanks for bringing your wonderful children into the world and to our family. I love you, Lori.

Finally, to the many patients whose stories are shared within these pages I express my gratitude for inspiring my life and, hopefully, the lives of those who will read this book.

Contents

Foreword	xiii
Introduction	xv
I: Your Body-Mind Energy System	**1**
Chapter 1: Clinical Kinesiology	3
Chapter 2: Acupuncture: The Healing Energy	24
Chapter 3: Energy and Emotions	54
Chapter 4: Divine Energy: The Chakras	73
II: Energy and the Immune System	**91**
Chapter 5: Energy and Food	93
Chapter 6: Energizing the Immune System	112
Chapter 7: Candida: Causes and Treatment	124
Chapter 8: Leaky Gut and Your Digestion	143
Chapter 9: Unfriendly Energy: Electromagnetic Pollution	162
III: The Energetic Systems of Women, Men and Children	**179**
Chapter 10: Premenstrual Syndrome	181
Chapter 11: Natural Menopause	200
Chapter 12: The Male Energetic System	215
Chapter 13: Optimizing Your Children's Health	236
IV: The Medication Dilemma	**277**
Chapter 14: Drugs: Just Say *No Thanks!*	278
V: Additional Resources	**345**
Afterword	346
Appendix: Associations and Referrals—Resources and Product Guide	349
Endnotes	356
Index	362
Contact Information	366

Foreword

The story of Clinical Kinesiology (CK) is the story of Alan G. Beardall, B.S., D.C. It begins in 1968 when Dr. Beardall graduated from the Los Angeles Chiropractic College. His desire to offer his patients the most effective technique for their particular problems led him to advance his study at over 100 different technique seminars. Each technique seminar was designed to teach the methods of dealing with one or more conditions of the body—low back pain, for example. Despite his vast range of skills, however, Dr. Beardall became increasingly frustrated by his inability to determine precisely which Chiropractic technique to use for an individual patient's needs, since many had complaints for which the generally recommended technique would do little or nothing.

Clinical Kinesiology is the outgrowth of the failure of any one system of treatment to solve all problems, since it gives the doctor and the patient the ability to determine the appropriate technique, as well as the appropriate time in which to administer it. (The most important criteria is timing. There is a "... time for every purpose ..." as the great prophet wrote.)

Clinical Kinesiology looks upon the body as a living biological computer—one with numerous complex biological functions and enormous stores of memory. Meticulously observing the blueprint of the body, the Clinical Kinesiologist searches for the underlying causes of the apparent symptoms. Once finding the "errors" at the causal level and examining the ways in which the body has adapted based on those errors, a technique can then be chosen to specifically treat the underlying cause.

In treating underlying causes, Dr. Beardall developed the most extensive research, to date, on the proper functioning of 576 muscles of the human body, together with specific methods of testing each muscle. He has invented more than fifty Core Level ™ nutrients to address nutritional deficiencies. Dr. Beardall is further credited with the development of over 300 handmodes and seventy therapies specific to Clinical Kinesiology, and has authored ten books on the subject, all for physicians.

The book you are about to read is about Clinical Kinesiology. Susan Levy, D.C. has here produced one of the finest texts on the subject. I recommend it as a "must have" for any person interested in Clinical Kinesiology.

—Christopher Beardall, B.S., D.C., L. AC

Introduction

A strong jolt and the sound of crunching metal shattered my peaceful morning drive. I knew instantly I'd been rear-ended. Being a doctor, of course I hopped out to see if the driver of the other car had been hurt. Luckily, she was fine, so I proceeded on to my office and a full day of treating patients.

As the day wore on, however, I began experiencing a bit of neck and upper back pain, so I scheduled some basic Chiropractic treatment that addressed the spine and muscles. I felt confident the problem wasn't serious. I was wrong. The pain persisted on and off for the next five years! Many times, by the end of a long day of treating others, areas in my middle back were spasmed and burning. I kept treating and hoping.

Then, in 1989 during an acupuncture seminar, I met a colleague who gave me new hope. Dr. Burt Espy had trained for four years with Dr. Alan Beardall, the originator of Clinical Kinesiology energetic muscle testing. Although I had previously observed at Dr. Beardall's clinic, I'd never been evaluated with the technique.

When he heard my symptoms, Dr. Espy offered to assess and treat my mid-back pain. With Clinical Kinesiology testing, he "asked" my body what was wrong and my body talked back. Based on what my body "said," Dr. Espy quickly determined that my problem didn't truly stem from the accident but from an underlying heart imbalance. That discovery marked the turning point in my recovery and the beginning of my personal experience with this amazing method for accessing the body's wisdom known as Clinical Kinesiology.

In a few months of treatment I fully regained the health I had lost five years before. My quick recovery inspired me to begin learning this intriguing technique for myself. With my condition dramatically improved, and new knowledge gained, I was so impressed with Dr. Burt Espy that I married him!

For many years prior to my experience with Clinical Kinesiology, I'd integrated a holistic viewpoint into my Chiropractic practice. I'd conducted numerous classes, including weekly lectures and day-long seminars for my patients, the public, special groups of nurses and even medical doctors—which enabled me to educate others on wide-ranging topics involving alternative healthcare.

After a year of extensive study with Dr. Espy and others trained in the method, I began incorporating Clinical Kinesiology evaluation, processing and testing procedures into my practice. I also began educating my patients on this new method, hence the creation of an all-new manual.

The message of this book is simple: "Yes, there is help. Yes! You can solve your health problems. And yes, Clinical Kinesiology can help you to hear what your body already knows about health and well-being."

OVERVIEW

PART I – How Your Body Talks

The initial chapters of the book serve as an introduction to the energetic system that links mind and body. In Chapter 1, learn how the body can talk, and therefore be used as a diagnostic tool to measure body "function," along with specific treatment modes that heal energetic imbalances.

In Chapter 2, discover how Clinical Kinesiology expedites the application of acupuncture and facilitates realignment of energetic imbalances.

Chapter 3 will help you understand the critical role emotions play in maintaining physical health by presenting the Chinese Five Element theory, which interprets organ/emotion relationships.

In Chapter 4, learn how Clinical Kinesiology diagnoses and allows healing of Chakra imbalances through the use of Bach Flower Remedies.

Part II – Hearing Your Body's Cries for Help

Armed with a deeper understanding of your body's multileveled energetic system, Chapters 5 through 9 will offer specific methods of fighting disease through a healthy and well-functioning energetic system and a fortified immune system.

Chapters 5 and 6 show how Clinical Kinesiology diagnoses energy sensitivity to foods, along with ways of protecting the immune system from unnecessary drugs, antibiotics and immunizations, which further undermine immune function.

Rebuilding the body's ecology following an overgrowth of unhealthy bacteria or Candidiasis is the focus of Chapter 7. Chapter 8 deals with the increasingly recognized condition of Leaky Gut (increased intestinal permeability), which often manifests as a variety of confusing symptoms. Chapter 9 provides recommendations for maintaining the integrity of the energy system through minimizing exposure to unhealthy electromagnetic fields, or EMFs.

Part III – Your Body's Messages

The next four chapters are specifically devoted to optimal health for female, male, and children's energetic systems. Chapters 10 and 11 for women address solutions to premenstrual syndrome and a healthy transition to menopause through natural balancing of body cycles. Chapter 12 educates male readers, giving them steps to maintain overall health throughout life.

Chapter 13 is practically a book in itself. This Children's Chapter discusses the beginning of life, and illustrates a road map for giving your children (and children yet to come) the best potential for optimal health. This chapter truly educates you with valuable data about lifestyle choices to optimize health, and treatment choices to minimize side effects and trauma.

Self-testing instructions and treatment recommendations for unique health problems may be found at the end of each chapter.

Part IV – The Medication Dilemma— What Does Your Body Say?

Chapter 14 presents information on both sides of the critical issue of medical drug use. The purpose of this chapter is twofold: first, to acquaint you (more specifically) with how your body actually functions; second, to share an array of natural remedies to enhance your awareness of your many non-drug treatment choices.

Few people appreciate the miraculous intricacy of the body's special innate functions—such as its own blood pressure regulation, blood sugar balancing, and sleep cycle. I will be encouraging you to celebrate your very intelligent body, seeing it as a synergistic, well-designed miracle. All of its components and systems have sophisticated methods of communicating and coordinating. I will be stressing that superimposing synthetic medications over your body's incredible design can overwhelm and unbalance many vital functions.

Self empowerment is a primary goal of this chapter, which is why I will present you with detailed charts listing different approaches and options other than pharmaceutical drugs for handling the most common disease and imbalance conditions.

Part V – Additional Resources

A Resource and Product Guide contains a list of products that complement the Clinical Kinesiology diagnostic method and are especially appropriate in the healing process. An Association and Referral Guide provides a list of organizations from which interested readers can help locate Clinical Kinesiology practitioners, or alternative healthcare providers who use similar or related diagnostic techniques and non-invasive treatments. Endnotes are also provided for cross-referencing purposes and to identify the sources used in writing the book. Additional book lists of suggested reading are also available at the end of each chapter.

* * *

I am so thankful for this wonderful legacy of Clinical Kinesiology left by Dr. Alan Beardall—the "daVinci" who has painted a portrait of the human body, the intricacies of which we have only begun to discover. Tragically, Alan Beardall was killed in an automobile accident on December 1, 1987 while on a teaching assignment in England.

For practitioners and their patients searching for long-awaited answers to renewed health, Dr. Beardall's method lives on deep within our bodies. By inspiring you to learn the language in which your body can talk, and thereby get in touch with your body's own unique energetic system, we hope you will begin to use that system for new understanding, new energy and new hope for a healthy future. May you help pass this wisdom on to future generations.

—Susan L. Levy, D.C.

PART I

HOW YOUR BODY TALKS

CHAPTER 1
Clinical Kinesiology

Carla, a forty-year-old mother of four, was desperate. She firmly believed she wouldn't live to see her children become adults. On the day she hobbled into my office she was taking no less than twelve prescription drugs. Over the years, several different doctors had "diagnosed" her condition as everything from rheumatoid arthritis to Lyme disease to lupus. Despite the diagnoses and medications, her swollen joints and excruciating knee pain quickly progressed from bad to worse. Carla came to my office as a last resort before ordering a wheelchair.

I gathered her history and long list of symptoms, then asked her to lie down on my treatment table, raise one arm and resist the pressure I applied to that arm as I attempted to muscle test her normal strength. I instructed Carla to place the open palm of her other hand over her painful knee area as I performed the muscle test a second time. This time, Carla's previously strong arm muscle responded helplessly weak.

More simple tests followed. Within minutes I pinpointed Carla's "knee" problem as stemming from a chronic kidney imbalance. Her medications and unhealthy diet had compounded the stress to her energy-depleted organs. Left untreated, the imbalance had reached the point where Carla could barely walk.

With the problem identified, I performed two or three more tests and quickly determined the appropriate treatment. The plan for Carla would involve acupuncture; vitamin, mineral, and herbal support for the kidneys; simple detoxification and additional treatments for symptom complexes relating to other organs.

Today, the idea of Carla in a wheelchair is unthinkable. Symptom-free and medication-free, she exercises, takes care of her four children, prepares healthful meals, and provides informational tours of her neighborhood health food store. With a renewed sense of self-confidence, Carla now trusts her body's power to heal itself. She is one of many who have experienced the healing benefits of Clinical Kinesiology diagnosis and treatment.

WHAT IS CLINICAL KINESIOLOGY?

On the frontier of the healing arts, Clinical Kinesiology muscle testing (the simple "straight arm" test described above) applies non-traditional, bio-energetic methods which allow you to unlock or ascertain your body's hidden messages, and obtain insightful answers to health problems you've been searching for through more traditional approaches.

Through this unique feedback system of muscle testing, you can learn how to interpret your own special "body language." Your body can "talk" simply through changing the response of the muscle test. Ask the body specific questions and you can get answers to growing health concerns, and gain valuable information which cannot be attained through traditional types of laboratory testing or symptom analysis.

Clinical Kinesiology taps into an early warning system that displays changes in body *function* before they appear physically. This new diagnostic method evaluates energetic imbalances or dysfunction "before" heart disease, cancer, or other serious disorders have the chance to develop. Using this simple noninvasive energetic-based information, a practitioner may look into the pre-disease stage and gain insights into the changes necessary. Meanwhile, traditional lab tests and physical symptoms may still be showing up normal.

Clinical Kinesiology also indicates changes necessary to pinpoint specific modes of treatment such as acupuncture, magnetic therapy, nutritional recommendations, and other holistic protocols which strengthen, cleanse, or rebalance the energy system of the body, thereby "releasing" the energy and abating any impending physical change or symptom. Since your body works like a powerful "living computer," each microscopic cell and bit of energy within that cell contains intelligence regarding body function. This vibrating energy alone exerts tremendous power to produce solutions to complex problems in the body. Clinical Kinesiology employs simple ways to tap into these same electrical connections that run the "software" system in your body.

The Origins of Clinical Kinesiology

Clinical Kinesiology monitors and tests the energetics of the body. The word Kinesiology or *kinetics* originates from the study of muscle and joint movement. From original muscle response research called Applied Kinesiology, developed by Dr. George Goodheart, D.C, in 1964, simple body movements (especially muscle movements) were used to evaluate physical functioning. Over fifty-four muscle tests were discovered and correlated to other reflex (related) points to organs and spinal segments.

In 1968, Dr. Alan Beardall, a graduate of Los Angeles Chiropractic College, became one of Dr. Goodheart's most brilliant protégés. While treating a famous marathon runner, Beardall discovered that individual muscles did not function as one unit. Through study, personal observation and testing procedures, he identified functional divisions *within* muscles, and went on to isolate reflex points which further differentiated those muscle divisions. Beardall's first paper presenting his exciting new findings was published in "Selected Papers of the International College of Applied Kinesiology."[1]

In 1975, Beardall began innovating and testing the Clinical Kinesiology method, discovering over 250 specific muscle tests while concentrating primarily on related muscle *reflexes*.

Following his first paper, Beardall also published five muscle testing instruction books from 1980 to 1985.[2] His new diagnostic method would thereafter be officially known as Clinical Kinesiology.

In 1983, while conducting a muscle test on a patient, Beardall noticed a unique phenomenon. The patient touched a painful area with an open hand and the muscle test indicated weakness. In a second test on the same injury, the patient shifted the position of his thumb and small finger. As a result, the muscle registered strong. Beardall instantly saw an exciting relationship between the hand and finger positions (*handmodes*) and the body's reaction.

This discovery allowed Beardall to further modify Clinical Kinesiology and extend his method of diagnosis to discover deeper, more underlying imbalances in the body's energy patterns. Today, many hundreds of handmodes have been discovered as "words" in a new body language.

Dr. George Goodheart had contributed all of the groundwork on Applied Kinesiology muscle testing from the Chinese acupuncture philosophy. By 1975, Goodheart became so inundated in other research projects that Beardall undertook personal research efforts himself which achieved a new measure of understanding eventually surpassing previous information from muscle testing research. Drawing from a vast education, experience and intuition, Dr. Alan Beardall integrated all major chiropractic techniques, numerous adjunctive therapies such as acupuncture, nutrition, and homeopathy, including Flower remedies and Chinese Five Element diagnostics into his verification research of Clinical Kinesiology.

"Health," according to Dr. Beardall, "may be regarded in a general sense as a robust existence, a feeling of optimum vitality and strong resistance, a state of alertness and awareness." He liked to think of it as "being able to do physically whatever you envision for yourself mentally."[3]

Clinical Kinesiology provides a new and fascinating way of communicating and healing through the inseparable energy linking mind, body and spirit.

BODY LANGUAGE: WHY CLINICAL KINESIOLOGY WORKS

In the Chinese system of acupuncture, every reflex point on your body contains electrical potential. Through stimulation of acupuncture points, the treatment re-aligns the energy in the body.

Dr. Alan Beardall's Clinical Kinesiology method also relies on the extremely precise energy connection between mind and body. Your body has been pre-programmed to sustain life. Each cell, body part, organ and energy system is genetically encoded to work for continued survival of the organism. Your brain acts as a giant "switching" center to channel this energy into action to maintain body function, coordinate messages, store data and retrieve information. As connections are made, energy flows and intelligence is communicated. Your body "talks," thus the "tapping in" to this communication through muscle testing "works."

The Brain and the Body Work Together

The brain processes information precisely like a binary (functioning on a system of "two") computer systematically turning "on" or "off" in relation to any given subject, or perception. Based on the Clinical Kinesiology test, we're looking for a "lock" or neurological reflex that's "on" or "off." This makes a muscle test that is

> ### Help for Your Health
>
> Many Clinical Kinesiology practitioners utilize the manual therapy systems developed by Dr. Beardall. These include very specific correlations between muscles, muscle divisions, neurolymphatic reflexes, organ, acupuncture, and various bony structure correlations. The study of this specific manual therapy approach is much too complex to present in *Your Body Can Talk*. A well-trained Clinical Kinesiologist will be able to design your treatment program by exploring these facets of your health concern.

strong (on) or weak (off) a simplistic, yet invaluable diagnostic tool.

If I say to you, "Don't think about pink elephants," you have to think about pink elephants! I just turned "on" the pink elephant switch in your brain. It will stay on until your brain determines the next priority, or the next important thing that it needs to think about. Then, you'll drop the "pink elephants" and move on.

When a practitioner of Clinical Kinesiology taps into your body's software system by testing a designated muscle, the muscle responds either "strong" or "weak;" the brain's way of saying "on" or "off." If a muscle proves weak during the testing of a problem area or the touching of an acupuncture point, you've uncovered a relationship which may be a clue! Many underlying stimuli cause your muscles to react as they do.

All messages from your sensory, visual, auditory and other nerve endings, including all thoughts, are processed through the brain. The brain must immediately decide, "Yes, that's important," or "No, that's secondary. Let's file that information in the subconscious in case it's needed later." (Relax, it doesn't really matter that you retain every detail in your conscious mind. After all, who reads all the junk mail?)

The part of your subconscious mind which regulates the special software program in your body is called a Reticular Activating System. While not something you have to remember or think about very much, the Reticular Activating System functions as a filtering system—working to filter data into either your conscious or unconscious mind as needed.

Imagine getting dressed each day, feeling your clothing briefly on your skin. Now, imagine having conscious and intense awareness of that cloth all day long? Imagine "feeling" all your body functions—the cellular processes, or the coursing of blood through your veins? You'd constantly be distracted and couldn't function well. Mercifully, your brain filters the unnecessary information into your unconscious mind—storing the data in your Reticular Activating System. Needed information lies just below the surface for recall and, specifically, to monitor the body. If the system records an imbalance, you're notified immediately—the body-mind works together to create a symptom.

The Right Test

In studying symptoms, Dr. Alan Beardall searched for truth and found that the key to diagnosing any problem with Clinical Kinesiology depended on the energy feedback from each individual's unique body. Dr. Beardall monitored "yin" and "yang," two forces of opposing energy in motion, taking into account each person's changing balance. The essence of treatment, he concluded, must be appropriate to the current state of the body at the time of testing. Beardall discovered this uniqueness through testing and monitoring the energetic activity of the body, rather than drawing conclusions from staid academic observation or what he "thought was needed" based on initial symptoms. Alan Beardall believed that the body knows what's going on internally, what is needed and how to heal itself.

Unfortunately, many people today spend huge amounts of money on various laboratory tests, including CAT scans, blood tests, MRIs, and virtually every other known test in the medical repertoire. Even then, most never find the true solution to "functional" problems which go undetected by modern medicine—because these tests do not take into account the energetic patterns that precede the physical—until they become full-blown pathology or disease.

Clinical Kinesiology includes the testing component for each individual which translates what is going on energetically in the body. The Reticular Activating System continually evaluates, sorts, and prioritizes possible danger, which becomes the feedback or "body language" interpreted through the muscle test. It is simple in concept and design. No longer must you depend on chemical drugs or questionable surgery to obtain answers. Your body can talk, so, simply ask it! Information from your software system relays hidden, energetic messages to the surface for consideration and indication of healing through Clinical Kinesiology muscle testing.

SYNERGY OF THE BODY

Like a jigsaw puzzle, each "piece" of your body connects to another "piece." However, modern medicine believes it can extract a piece here or there and simply discard that piece without problems. In contrast, Clinical Kinesiology relies on the synergy (the combined action or function) of all parts of the body, and recognizes that there are no "quick fixes" to maintaining your whole body. Everything affects everything else.

Only by learning the principles of how your bioenergetic system works can you happily and healthily resolve that *you are much more than just individual body parts*! Clinical Kinesiology reveals the link between pain or symptoms in one part of the body and the underlying cause of that pain or symptom. Often, the cause may not lie in the same area where the symptom manifests.

For example, think about your organs. While their functions are vitally important, they contain few pain nerve fibers. The majority of pain fibers rest on the surface of the body. Consequently, most people feel more in touch with the outer rather than the inner body. On one hand, too much conscious awareness of the body's organs would be distracting. On the other hand, the organs have so few pain and sensory fibers that one could remain unaware and detached from recognizing energetic imbalances affecting the organs.

All unbalanced organs refer pain externally to corresponding energy meridians on the surface of the body. The locus of pain depends on the segment of the body from which that particular organ developed embryologically. Theoretically, internal organs in the lower half of the body refer pain to the surface of the lower body. Upper organs refer pain or symptoms externally to the upper body.

Expressions of the Heart

The heart represents one of the body's most important organs. Dr. Burt Espy, former colleague of Dr. Beardall, confirms that during body development in the womb, the heart originated in the neck and upper thorax. Thus, the heart refers energy mainly to the base of the neck, over the shoulders, to the pectoral muscles, down the arms, and directly beneath the sternum.

In the same way, according to Dr. Espy, minor or sub-clinical heart imbalances refer pain throughout the neck, shoulder, arm, wrist, elbow or any point on the heart meridian. Pain may also be experienced in the chest itself.

Many times, heart "functioning" may be out of balance, without signaling pathology or disease. To explain further, if over half a million people in the United States die each year of heart attacks, with statistics indicating that fifty percent of them had "no previous symptoms," does that mean they had no symptoms, or that no one knew what those symptoms were?

It is unreasonable for a person to live healthily for many years with no apparent heart problem and then suddenly suffer a fatal heart attack. Does a car wear out in one day? No, it's a lengthy process. Your body doesn't wear out in one day either, and neither do any of its parts.

Many people experience chest pain but simply brush it off. "Oh," they say, "it's just indigestion." Their doctors may even concur. Undiagnosed, they go on thinking their pain is indigestion until they suffer a heart attack.

Many times, when doctors perform an EKG and a blood test for heart problems and nothing shows up, they automatically rule out the heart. Take caution: if your ongoing symptoms don't medically show severe heart pathology, look at what else they could mean.

Dr. Espy discovered that many people experience common symptoms such as fatigue, mid-back pain, numbness, swelling, wrist pain (medically known as Carpal Tunnel Syndrome), yet are not uncomfortable enough to seek treatment. However, few realize the potential seriousness of the symptoms until it's too late.

George's Story

One morning, a vague *inner knowingness* stirred in George, a fifty-five-year-old executive. He abruptly informed his wife Flora, "I think I'd better get a checkup." His doctors promptly scheduled an entire cardiac workup including stress EKG, cardiac enzyme evaluation, blood test, and chest x-ray. The results came in and all were "normal." Sadly, a few weeks later, George suffered a fatal heart attack.

Were George's medical doctors correct in assuming there was no problem prior to his heart attack simply because all his tests came back "normal"? Or, did they miss something? Let's assume we look at George's medical history for clues leading up to his fatal attack; clues that no diagnostic machine could possibly detect. No machine, that is, except for the most sensitive diagnostic tool ever created ... the human body!

Fifteen years ago, George played several rounds of golf each week. One day, he developed elbow pain. Unbeknownst to him, his heart was already energetically out of balance. The lack of sufficient energy running through his heart meridian, and added muscle stress from golfing, further compounded George's elbow pain. He decided then and there to "quit playing golf." With his elbow no longer physically stressed on top of his heart imbalance, his elbow pain eventually faded out.

Five years later in a serious car accident, George suffered a whiplash injury which resulted in a great deal of neck pain and stiffness. "Well," George reasoned, "it may take awhile, but this pain will go away too." What George didn't know was that the whiplash injury superimposed over his weak or unbalanced heart meridian would become much more serious and longer lasting than a trauma to an area with no previous imbalance.

Consequently, George's whiplash pain and his aching, stiff and burning muscles continued for two or three more years. He could have chosen any number of treatments, but finally decided he'd "... take a few aspirins every day." Afterwards, George didn't notice the pain quite as much.

George suffered four or five episodes of fairly severe chest pain in later years. Again, he chalked it up to "... just something I ate!" Thus, George battled a whole string of symptoms over the years, yet no one picked up on them; and George himself had never been taught what those symptoms meant, or how important they really were as precursors to a heart condition.

Symptoms Unnoticed

Millions of people trained in CPR (cardiopulmonary resuscitation) know the referred pain patterns of the heart meridian. CPR students are taught that prior to a heart attack the victim might notice shoulder, elbow, arm or neck pain. They may also experience upper back or jaw pain, headache or nausea. The heart meridian continuously sends energy to all those areas. However, most CPR certification classes do *not* teach students to look more broadly at what those symptoms mean throughout life.

Imagine how George's life might have changed if he or someone else had been able to diagnose these symptoms early. George might have made the necessary changes that would have allowed his heart to grow stronger instead of weaker.

Your heart, your body, and your spirit communicate with you. If you can only begin to understand its language you won't miss those early warnings that may one day save your life.

If Clinical Kinesiology testing had been widely used since the time of its development, thousands of people like George would not have died from heart attacks. Most would have known how to read their symptoms and heed the messages being sent. In correcting and making changes in these seemingly minor afflictions, they would have lessened and even dissipated their pain; their bodies would have changed to grow stronger; and their lives made longer and healthier.

ENERGETIC AND PSYCHOLOGICAL THERAPIES AND TREATMENTS

Your body contains the information for what's wrong—along with what's needed to cure it. When an initial imbalance is confirmed, Clinical Kinesiology testing may also be used to determine which aspects of treatment will be most helpful. Dr. Beardall identified three main categories of treatment based on a chemical, structural, or electromagnetic response model of the body.

Chemical

Imagine an island floating in a vast ocean. The whole ecology of the island, including the water, coral reefs, fish, trees, air, sun and sky is interdependent. Each element complements and sustains every other element. Ecological balance and survival requires the synergism of all. Your body is like this island. Its survival depends upon a balanced ecology: all nutrients working together to support the whole.

Daily, the body faces problems which reflect inadequate nutritional support. Such deficiencies promote a wide range of biochemical reactions. Chemical imbalances diagnosed through Clinical Kinesiology testing require treatment of biochemical components in the body. Diet changes and the addition of appropriate nutrients will support the body's survival.

Since all nutrients work in a synergistic relationship with the body, Beardall developed Nutri-West® Core-Level™ nutrients to strengthen the body. (These nutrients are unique because Clinical Kinesiology testing was used to formulate ingredients and dosage.) When the body chemistry tests out of balance, a Clinical Kinesiology practitioner will recommend specific nutrients to rebalance it. In addition to the Core-Level™ nutrients, other supplements such as specific vitamins, minerals, glandulars, enzymes, herbs or amino acids may be required depending on what the body is "asking for" to heal itself. (See Product Guide.)

Structural

A variety of Chiropractic treatment methods may be used to address imbalances in body structure, which include the bony joints, muscles, tendons, and ligaments. Insufficient energy balance during the fetal stages of body development often affect the body's muscular and skeletal structure, specifically in cases of spinal abnormalities such as scoliosis (a curvature of the spine).

Clinical Kinesiology identifies the structural imbalance and pinpoints the specific areas and types of tissues involved and what is needed to changes these imbalances. Structural treatments involve gentle chiropractic adjustments, muscle work, therapeutic massage, and others.

Electromagnetic

Many times, Clinical Kinesiology diagnosis indicates an electromagnetic or energetic imbalance in the body. Electromagnetic imbalances usually implicate the organs and acupuncture meridians. Different treatment methods can bring about specific results, however, Clinical Kinesiology electromagnetic considerations rely primarily on acupuncture, herbal and homeopathic philosophies of treatment (see Chapter 2). Therapeutic magnets may also be used to realign body energy, along with laser therapy and Neuro-emotional remedies (see Chapter 3) or Flower remedies—including Bach (see Chapter 4), petite, California and Western. These particular remedies work on an energetic level rather than a chemical/nutrient level. (Homeopathic remedies, which are taken under the tongue, are absorbed directly into the bloodstream without digestion. Although synergistic with the body, they are assimilated and function differently than nutrients.)

Psychological Kinesiology

It's widely thought that more than half of all medical complaints contain a strong emotional or psychological component. Identifying and reprogramming such components is the goal of Neuro-Linguistic Programming (NLP) practitioners.

Robert M. Williams, M.A. of Psych-K Centre™, in Colorado, has merged Neuro-Linguistic Programming and a branch of Kinesiology called Psychological Kinesiology to provide training courses in stress management.

NLP practitioners like Williams help people tap into unconscious thought and behavior patterns in an attempt to alter psychological responses which aid healing. Incorporating Kinesiology muscle testing, Williams utilizes NLP, auditory, kinesthetic, and visual inputs to reverse negative belief systems.

MUSCLE TESTING RESEARCH TODAY

Other recent research on muscle function as it relates to muscle testing has been completed by Dr. Craig Buhler, D.C. at the University of Utah. Dr. Buhler, the primary research associate who helped create Dr. Beardall's early muscle testing books, was the team Chiropractor for the professional basketball team, Utah Jazz for twenty-nine years, ending in 2008. During that period of time, the Utah Jazz had the lowest injury rate of any professional sports team in America.

Today, there are upwards of one hundred Clinical Kinesiologists in the United States. There are about 600 Clinical Kinesiologists throughout Europe and another 200 in Australia. Dr. Alan Beardall's son, Dr. Christopher Beardall, developed modifications of his father's original work and offer training classes for other doctors.

While it requires much study to become a fully trained, professional Clinical Kinesiology practitioner, limited self-testing may be performed by interested laypersons and others. This book will teach you some simple and immediate methods which you can use to get your body to talk about what it knows and needs for health and happiness.

LISTEN TO YOUR BODY TALK

A. Listen to Your Symptoms

The first step in using Clinical Kinesiology is to begin listening to your body by recognizing the importance of your symptoms. Remember, every symptom in your body constitutes a signal—a warning that something is not quite right.

Imagine driving your car when the oil warning light goes on. If you pay attention to the "symptom," you will stop, check the oil and supply more oil if necessary. After taking the appropriate steps, you're able to keep driving as usual.

But, if you ignore the "symptom"—or worse yet, try to cover it up by unhooking the wire that makes the oil warning light work, you'll only cover up or ignore the message. If you continue to drive, you may also ruin the engine of your car.

When you notice a symptom, it's your body computer flashing its warning light signaling that you may need to make some changes. Somewhere, something needs to be improved, balanced, or regulated. Allopathic medicine often says, "Symptoms? That's all there is to the problem! Let's get rid of them." To modern medicine, symptoms lie only on the surface, and are routinely eliminated with drugs or surgery! In essence, from the viewpoint of Clinical Kinesiology, *symptoms* are your friends—little warning messengers that should be listened to. Pay attention to your symptoms and regard them as clues. The more carefully you listen to your "body language" the more you will come to know what those symptoms mean and how to treat them. Clinical Kinesiology will show you how—through muscle test changes and handmodes related to the symptoms. With Clinical Kinesiology you can begin to achieve real insights about the interconnectedness of problems; opening and creating the opportunity for a new and balanced state of health by making the changes indicated instead of merely covering up your symptoms.

Observe your symptoms cautiously. What appears on the surface may be an important indicator of unseen problems beneath the surface. The size of most icebergs in Arctic waters can be deceiving. Ninety percent of a massive iceberg may float silently underwater, while only ten percent appears in view.

Generally, the problem is not where the pain is, as we saw earlier in George's case. Classically, acute problems are of local origin. Chronic problems manifest distantly from the pain site.

Clinical Kinesiology testing perfectly utilizes your mind-body computer in uncovering underlying causes of symptoms; it's simply the tool relied on to detect pre-stage dysfunction to disease, which your symptoms represent.

B. Listen to the Strategy of Adaptation

The second step in using Clinical Kinesiology is to recognize that your body's primary method of survival often requires that it alter its own state of physiology from time to time. Lacking adequate energy to support the body, the body's living computer develops adaptive strategies to continue operating at reduced efficiency and robustness, Dr. Beardall discovered. When unable to operate at optimal function, the body performs an "adaptation," the process of removing current energy patterns from affecting current body functioning rather than allowing itself to become open to disease. Clinical treatment of such a reaction entails healing indirectly by removing layer upon layer of adaptations until your body's own innate intelligence is once again able to heal itself.

An oyster represents a good example of an adaptation. In order to tolerate the tiny grain of sand in its shell, the oyster makes its situation livable by secreting a substance known as mother of pearl. By surrounding the grain of sand, the oyster successfully adapts to a potential problem that once threatened its life by creating a pearl as its adaptation. The body performs the same action through rechanneling energy, changing posture or eventually accepting disease.

Treating a series of adaptations in the human body requires dissolving or breaking through those many layers of protection. Lori's story explains how Clinical Kinesiology does this.

Lori: Case Study of an Adaptation

During one of many educational seminars, I tested Lori, an audience participant with a pain complaint in her left shoulder. As instructed, Lori lay down for testing, raising her right arm perpendicular to her body. I firmly pushed against her arm while she resisted. Confirming the apparent strength or strong response of Lori's right arm as an "indicator" muscle enabled me to use it to perform further testing.

Lori identified her left shoulder as her major area of complaint. Touching the painful area with her free hand activated Lori's "on" button in her brain. (Remember pink elephants?) Now, Lori could not avoid thinking about her painful shoulder and her "indicator" muscle instantly tested weak. In this way, her body confirmed the shoulder problem.

Lori's weak muscle response indicated an insufficient flow of available energy to one of her meridians; *thus her inability to maintain enough strength for resistance.* Her Reticular Activating System channeled the most important information, her painful shoulder, and communicated it through the Clinical Kinesiology muscle test. At this point in time, Lori's shoulder pain represented only her most noticeable symptom.

To form a complete diagnosis, I needed more specific data to move into the root of her problem. Why was her shoulder really hurting? What inner problems radiated such pain to the surface? What adaptations needed to be treated?

Each test supplied more and more data—more hidden information.

Dr. Alan Beardall, as mentioned earlier, developed specific finger positions known as handmodes, which serve as messengers or electrical connections to the brain. I instructed Lori to touch her fingers together in certain ways, and change the position of her arm. This triggered energetic reactions which enabled me to categorize Lori's problem as structural, biochemical, or electromagnetic.

I continued the investigation through a process of elimination, monitoring her body muscle responses, loading and re-loading data, and saving information in Lori's marvelous "living computer."

Using the specific handmode for organ imbalance, I instructed Lori to curl three fingers into her palm along with her index finger touching her thumb.

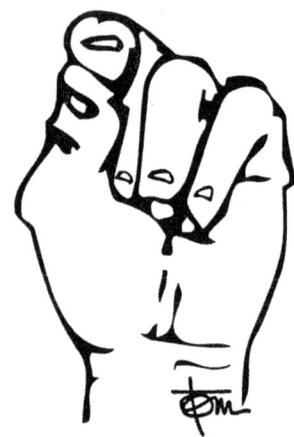

HANDMODE FOR TESTING ORGAN IMBALANCE

Weakened and wobbly, Lori's muscle reaction indicated that her shoulder pain was connected to a specific organ in her body. But which organ was involved? I tested several.

With my help, Lori located her pituitary gland and placed her hand on the area. With her mind trained on her pituitary, I tested. Her indicator muscle remained strong. Next test? The thyroid. Again, her muscle held strong. Finally, the heart. Lori resisted, but her muscle instantly responded weak.

The pain energy had traveled somewhere else since Lori's heart lacked enough pain fibers to make it actually "hurt." And so, programmed to avert a serious heart problem, the pain/energy "stepped down" a notch on the heart meridian, localizing specifically at Lori's left shoulder. In this masterful way, pain diverted away from the affected organ serves as a warning signal. (An adaptation represents one or more ways the infinite intelligence of the body strategizes to produce solutions which allow survival or protection of life.)

Lori's heart was so energetically stressed that it wanted desperately to tell her something was wrong. Through her shoulder pain symptom, her body was crying out, "Stop, slow down, pay attention to me. This is your heart speaking!" Fortunately, by using Clinical Kinesiology muscle testing, interpretation of the heart's message didn't go unheard.

As in Lori's case, most challenging heart stress symptoms generally stem from inadequate diet, negative emotions, genetic weakness and prolonged mental or physical stress. Eventually, by cutting down stress, using acupuncture treatment, adding supplemental nutrients to her diet and realigning her body through chiropractic adjustments, Lori's body was rebalanced. This made her heart happy and re-energized enough that her left shoulder stopped hurting.

Listen to your body. Adept at hiding underlying or secondary problems, it is programmed to draw attention to the most critical problem first in locations or ways you may not expect.

APPLY CLINICAL KINESIOLOGY RIGHT NOW

When people first see the Clinical Kinesiology muscle test being performed they often experience shock and disbelief. Reactions to the procedure range from, "It looks kind of weird!" to "There has to be some trick!" Or, they challenge that the "testers" are not testing the muscles with consistent strength.

The principles of Clinical Kinesiology testing remain simple:
- The person performing the testing asks questions and tests the body's response through strong or weak indicator muscles.
- The individual being tested communicates the reservoir of data (all the internal information about his or her particular body function) through the language of muscle responses.

Through self-testing you can discover:
- Which specific energetic imbalances or chemical sensitivities exist in your body.
- The health status of various organs, acupuncture points, and meridians.
- The specific and ideal treatments which will enhance your health.

Pre-Conditions for Accurate Testing

Before beginning the Clinical Kinesiology muscle testing procedure, certain checks and balances may be required to optimize the accuracy of your test.

1. *Make sure the person being tested is not distracted by any other activity.*

    A simple activity such as gum-chewing can divert the conscious mind, adding an unwanted stimulus into the temporomandibular jaw joint (which holds many nerve endings leading to the brain). If a test subject had a history of problems with the jaw joint or bite function, a negative input might be sent into the brain, resulting in a weak muscle test. The results of this test would not reflect a "true" response from the muscle.

2. *Put aside any items which may cause a negative influence on the test-subject's electromagnetic system.*

    The body's electromagnetic system is extremely sensitive. A conflicting influence in a subject's energy field, such as a bottle of prescription medication or pack of cigarettes in his or her pocket, would disturb normal muscle test results. Absolutely avoid having cellular phones or other electronic devices in the testing area.

Items such as wristwatches need to be removed. Other jewelry items are rarely suspect, but it's good to keep these checks and balances in mind as jewelry may interfere with testing.

3. *Make sure the test-subject is properly hydrated prior to testing.*
Following a sequence of tests, you sometimes find a person's arm wobbly when it should be strong (especially during a simple preliminary indicator test). Several influences may be involved, but dehydration is the primary problem to look for. It's always a good idea to have a test-subject drink some water prior to testing.

4. *Maintain a healthy atmosphere for accurate testing by eliminating interfering factors.*
Performing Clinical Kinesiology muscle testing in a building with extreme electromagnetic disturbances may affect the test. (Later, we'll explain how you can test a person for his or her sensitivity to electromagnetic fields.) Always be wary of any testing in a high-voltage electrical power line area or within a building that contains a great deal of high-technology equipment such as computers, programmable controllers, Wi-Fi, wireless security systems, and other uninterrupted electric power supplies. Choose another location, or improve the electromagnetic condition of the area by turning off all electrical appliances before you proceed.

A private atmosphere affording complete relaxation is much more desirable than the middle of a busy cafeteria. Avoid places where testing becomes a spectacle; where hoards of people become interested and want to watch. The onlookers may learn something, but the person being tested may become nervous or self-conscious. Such conditions do not allow the most accurate testing to occur.

Also avoid loud music, disturbing noises, traffic sounds, noxious or industrial smells, chemical odors and other disruptive sources of input which may affect your test. Bright lights are a negative factor, especially if the test-subject is light sensitive. Use dim lighting or a table lamp rather than fluorescent lights to cut down on stress from electromagnetic output.

5. *The Mind Set*
Be emotionally and intellectually neutral to avoid interference with your test. Keeping your mind neutral and unattached to the outcome is most important. Your thoughts and preferences could alter the test. Periodically remind yourself to be neutral. Remind yourself to "search for the truth," as Dr. Alan Beardall often counseled his students. (Your practice training described below may seem to contradict this principle. After some practice runs, reinstitute mental neutrality.)

6. *The Testing Instrument*
Carefully calibrate the testing instrument (yourself). After assuring that the five previous conditions are met, perform a few "trial runs." Perform a few simple practical tests that have easily anticipated outcomes. For your practice tests, you will be testing to feel the distinct difference between a strong muscle response (a yes) and a weak muscle response (a no). For a practice or

calibration test, you could test for compatibility of various household items to see how they affect your energy field, or the field of the person you are testing. Here are some examples of items to consider using: fruit or vegetables (organic is always best) to which you or your subject have no known allergy or sensitivity, motor oil, dish soap, or anti-freeze. Another method is to verbalize a truthful statement, saying "the sky is blue," and an untruthful statement, such as "the sky is polka-dotted." By doing these practice tests that have obvious outcomes, you are actually discovering how the muscle responds, and you can begin to feel the difference between a strong response and a weak response.

Below is a concise chart of sample options for your preliminary testing.

HOW TO MUSCLE TEST

The Technique

1. The Best Position:

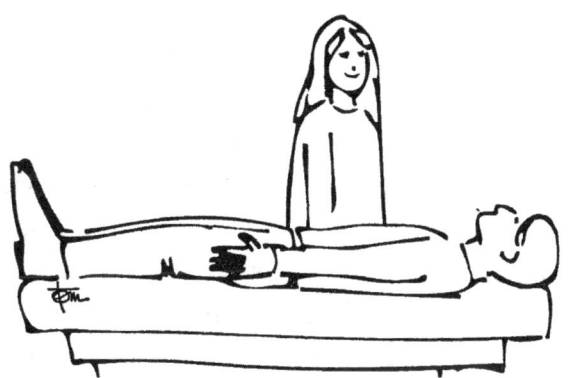

The typical Clinical Kinesiology muscle test utilizes a group of muscles which support the shoulder. For accurate testing, the person being tested should lie down. This position increases the chances that all other muscles of the body remain relaxed.

If it's inconvenient to test an individual who is lying down, you may test the subject by having him/her sit up or stand. Seated is preferable to standing, however, because in standing the body is more likely to become off balance, resulting in an inaccurate test. A person standing can also widen his or her stance, thereby gaining firmer support than normal. Tightening muscles throughout the body or recruiting other muscles will skew the test results.

2. The Elbow Straight:

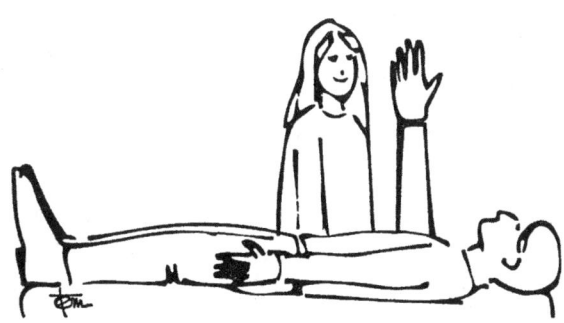

Only the shoulder muscles are needed to secure an accurate test. Of course, the more comfortable and relaxed the person, the more reliable the test.

The person lying down raises her or his dominant arm (for most people, the right arm is stronger) at a ninety-degree angle perpendicular to his or her body. The arm should be held stiff,

Chart of Sample Options for Preliminary Testing.

Anticipated STRONG or YES Response	Anticipated WEAK or NO Response
• Purified drinking water • Fruit or vegetable • Statement: "The sky is blue" • Statement: "This is yes"	• Soda pop • Motor oil, antifreeze, or dish soap • Statement: "The sky is polka-dotted" • Statement: "This is no"

but not rigid. The elbow must be straight, or otherwise functional changes in the arm muscles can cause inaccurate and unreliable test results.

3. The Push and the Resist:

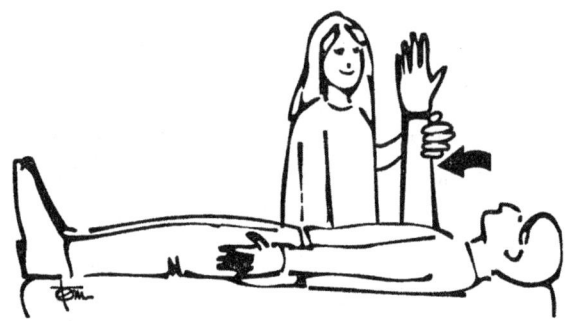

The tester should stand at a forty-five degree angle facing the test-subject's right side and may use either arm to perform the test. One arm's length from the test-subject's upright arm should assure a comfortable position.

Once assuming the correct positions, the tester places the flat or palm of his or her hand at the top of the wrist of the person being tested and performs the muscle test by pushing down toward the subject's feet. Begin by commanding the subject to gently "resist" the tester's push.

An alternative method for testing a subject in a sitting position requires the person to hold his or her arm directly out in front of the body, parallel to the floor. The tester then exerts pressure with an outstretched palm against the wrist of the subject, bearing downward while the subject resists.

If the person being tested is physically weak or unsure of the level of pressure to apply, encourage him or her to exert more energy or strength. It's a good idea to take several "trial runs" or practice tests with a new person to guide them in facilitating the test.

4. The Monitor:
Always monitor the accuracy of the arm position as the tests are administered. Most people tend to drop the arm back toward the head which results in more of a mechanical advantage. They unknowingly become stronger by utilizing extra muscles which support the backside of the shoulder. As always, correct positioning is imperative in performing an accurate Clinical Kinesiology muscle test.

5. The Muscle Response:
Some testing situations prove more difficult than others to ascertain whether a weak or strong muscle response is being given. This happens for a few reasons and may be remedied by the following appropriate steps.

Watch for significant differences in strength between the tester and test-subject. Frail, ill, elderly persons or small children require less force than a strong or robust person. In this case, a tester may need to use only two fingers instead of the whole palm of the hand during evaluation.

In opposite cases, a test-subject (a muscular body builder, for example) may be much stronger than the person doing the testing. Lowering the testing table often helps in this situation. Or, begin by testing a particularly "toxic" substance (such as sugar), which renders *everyone* weak. Test at various table heights until a comfortable and accurate testing position is determined.

In confusing situations, it's also helpful to lower the test-subject's arm to between a forty-five and ninety degree angle as opposed to the standard ninety degree angle. Experiment with finding a different angle which allows the tester a little more leverage, while not overpowering the test-subject.

If the test is unclear, *retest, retest, retest*! Change the conditions. Assess the test-subject's comfort level, the tester's position, and both persons' relative strengths. Determine such incompatibilities with good testing procedures and then test several times to find the most consistent (and most accurate) answer.

6. Surrogate and Self Testing:

These techniques are most utilized when you have no testing partner, or need to test for someone who is unable to fully participate. Surrogate testing is a good choice when testing someone too weak or injured to perform a test, or when you need to test an infant or young child. You can even use surrogate testing for your pets. When surrogate testing, you often include another unimpaired person who touches or holds (for children) the test subject. The surrogate must keep a neutral mind and look at and focus on the subject being tested. From an electromagnetic viewpoint, the surrogate is simply an extension cord for the electrical system of "energetic current." The person performing the test uses the straight arm of the surrogate. The tester focuses on the subject as well. Surrogate testing is mentioned and illustrated in Chapter 13: *Optimizing Your Children's Health*.

Self testing is best performed by an individual testing one of his/her own limbs, rather than doing a finger test. I feel that the finger-only testing method is not as accurate or reliable as using a limb. The arm or leg is a long lever compared to a finger, and is less likely to fatigue or "give out."

Use either your arm or leg in the sitting or standing position. If sitting to test yourself, sit comfortably on a sturdy chair, not a swivel or rocking chair. To self test using your leg while standing, brace yourself or lean against a counter or wall. Otherwise the instructions for testing while sitting or standing are the same. To test your leg strength, elevate your right knee (and therefore thigh) so that your right foot is about four to six inches off the floor. Attempt to firmly hold your thigh up, basically parallel to the floor. Hold the item to be tested in your left hand. Place your right hand directly on your right thigh, keeping the palm and fingers flat, and push down (toward the floor).

For testing arm strength, hold one arm straight forward at shoulder height, parallel to the floor. Place the outstretched fingers on the other hand just slightly above the wrist of your testing arm. Keep the palm and fingers of the testing hand flat, just resting above the other wrist, not clutching it. Firmly hold the testing arm stationary as you then push down or toward the floor with the other (the pushing) hand. If you want to test yourself for compatibility with a food or supplement, hold the item in your testing arm (the straight arm), or place it in your pocket. You should be able to discern between a weak and a strong muscle response. I strongly advise doing several practice tests to get the feel of the process.

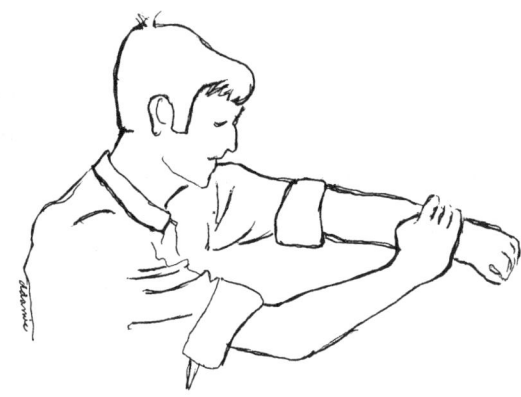

In the event your responses are not as described, you may have an energetic switching or brain balance problem. These are easily remedied, but must be addressed before accurate testing can be performed. The first step to remedy a switching imbalance is to vigorously rub the Kidney 27 acupuncture points (K27). Be sure to rub both the right and left points as shown on the Kidney Meridian illustration in Chapter 2: *Acupuncture: The Healing Energy* (page 39). The second step to remedy an energy switching or imbalance is to drink a glass of water, and to be sure you and the subject are hydrated. Recheck your technique, steps 1-5, and keep practicing. If you still have difficulty achieving an accurate response, seek hands-on guidance from a Kinesiology practitioner.

The Indicator Muscle Test

In order to establish a baseline for comparing the strength of a test-subject's muscle, you need to perform what I call the "Indicator-muscle test." The second purpose of this test is to ask the body whether it is O.K. to proceed with the test. Remember to keep your mind neutral and detached from the outcome.

Either arm of the subject or tester may be used to check the initial strength of a test-subject's indicator muscle. If, of course, the test-subject has a painful arm or a problem with one or the other, refrain from testing that arm.

To confirm the strength of the indicator muscle, have the test-subject lie down and, for convenience, test the person's right arm, simply because many people are right-handed. Since you may want to perform a number of tests at one time, the dominant arm usually has more endurance than the other. Using the right arm is often more energetically balanced as well.

> Assume Test Position + Muscle test + Strong Indicator arm = Proceed with further testing

Therapy Localization

Therapy localization, or TL, is the diagnostic term used to evaluate problem areas through Clinical Kinesiology muscle testing. For example, using the therapy localization procedure to evaluate a test-subject complaining of knee pain requires the following:

Step 1: Always begin testing by first performing preliminary indicator muscle test.

Step 2: Instruct test-subject to place his/her left hand on the painful knee area, while tester performs the muscle test on the subject's right or opposite arm.

Step 3: If the muscle test renders the arm weak, it's an indication that a problem exists in the knee.

This diagnosis is referred to as a positive TL or positive therapy localization. The pain or imbalance has been localized and the patient can now seek correct therapy.

> Therapy Localization/(Touch Problem area) + Muscle test + Weak arm = Positive TL = See Chapter 2 for complete lists of symptoms associated with imbalances of each acupuncture meridian, along with suggested treatment alternatives.

Applied and Clinical Kinesiology are evaluation tools used by many Chiropractors as well as other natural healthcare practitioners, and other health-minded individuals. I use Clinical Kinesiology along with physical examination and palpation to pinpoint spinal misalignments or subluxation.

At the age of ten months, Joey had not mastered crawling. He tried and tried, yet when he went to propel himself forward on his right knee, he would fall to the right. I tested Joey, using surrogate muscle testing. It was obvious that his sacrum (tailbone) was torqued in a clockwise malposition. Gentle Chiropractic adjustment was applied to his sacrum to reposition it. The next day he was in a car seat all day, going home (several hundred miles away). The following morning, when he had floor space to explore, Joey crawled as if there had never been an issue. Joey's parents and grandparents were overjoyed, and perhaps a bit surprised about the results of his treatment. When they called to report the wonderful news, I was pleased, but in no way surprised—I fully expected this outcome!

Therapy localization may be used as a screening test to determine imbalances in the body's organs. Some of the more important and more commonly affected organs in the energetic system are the heart, lung, liver, kidney, and pancreas.

Heart Test

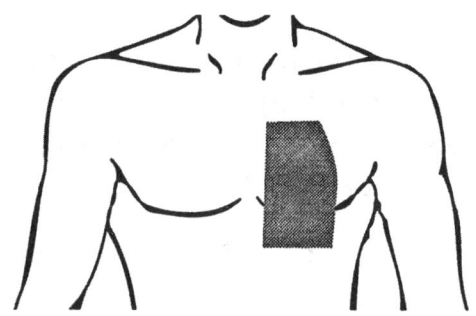

Therapy localizing for the heart has been determined by the pathway in which the heart energy projects onto the surface of the body. While anatomically the heart rests mostly mid-line in the upper body, its energy pathway radiates slightly to the left side of the chest. To therapy localize, the test-subject lays his or her hand palm down to the left of the sternum or breastbone (instead of directly on the body mid-line).

> Heart TL (Touch over heart) + Muscle test + Weak arm = Heart imbalance = Seek guidance from an alternative healthcare professional.
>
> Heart TL (Touch over heart) + Muscle test + Strong arm = Heart balance

Analyzing Heart Test Results

Immediately following a weak muscle test, you will still not have enough information to determine if a heart imbalance is mild, moderate, or severe. However, on the first test, you will know an imbalance of some type exists. For most people, the heart test proves mild or moderate. In comparison, the test of someone with a documented heart problem may prove extraordinarily weak.

> ### Helpful Hint
>
> One caution: Following a weak heart test, do not be frightened into thinking you are about to suffer a heart attack or heart disease. A weak test simply alerts the test-subject that the heart may be out of balance and require follow-up testing by a knowledgeable practitioner. The practitioner then uses more advanced Clinical Kinesiology techniques to further evaluate the problem and recommend treatment.

Lung Test

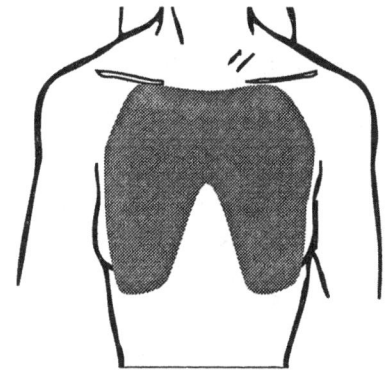

To locate the lung for muscle testing, the person being tested should first outstretch the fingers of the opposite hand from the arm being tested, then place the outstretched hand from the mid-line of the sternum and over the right side of the chest. Try to avoid touching the heart area (on the left) to avoid getting crossed information.

Do not use the back of the body for testing the lungs because of its conflicting and close contact to the ribs and the spine. Lung energy is better projected through the front of the body.

> Lung TL (Touch over lung) + Muscle test + Weak arm = Lung imbalance = Seek guidance from an alternative healthcare professional.
>
> Lung TL (Touch over lung) + Muscle test + Strong arm = Lung balance

Lung balance depends on several factors. If the person being tested smokes currently, or has been non-smoking only one to three years, more than likely the lungs will prove weak during therapy localization. In addition, anyone who suffers from asthma or bronchitis will probably prove weak during the muscle test.

Helpful Hint

It is unnecessary to take a deep breath, or to stress the lungs in any way during the muscle test. In some cases, where a very mild lung problem has been diagnosed, or reasonable, natural treatment has been pursued, the lung may still prove strong. However, it's best to refrain from running up a flight of stairs before the test—or the test may turn up weak.

Liver Test

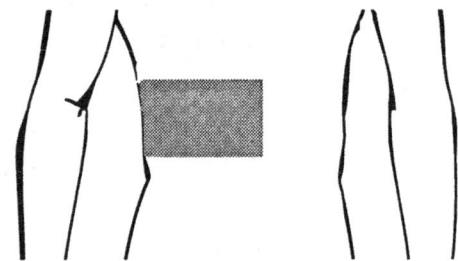

Large and floppy, the liver covers nearly one quarter of the upper abdomen. During therapy localization, the liver may be evaluated by the test-subject laying one hand over the lower-right rib cage, with the remaining arm free for testing. Normally, the lower four to five ribs contain the liver.

> Liver TL (Touch over liver) + Muscle test + Weak arm = Liver imbalance = Seek guidance from an alternative healthcare professional.
>
> Liver TL (Touch over liver) + Muscle test + Strong arm = Liver balance.

If the correctly performed muscle test results in a weak arm, therapy localization has determined that the liver may be out of balance, under too much stress, or not functioning correctly.

Helpful Hint

Therapy localization over the liver also means touching the gallbladder area or energy field. If a weak muscle test is determined in this area, consult with a natural healthcare practitioner for further guidance on whether the test is linked specifically to the liver, the gallbladder or both. A well-trained Clinical Kinesiologist will quickly determine the root issue by properly using organ finger modes. In either case, give special attention to your diet; avoid toxins such as additives and preservatives; reduce excess fats, and lessen environmental pollution.

Kidney Test

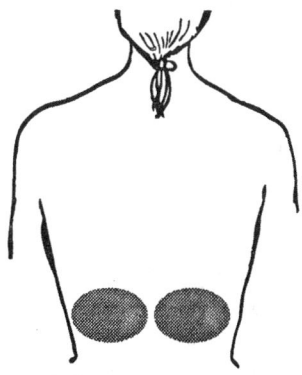

The kidney is another important organ commonly found to be out of balance in many people. Therapy localizing for the kidney is performed on the posterior of the body. The kidney's center line rests more toward the back of the body than the front and is deep to the skin, ribs and muscles.

To test the kidney, the test-subject uses the flat palm of the hand laid over the lower back, or, the lowest four or five ribs. Each kidney should be tested separately. Generally, the kidneys function together; the right and left kidney meridian and the two kidneys combine as one energy circuit.

Kidney TL (Touch over kidney) + Muscle test + Weak arm = Kidney imbalance = Seek guidance from an alternative healthcare professional.

Kidney TL (Touch over kidney) + Muscle test + Strong arm = Kidney balance.

I've treated two patients who each had one kidney removed. The first patient, Ermalinda, had a tumor, while the second, Eddie, sustained a damaged ureter (the drainage tube that runs from your kidney to your bladder) and had the kidney removed as a child. When I therapy localized over the area of the missing kidney in each, obviously the body registered an energetic disturbance. Automatically, both patients' arm muscles were rendered weak.

Upon testing the opposite kidney in each, I found another weak arm test. Because of the energetic balance of the kidney system, the whole circuitry had been disturbed. The remaining kidney in each patient was working double time.

Many people do live a full, long life with only one kidney. However, that kidney probably is working very hard. Try to test both kidneys to

Helpful Hint

If the kidneys test out of balance, it's very important to begin drinking a great deal of good-quality water. The amount of water to drink equals the amount which makes your urine appear practically clear. If you take B vitamins, for the next few hours your urine will appear bright yellow. Once the excess is excreted, the urine should become clear. In addition, the darker the urine, the more dehydrated the body. Of course, leaving out soda pop, coffee or other similar stressors on the kidney will also facilitate a better balance.

If you or a family member is dehydrated, consider using the following electrolyte replacement drink.

Mix together:
1 quart of water
½ tsp of sea salt
½ tsp of baking soda
½ cup of freshly squeezed fruit juice
  for flavor (optional)

determine any kidney imbalance in the body's energetic system.

Pancreas Test

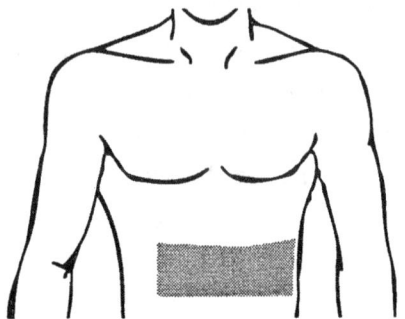

A pancreas imbalance may be present in someone with hypoglycemia or diabetes. In either case, the area used for testing the pancreas may be found by locating the spot directly in the middle of the inverted V between the right and left halves of the rib cage.

Using only fingertip touch, locate the pancreas—a long, horizontal organ which overlaps the lungs, small intestine, and stomach. Attempting to cover the entire pancreas with your hand may result in a weak muscle test, which may be inaccurate since you may actually be testing the other organs in close proximity.

To avoid overlapping of other organs, touch the tiny space in the narrow V between the ribs. Approximately two inches down from the apex of the inverted V you'll find the pancreas. It's important to therapy localize with only fingertip contact, even though the pancreas is a large organ.

> Pancreas TL (Touch over pancreas) + Muscle test + Weak arm = Pancreas imbalance = Seek guidance from an alternative healthcare professional.
>
> Pancreas TL (Touch over pancreas) + Muscle test + Strong arm = Pancreas balance.

> **Helpful Hint**
>
> Following any weak muscle test response, be sure to avoid sugar and refined carbohydrates of all types. To strengthen the pancreas, you may need additional B vitamins and trace minerals as well as further help through acupuncture, nutrition and lifestyle adjustments.
>
> Anyone with undiagnosed, severe hypoglycemia in younger years who continues on the same dietary path, will risk becoming a victim of a much greater health consequence—adult onset diabetes.

YOU ARE THE EXPERT

The Afterword of this book contains a valuable Organ Meditation exercise which will guide you in balancing and strengthening each of your organs. Take a minute now to locate (page 346-348) and read the Organ Meditation. As you read through each of the book's chapters feel free to incorporate all or part of the Organ Meditation in your healing work on specific organs or for other daily health challenges.

Your magnificent mind-body computer is the expert on energetic diagnosis, treatment and healing. The body knows which organs or systems are out of balance and which treatments help to rebalance. With Clinical Kinesiology you ultimately take more responsibility for your health and well-being.

Improving the chemical, structural, and electromagnetic balance in your body restores energy flow to all of these systems, while also giving relief to the organs that share those systems. Restored energy affects the entire mind-body balance. Consequently, you think and feel differently. Your healing has begun.

You've now learned how the body can "talk," and therefore be used as a diagnostic tool to measure body "function." In addition to discovering the history and principles of Clinical Kinesiology, you've also practiced how to apply the method. In Chapter 2, *Acupuncture: The Healing Energy*, I'll introduce you to *specific* treatment modes that heal energetic imbalances and show you how to answer your body's own unique "alarm" system that can help deactivate illness in your body's energy system.

CHAPTER 1 SUGGESTED READING

Diamond, John, M.D. *Life Energy: Using the Meridians to Unlock the Hidden Power of Your Emotions.* New York: Paragon House Publishers, 1998.

———. *Your Body Doesn't Lie: A New Simple Test Measures Impacts on Your Life Energy.* New York: Warner Books, Inc., 1983.

Frost, Robert, Ph.D. and George J. Goodheart, Jr., D.C. (Foreword). *Applied Kinesiology, Revised Edition: A Training Manual and Reference Book of Basic Principles and Practices.* Berkeley, Calif.: North Atlantic Books, 2013.

Goodheart, George J., D.C. *You'll Be Better, The Story of Applied Kinesiology.* Geneva, Ohio: AK Printing, 1989.

Hetherington, Michael, L.Ac. *The Art of Self Muscle Testing for Health, Life and Enlightenment.* Brisbane, Australia: *www.michaelhetherington.com.au*, 2013.

Holdway, Ann. *Kinesiology: Muscle Testing and Energy Balancing for Health and Well-Being.* Rockport, Mass.: Element Books Ltd., 1st edition, 1997.

Lepore, Donald, N.D. *The Ultimate Healing System: The Illustrated Guide to Muscle Testing & Nutrition.* Salt Lake City, Utah: Woodland Publishing, 1998.

Ornish, Dean, M.D. *Dr. Dean Ornish's Program for Reversing Heart Disease: The Only System Scientifically Proven to Reverse Heart Disease without Drugs or Surgery.* New York: Random House, 1996.

Rich, Mark. *Energetic Anatomy: An Illustrated Guide to Understanding and Using the Human Energy System.* Dallas, Texas: Life Align, 2004.

Shepard, Dr. Stephen Paul. *Healing Energies.* Provo, Utah: Woodland Health Books, 1983.

Thie, John, D.C. and Matthew Thie, M.E. *Touch for Health* 2nd Ed. Camarillo, Calif.: DeVorss & Company, 2012.

Whitaker, Julian M. *Reversing Heart Disease, Revised Ed.* New York: Warner Communications Co., 2002.

Williams, Louisa L, M.S., D.C., N.D. *Radical Medicine: Cutting-Edge Natural Therapies That Treat the Root Cause of Disease.* Rochester, Vermont: Healing Arts Press. 2011.

Valentine, Carole and Tom Valentine. *Applied Kinesiology: Muscle Response in Diagnosis, Therapy, and Preventative Medicine (Thorson's Inside Health Series).* Rochester, Vermont: Healing Arts Press, 1985.

CHAPTER 2

Acupuncture: The Healing Energy

One of the first myths surrounding the development of acupuncture retells the story of a young warrior in ancient China. The warrior had been plagued with an ongoing physical disorder for many years. One day, in the midst of a brutal battle, the young warrior suffered a spear wound to his body. Miraculously, when he recovered from the spear wound he discovered that the previous disorder was healed as well. As the theory goes—that spear puncture stimulated a blocked energy pathway in the warrior's body, and the released energy, or *ch'i*, was enough to cure him!

WHAT IS CH'I?

It's been over five thousand years since the ancient Chinese discovered a subtle energy in the body that cannot be seen, felt or found in any way with the senses. Philosophers believed that two opposite ends of the spectrum—*yin*, the energy of earth and *yang*, the energy of heaven—combined with the human to create this vital energy.

From that discovery, the Chinese identified the "Twelve Branches" or the twelve acupuncture meridians along which this energy travels in the human body. Call it *spirit*, the *enlivening spark*, *life essence* or whatever you choose. The ancient Chinese call it *ch'i*—the pure, harmonizing and free-flowing energy that sustains all of life.

Various Chinese sages have philosophized over the healing properties of this unique and mysterious energy. Throughout history, many different views and approaches have evolved from the wise Chinese about how to perfect physical health.

CLINICAL KINESIOLOGY AND ACUPUNCTURE

Dr. Alan Beardall integrated the philosophies of anatomy, physiology and acupuncture in the development of Clinical Kinesiology.

The Chinese were especially concerned with eliminating energy blockages in the energetic body channels. They created intricate maps of the body's energy system, and used acupuncture needles to draw awareness to specific areas or points where energy blockages occurred, thereby rebalancing the channels. Clinical Kinesiology energetic testing utilizes this significant tool of treatment in correcting energy imbalances in the body's structural, biochemical and electromagnetic systems.

This chapter will be devoted to the electromagnetic aspect of healing explaining the basic importance of maintaining balanced energetic health through the introduction of the energy or *ch'i* that circulates throughout the body, much like an electrical system.

Clinical Kinesiology taps into your system of flowing energy, monitors its activity, accesses vital information, and retrieves it. Clinical Kinesiology incorporates practical aspects of acupuncture theory as an early warning response system for discovering energetic blockages in the body. Familiarization with the different pathways of body energy helps further identify the symptoms that signal deep energetic imbalances.

The material presented in this chapter will help you to:

- Gain new understanding of how acupuncture treatment corrects depleted, excessive or imbalanced energy supplies, making it possible to achieve new healing.
- Recognize the connectedness of each organ/meridian. Use the Acupuncture-Energy Body Clock to assess the symptoms of specific imbalances.
- Compare various therapies designed to treat organ/meridian imbalances such as—acupuncture, acupressure, laser and magnet treatment.
- Improve the energy related functioning of your body through self-testing of acupuncture alarm points.
- Determine existing energetic imbalances in your own body.

YOUR INVISIBLE ENERGY SYSTEM

Ch'i circulates along acupuncture pathways or energy channels in the human body (referred to as *meridians*) in a similar way that radio waves travel through space. Although they go unnoticed, radio waves jam the room in which you are presently sitting. Turn a radio on and tune it into one of the bands that conducts radio transmission, and the radio plays!

Acupuncture meridians are like an electrical energy system running throughout the body. Although imperceptible, like radio waves, electricity moving faster than the speed of light continuously charges the body. Your nervous system contains a "visible" set of electrical "wires," while the acupuncture system channels an invisible set. But, watch out! Even though no physical wires appear to identify meridian location, when acupoints are stimulated sparks may fly!

Matter Is Energy

Imagine the nucleus or center of an atom with electrons flowing around the center. As the electrons move, they emit energy, which spins off from the atom. This energy radiates away from the current, producing an electromagnetic field containing both magnetic and electric force.

Science affirms that solid matter—a table, lamp, even the human body—is comprised of mostly empty space, i.e., the space between the atoms and their components. Matter simply consists of focused or *kinetic* energy.

Try tossing a ball back and forth. While the ball sits immobile, it expresses stored or potential energy. Toss the same ball through the air and watch its energy become activated. Now, imagine an arc of energy flowing to the place where the ball was tossed. The arc symbolizes energy that has now dissipated in space—energy released from the movement—or kinetic energy. The same energy releases from every single atom at all times within your body and within every object around you. In short, you are a bundle of energy!

In *Your Body Doesn't Lie*, author Dr. John Diamond states that, "... all illness starts as a problem on the energy level."[1] In light of this theory, the more knowledge acquired about the movement or blockage of *ch'i* and the resulting energetic effects in the body, the greater advantage we have in learning to prevent illness and correct imbalances.

Measuring the "Invisible"

Dr. Y. Nakatani, M.D., the forefather of the modern-day Japanese electronics industry, developed the *Ryodoraku*, an instrument that may be used to scientifically validate *ch'i*, an energy that remains elusive and etheric.

The *Ryodoraku* supplies electrical output readings of human electromagnetic fields called Electro-Meridian Imaging, or an EMI exam. EMI is a term coined by Dr. John Amaro. Through the International Academy of Medical Acupuncture, Dr. Amaro teaches doctors to use

Sample energy reading of human electromagnetic field.

the *Ryodoraku* or Electro-Meridian Imaging procedures. Dr. Amaro is one of very few who teach this procedure in the United States. The *Ryodoraku* measures the specific energy level and balance in the body's twelve main acupuncture meridians.

Practitioners use a wet cotton swab attached to an electronic probe to touch certain acupuncture points. Each instrument reading is then written down and composed into an energy graph.

Although treatment does not rely solely on this information, the graph indicates an overall view of the body's health.

While acknowledging the *Ryodoraku* as an important "scientific" tool, the same diagnostic testing may be accomplished through Clinical Kinesiology muscle testing. If touching an acupuncture point on the body renders the "indicator" muscle weak, the body is talking— telling you that one or more meridians may be energetically out of balance and need help.

YOUR ORGAN/ENERGY SYSTEM

Using acupuncture energy pathways has led holistic healers through the ages to ascertain the body's inner workings. The ancient Chinese saw no differentiation between acupuncture meridians and corresponding organs. They never spoke of an organ (such as the kidney) and its meridian as separate components. They simply referred to both as one system.

The energy/organ system so intertwines that it's not unusual to experience knee pain, for example, when the kidney becomes unbalanced. The reason? The knee is located directly along the course of the Kidney Meridian (see chart of Kidney Meridian page 39). If an organ/energy pathway is blocked, off balance or "complaining" a bit, that condition is usually connected to a problem in the organ.

Energy Body Clock

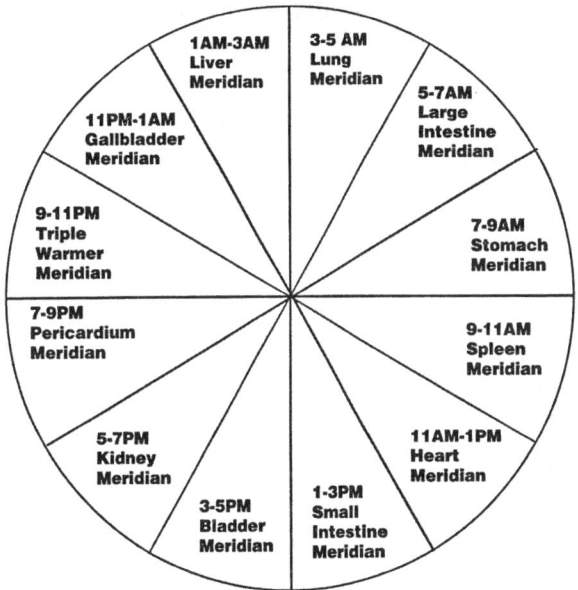

Energy Body Clock

According to Chinese theory, energy throughout the acupuncture meridians travels in a circular pattern or moving "body clock" of energy. Every two hours, the main supply of energy predominates in one of the twelve meridians. For example, from 3 to 5 A.M. the major energy in the body centers in the Lung Meridian. Two hours later, it moves to the Large Intestine Meridian and so on.

It's interesting when patients say, "At 3 A.M. I always wake up and have this symptom," or, "I experience low energy every day at 5 P.M." Significant symptoms may be identified from such statements. The meridian that requires energy and proves active at the time may not be sufficiently balanced and strong.

HEALING ... STRAIGHT AHEAD!

We are about to embark on an important trip through the body's energy highways. Remember, there are twelve major meridians, but no road signs. As we travel, consider the journey as a means to:

Daily Symptom Log

MERIDIAN	Sunday	Monday	Tuesday	Wednesday	Thursday	Friday	Saturday
3–5AM Lung							
5–7AM Lg. Intestine							
7–9AM Stomach							
9–11AM Spleen							
11AM–1PM Heart							
1–3PM Sm. Intestine							
3–5PM Bladder							
5–7PM Kidney							
7–9PM Pericardium							
9–11PM Tri-Warmer							
11PM–1AM Gallbladder							
1–3AM Liver							

- Help you recognize the energetic pathways of major organs and their connectedness to each body part.
- Provide you with a map of the territory of your self—along with easy instructions for use.
- Stimulate you to begin to question your own symptoms and how they might relate to other organs.
- Help you monitor any early-warning signs of energy roadblocks.
- Create new energy at your fingertips.

As you begin to locate the points on your own body realize that acupuncture meridian points follow much the same path on every human being. However, although anatomically similar, each body is also very, very different. According to charts, acupuncture points may typically be found at specific locations; nonetheless, on occasion one might have to probe slightly "off course"—a half-inch in one direction or another—to pinpoint the energy imbalance correctly.

As you follow along with the descriptions of the meridians:

- Try to identify each pathway in your body by tracing your finger along the route described. Note any areas of unexpected tenderness or tissue indentation you might encounter.

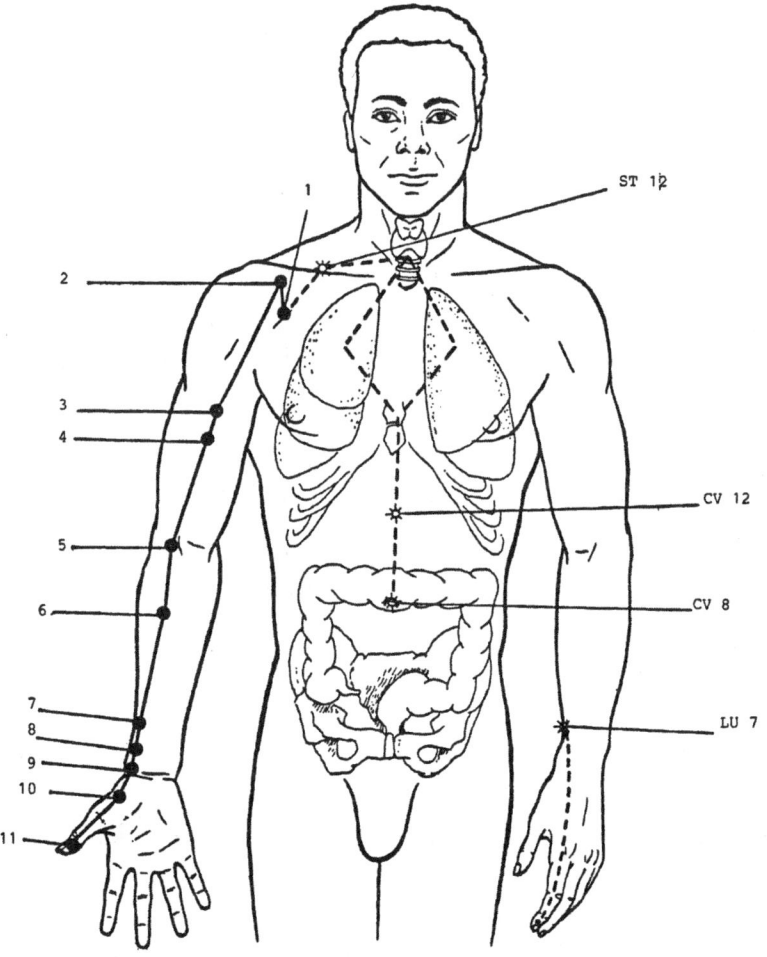

LUNG MERIDIAN
ILLUSTRATION COURTESY OF DR. JOHN AMARO,
INTERNATIONAL ACADEMY OF CLINICAL ACUPUNCTURE. COPYRIGHT © 1981.

- Begin to consider how your energy ebbs and flows throughout the day or season of year.
- Notice any instant feedback from your body, i.e., pressure on a point resulting in body sensation elsewhere.
- Refer to the sample body clock chart included in this section, and use the Daily Symptom Log to record any symptoms that occur at certain hours of the day. Review your symptoms after one or two weeks.

The Lung Meridian 3-5 A.M.

An early riser, the Lung Meridian represents the first meridian in the energy cycle. Originating by the shoulder, the Lung meridian progresses down the arm to the thumb. At first you may wonder how this meridian relates to the lungs when it travels a pathway down the arm. The energy of each organ and meridian system can be thought of as a circuit connecting joints, muscle areas and organs. Considering the embryological development of the human body also helps clarify the reasons why each energy pathway connects to its own distinct and distant areas. As the human embryo grew and stretched, its organ/energy pathways also developed and reached into distant parts of the body.

Study each acupuncture chart in this chapter closely. *You'll find that most of the major meridians also connect to one another deep inside the body.* On the surface of the body the meridians also circulate closely, within a half-inch to an inch of connecting with each other. Each meridian also runs on both sides of the body—mirroring itself.

Symptoms of Lung Meridian Imbalance

Quite simply, lung stress equals heart stress. The following symptoms may also implicate the Lung Meridian in other disorders:

- Throat or trachea soreness, vocal cord problems, coughing
- Sweating, shortness of breath, difficulty breathing, tightness of chest, bronchitis, asthma, emphysema
- Shoulder, elbow, or wrist pain, bulbous thumb (enlarged joint)
- Tightness of diaphragm
- Diarrhea, constipation, colitis

Jenny's Story

Jenny suffered from asthma since childhood. In a critical state, she used a minimum of two different asthma inhalers four times a day. After a particularly acute attack, her doctor prescribed a steroid drug. Continuing side effects finally convinced Jenny to pursue other options of treatment.

Clinical Kinesiology testing confirmed Jenny's lung imbalance, which was immediately addressed with acupuncture. Specific points on the lung meridian required stimulation. Additional Core-Level™ lung nutrients (see Product Guide) and other herbs and vitamins strengthened Jenny's lungs enough that she discontinued the use of inhalers. She has now been free of medication for many years. In fact, Jenny requested that I record in her file that she felt she no longer had asthma.

The Large Intestine Meridian 5-7 A.M.

The Large Intestine Meridian follows next in the circulation of energy or *ch'i*. The first, most obvious points on this meridian concentrate in the face and arm. The meridian flows from a point on the index finger from which the energy travels up the side of the arm to the shoulder and scapula. The energy then inches all the way up to the side of the nose.

Symptoms of Large Intestine Imbalance

In some cases, the following problems indicate an imbalance in the large intestine:

- Irritable bowel syndrome, intestinal noises, abdominal pain, swelling
- Constipation
- Teeth, nose, sinus problems
- Neck stiffness
- "Bursitis," shoulder or forearm pain, tennis elbow
- Stiffness of index finger, hand pain or weakness

The Stomach Meridian 7-9 A.M.

The Stomach Meridian originates directly under the eye, drops down the face, curves around the jaw, circulates back up into the head, then travels from the neck all the way down through the body to the second toe.

Symptoms of Stomach Meridian imbalances most often call for treatment of points on the leg for the following symptoms:

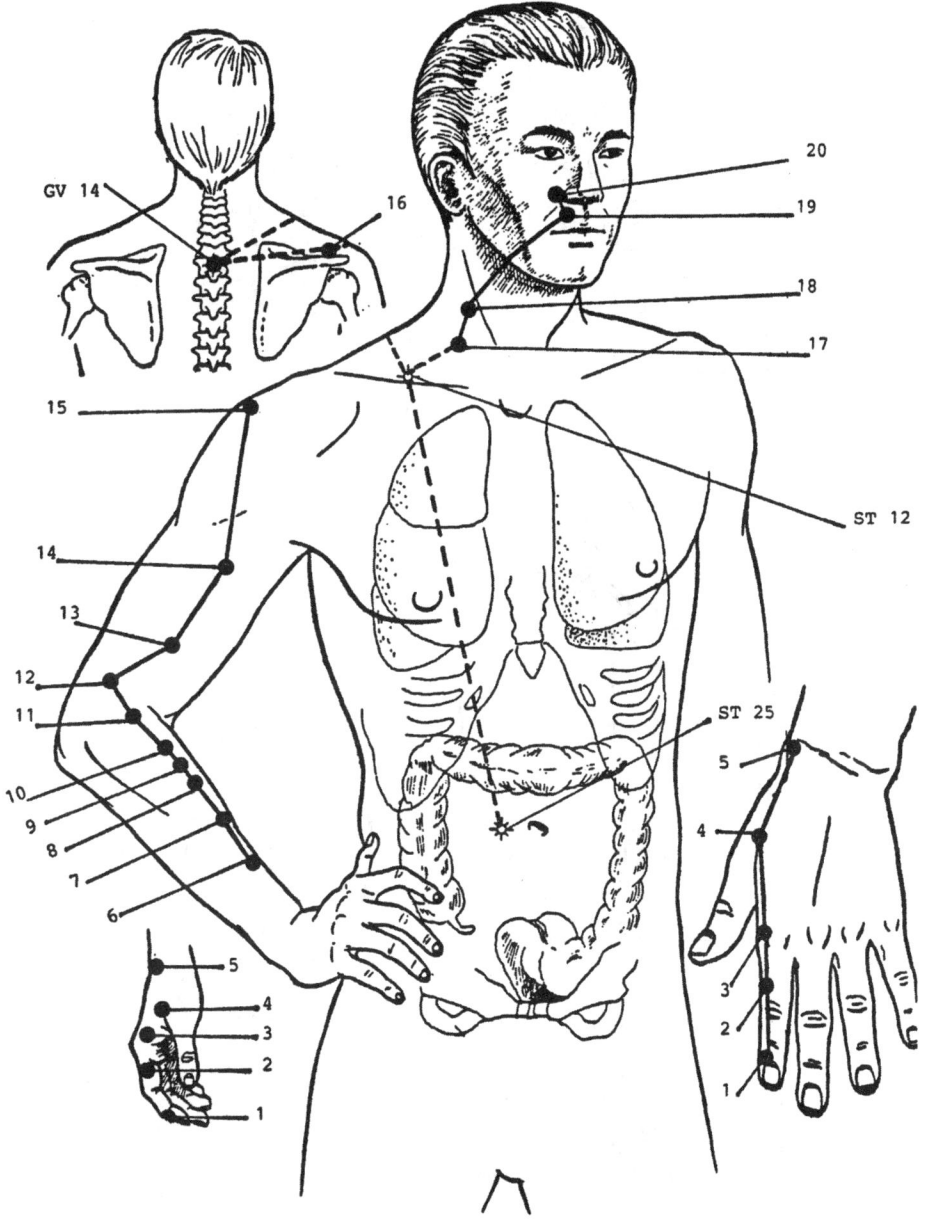

LARGE INTESTINE MERIDIAN
ILLUSTRATION COURTESY OF DR. JOHN AMARO,
INTERNATIONAL ACADEMY OF CLINICAL ACUPUNCTURE. COPYRIGHT © 1981.

- Headache, sinus or jaw pain
- Stiff neck, swollen throat
- Tightness of chest
- Stomach, digestive and gastrointestinal problems (hunger pangs, gastritis)
- Hiatal hernia, ulcers
- Pelvic, thigh pain
- Knee and shin problems

Many imbalances of the Stomach Meridian result from a lack of hydrochloric acid (or HCL) and other digestive enzymes in the body. Lack of HCL causes food to linger in the stomach for longer periods than normal, becoming an irritant. *More acid*, not less acid, may be needed. Clinical Kinesiology may be used to quickly evaluate such problems as well as to determine the dosage

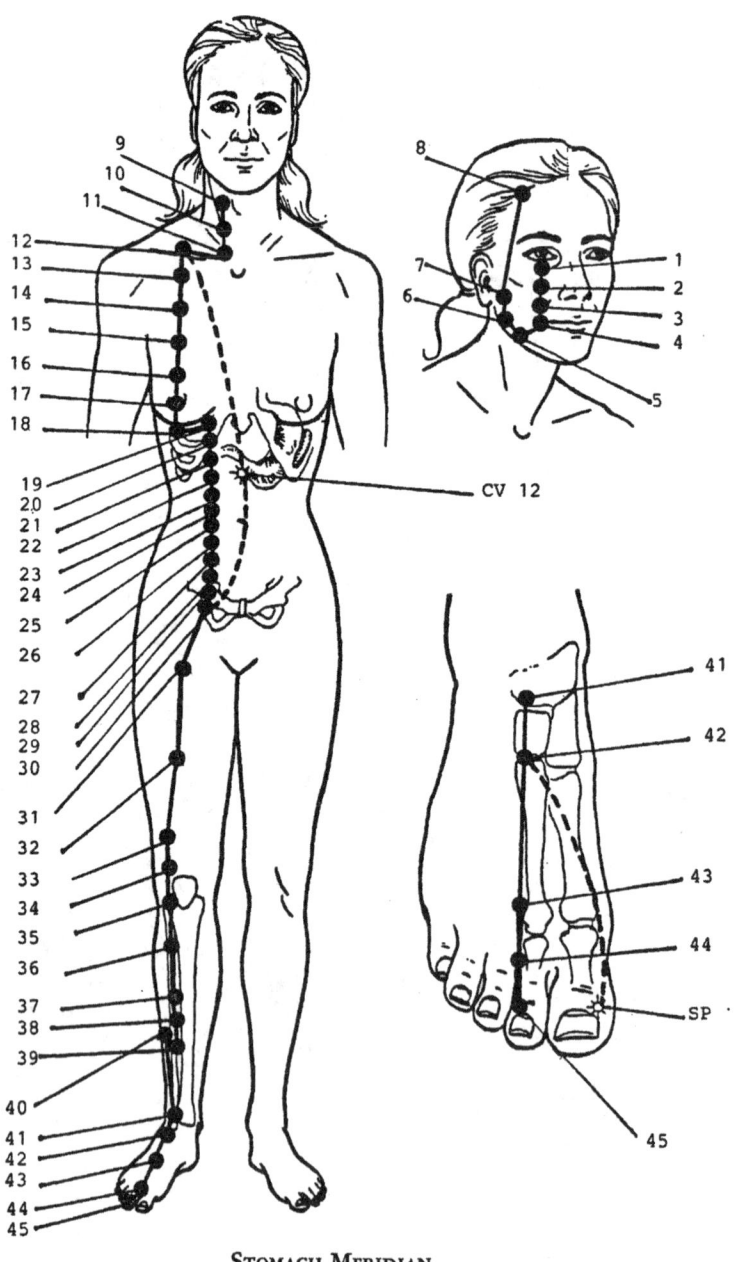

STOMACH MERIDIAN
ILLUSTRATION COURTESY OF DR. JOHN AMARO,
INTERNATIONAL ACADEMY OF CLINICAL ACUPUNCTURE. COPYRIGHT © 1981.

needed to correct the imbalance. Please refer to pages 109-110.

The Spleen Meridian 9-11 A.M.

The Spleen Meridian may be regarded as a priority connecting point for all the meridians. Its pathway zigzags up and down both sides and terminates under the arm on the side of the body. When an energy chart composed with the *Ryodoraku* indicates several meridians out of balance, treating the Spleen Meridian first proves helpful in beginning the rebalancing.

When I needed treatment for a heart imbalance following a car accident, Dr. Burt Espy

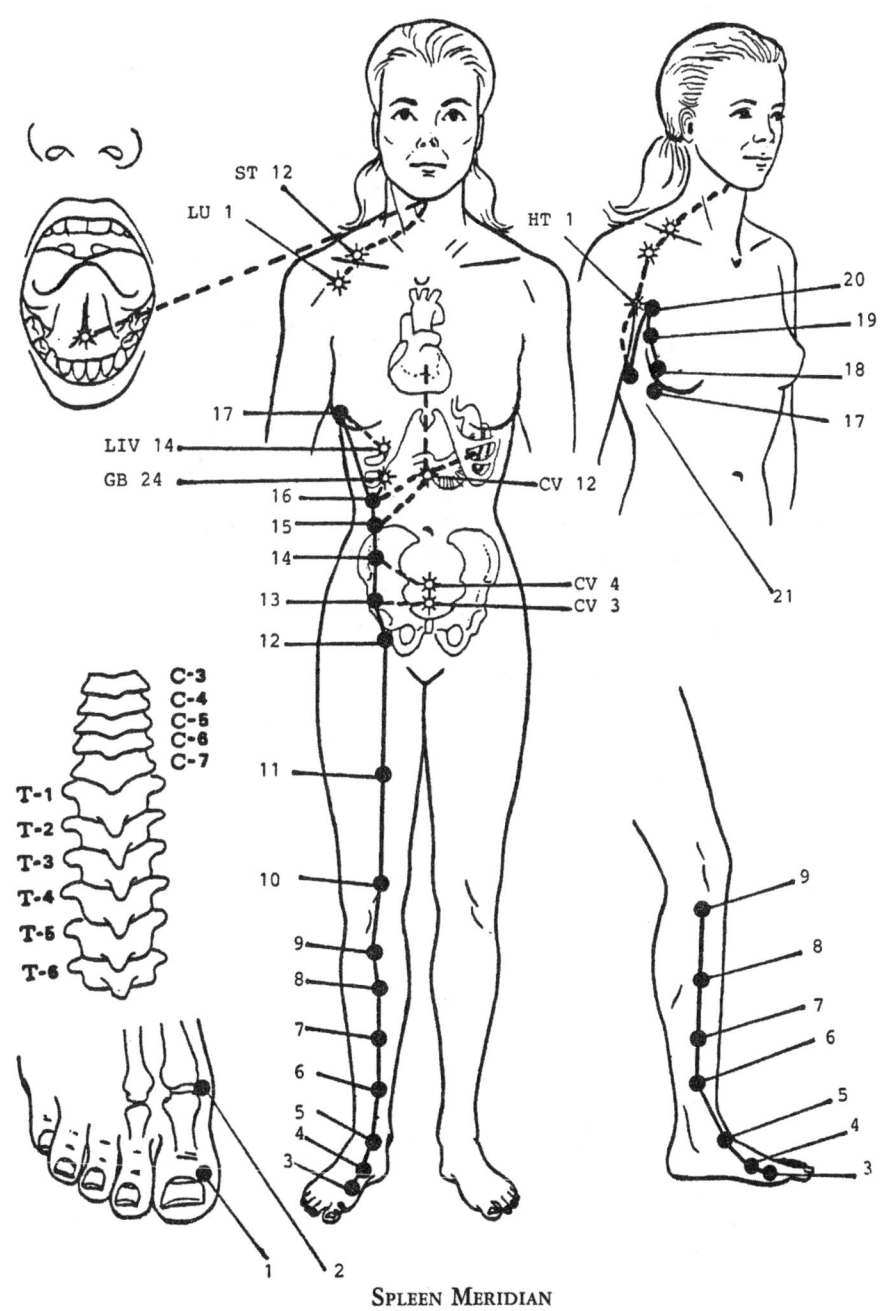

SPLEEN MERIDIAN
ILLUSTRATION COURTESY OF DR. JOHN AMARO,
INTERNATIONAL ACADEMY OF CLINICAL ACUPUNCTURE. COPYRIGHT © 1981.

treated my Spleen Meridian along with my Heart. The Spleen's internal points travel upward through the neck and directly cross over the Heart Meridian. In my case, Clinical Kinesiology testing results deemed this treatment necessary to expedite the healing process.

Symptoms of Spleen Meridian Imbalance

The spleen regulates the quality of blood in the body. Complaints that signal Spleen Meridian imbalance include:

- Lymphatic congestion
- Loss of appetite, nausea
- Abdominal pain, distention
- Stomach and/or pelvic problems, female imbalances
- Limb fatigue
- Leg, knee, thigh pain

The Heart Meridian 11 A.M.-1 P.M.

Because heart problems affect today's society so prominently, the Heart Meridian "reigns," perhaps,

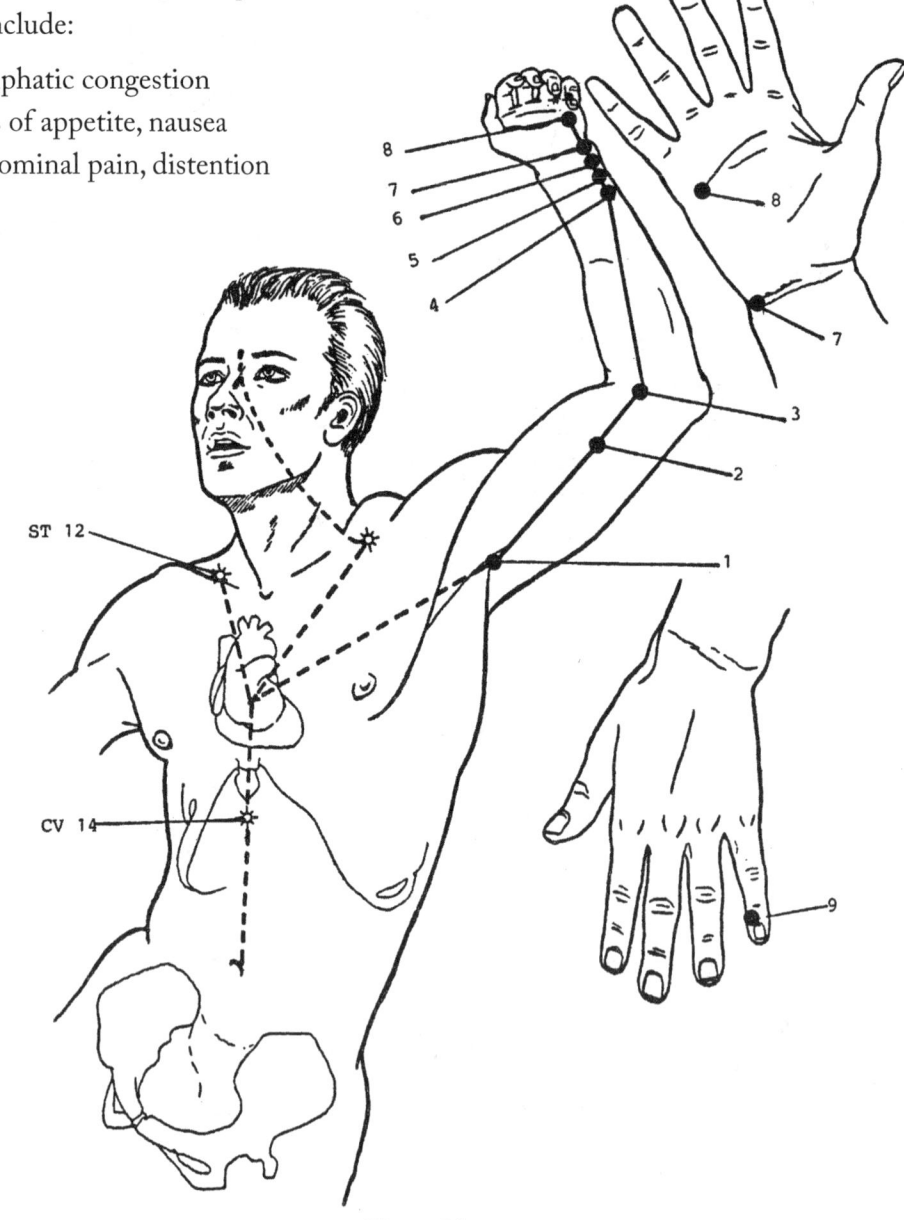

HEART MERIDIAN
ILLUSTRATION COURTESY OF DR. JOHN AMARO,
INTERNATIONAL ACADEMY OF CLINICAL ACUPUNCTURE. COPYRIGHT © 1981.

34 YOUR BODY CAN TALK

as the body's most important meridian. Its energy pathway commences under the armpit and wends down through the elbow and wrist, dissipating on the little finger. The very deep, internal part of the meridian extends into the heart itself, down into the digestive system, and finally, returns through the neck, head, jaw, and face.

Symptoms of Heart Imbalance Heart imbalances often manifest as:

- Headache, face pain
- Dry mouth, nausea
- Heart palpitations, chest pain
- Arm pain/ache, numbness
- Stiffness or pain of neck, forearm, elbow joint, small finger
- Mid-back pain or stiffness
- Weak wrists/carpal tunnel syndrome
- Digestive disorders, constipation, food allergies
- Swollen ankles
- Varicose veins

Vera's and Marian's Stories

Two women came into my office one day with the same complaint— aching pain along the crease of the nose. Vera accidentally bumped into a door. Three months later her pain still hadn't subsided. Marian was involved in a car accident. All of her resulting pain had cleared up except for the same nagging pain near her nose.

Interestingly enough, acupuncture charts show that the nose crease lies directly on the end point of the Heart Meridian. Clinical Kinesiology testing of each woman confirmed the need to treat the Heart Meridian of both after which their similar problems healed.

Heart Taboo

A strange taboo exists in our culture toward people acknowledging heart problems. While in nursing school, I presented a paper on this subject. Then and now, it's curious to me that people with any type of chest pain or other heart symptom seem bound and determined to deny its existence.

So many people say, "Me? Heart problems? No way! That wasn't chest pain, only indigestion." Even as children, we're trained not to acknowledge the true feelings or genuine expression of our hearts. Consequently, the stifling of the heart in this culture manifests even more heart problems. The word "heartburn" is generally a misnomer used to refer to an acid reflux condition involving the stomach. However, "heartburn" may be right on as a descriptor of this sad syndrome of heart "burnout" in our culture.

The Small Intestine Meridian 1-3 P.M.

The Small Intestine Meridian greatly influences the digestive system, in partnership with several other meridians. A great deal of the digestive process is accomplished in the small intestine.

This meridian springs forth from the side of the little finger, moves up the lateral or outer edge of the hand, forearm and elbow and then travels around to the back of the upper arm, shoulder joint, and across to the scapula. Here, it crisscrosses the upper trapezius muscle, winds around to the latter or back side of the neck to the cheek, and ends in front of the ear.

Symptoms of Small Intestine Imbalance

The Chinese refer to the end point on the Small Intestine Meridian as "listening palace." Symptoms of possible imbalance are:

- Ear problems, tinnitus, sore throat
- Sore temporomandibular joint
- Digestive difficulties, intestinal flu, diarrhea
- Abdominal pain
- Lateral shoulder pain, arm pain and stiffness

- Malabsorption of nutrients
- Crohn's disease

Alexa's Story

Sixteen-year-old Alexa was brought to my office doubled over in pain. Her mother reported that Alexa, overcome by nausea and vomiting, had been too sick to move. I helped Alexa lie down and stretch out slowly, and performed a Clinical Kinesiology muscle test. Immediately her body feedback signaled the appendix. Within seconds, acupuncture and laser treatments on the Small Intestine Meridian promoted a marked improvement in Alexa's color and severity of symptoms.

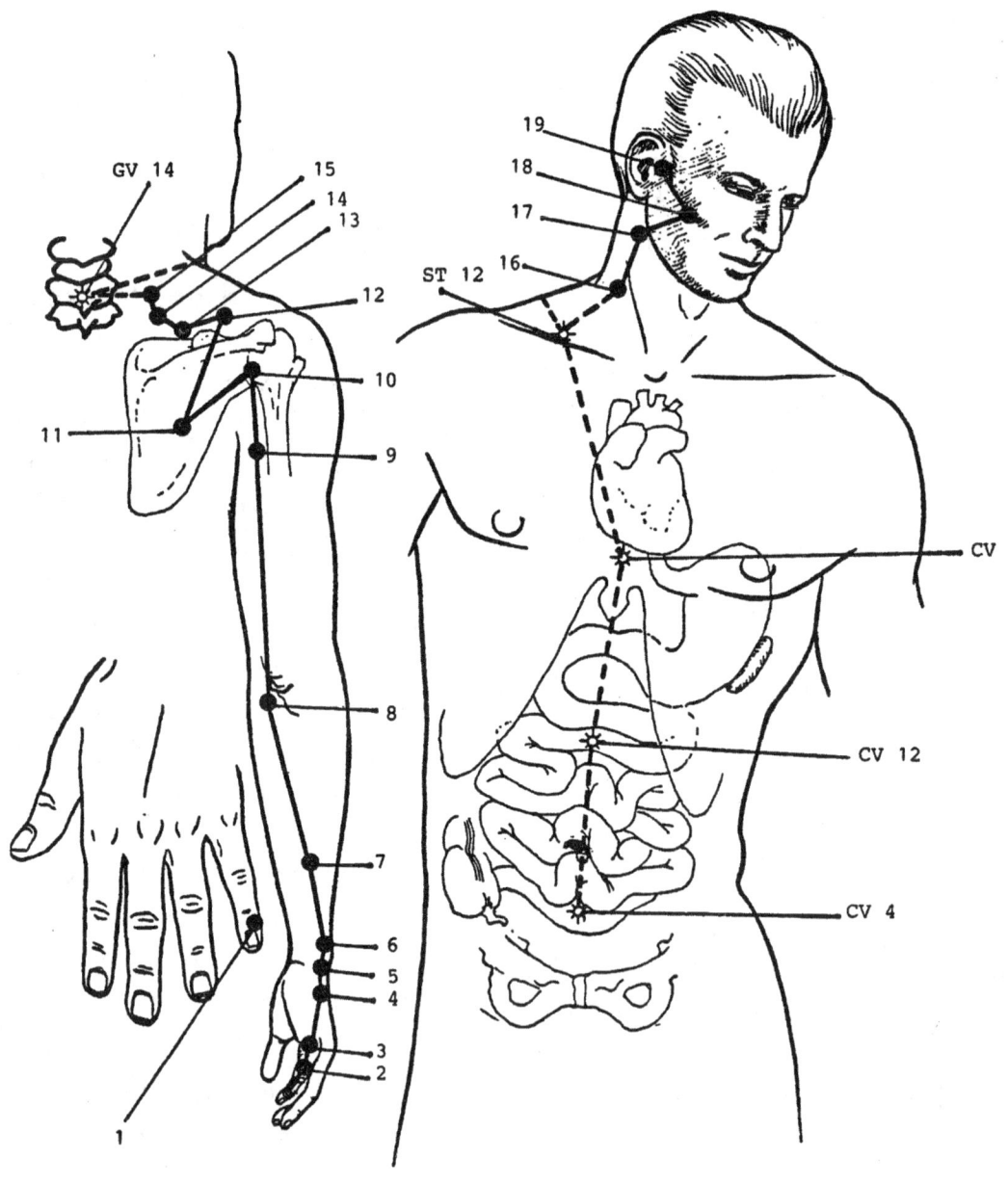

SMALL INTESTINE MERIDIAN
ILLUSTRATION COURTESY OF DR. JOHN AMARO,
INTERNATIONAL ACADEMY OF CLINICAL ACUPUNCTURE. COPYRIGHT © 1981.

The appendix is designed to perform specific functions in the body; therefore, *it must stay in the body*. Although Alexa's appendix had become swollen and inflamed, normalization occurred over two days of consecutive treatments. Poor diet and a propensity for Small Intestine Meridian imbalance often precipitate cases labeled "appendicitis." With more judicious diet choices, Alexa has had no further flareups in over nineteen years. She was young enough and healthy enough that the appendicitis had not reached "the point of no return," which does happen in many cases.

The Bladder Meridian 3-5 P.M.

The Bladder Meridian defines the longest meridian in the body. It contains sixty-seven acupuncture

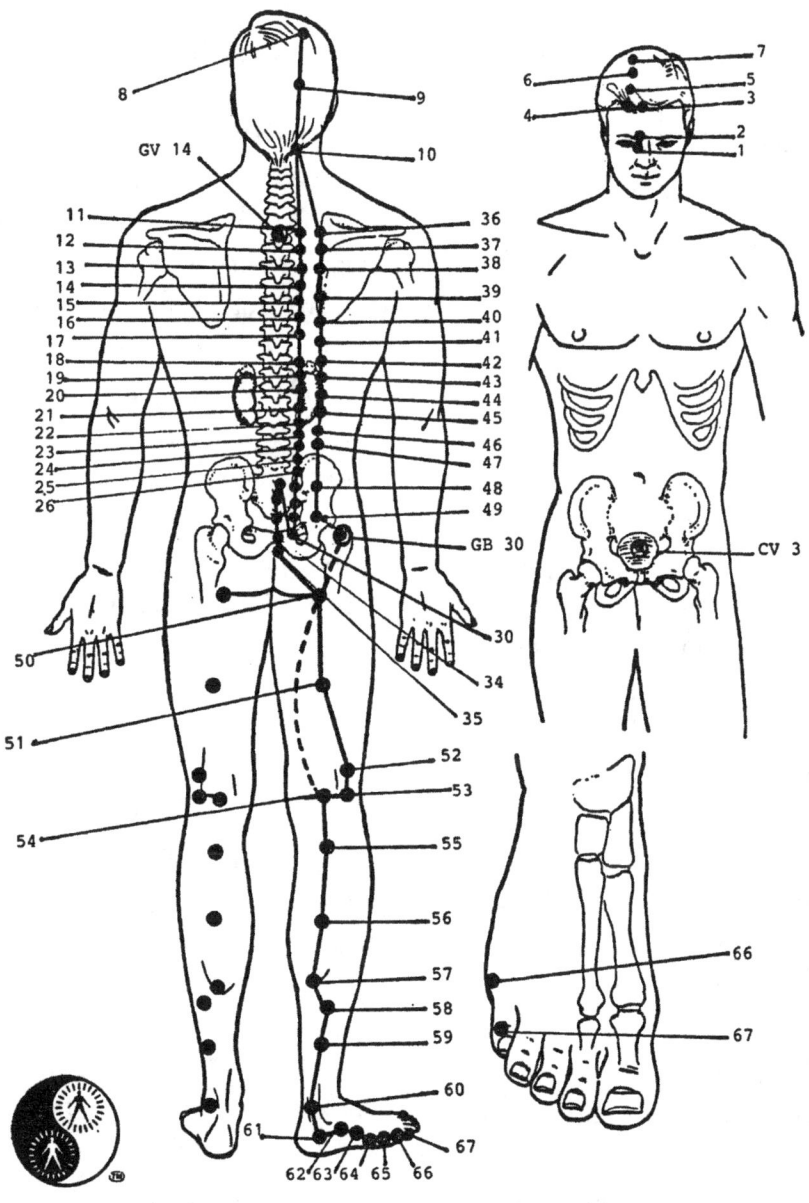

Bladder Meridian
Illustration courtesy of Dr. John Amaro,
International Academy of Clinical Acupuncture. Copyright © 1981.

points, as compared to the Heart and Circulation/Sex Meridians, the shortest meridians, which have only nine points. Bladder energy literally travels from head to toe, through the feet, backtracks up the body, flows back down once more, and finally settles in the little toe.

Symptoms of Bladder Imbalance

Normally, the bladder doesn't manifest serious problems, although it retains its own special relationships with other organs. Some complaints involve:

- Incontinence, painful urination
- Kidney, bladder infections, dropping bladder
- Spinal, low back pain or stiffness
- Hip and knee pain
- Leg ache
- Foot pain

Emma's Story

Emma, an eighty-four-year-old patient, came to me with the most unusual bladder problem I'd ever seen. Over forty years before, Emma's doctors recommended she undergo a hysterectomy. During surgery, the operating doctor accidentally nicked Emma's bladder. The surgical mishap resulted in chronic incontinence for which Emma could find no cure.

She underwent seven attempts to repair her damaged bladder, but all failed. In addition, Emma suffered so much scar tissue that, in the eyes of her doctors, nothing more could be done. Ironically, what finally brought Emma to my office was not her bladder problem, but rather, a seemingly unrelated ailment—excruciating pain in both of her feet.

Through Clinical Kinesiology testing, I discovered that Emma's bladder had been so damaged over the years—her imbalance so progressed—that her body began sending out energetic messages *through her feet*. Emma never guessed that her foot pain resulted from a "circuitry" problem which related to her previously damaged bladder.

Embarrassed by her incontinence, Emma also refused to drink water. Once I treated her bladder and kidney meridians, the excruciating pain in her feet subsided. Emma became healthy, her incontinence lessened, and with Clinical Kinesiology testing we had finally pinpointed her true problem.

The Kidney Meridian 5-7 P.M.

The Chinese name, "bubbling spring," refers to the ball of the foot where the Kidney Meridian originates. The Chinese created descriptive names for each acupuncture point, while Westerners have simply numbered the meridians. With hundreds of major acupuncture points, it would be quite a challenge for anyone, even the Chinese, to remember all those names.

For persons suffering from serious illness, "bubbling spring" often proves to be one of the best points to treat. It usually provides a wellspring of new energy. (Then again, it may not be the best point to treat, depending on what the body has to say during Clinical Kinesiology testing.)

The Kidney Meridian curlicues around the ankle and ascends through the inner knee. The internal part of the meridian circulates directly through the lumbar spine and sacrum, to the bladder and on to the kidney. There, it hooks up with energy that flows to the torso.

Symptoms of Kidney Meridian Imbalance

Disorders that stem from Kidney Meridian imbalances are listed as:

- Dry mouth
- Lung congestion
- Kidney, low back, hip pain
- Disc protrusions, ruptures

- Knee, ankle pain or soreness, proneness to injury
- Incontinence
- Foot or ball of foot pain, proneness to injury
- Hemorrhoids, hernia, tailbone pain

Hernia and Hemorrhoids

Dr. Burt Espy has treated several cases of hernias which directly related to the Kidney Meridian. Often, hernias and hemorrhoids stem from kidney imbalances because of the deep, internal energy that travels directly through and affects the sacrum or tailbone area of the body.

Jeff, one patient of Dr. Espy's, had already consented to surgery for a hernia. Following successful treatment, Jeff's hernia receded and he cancelled the surgery. Jeff went on to live a relatively normal life, being careful to avoid

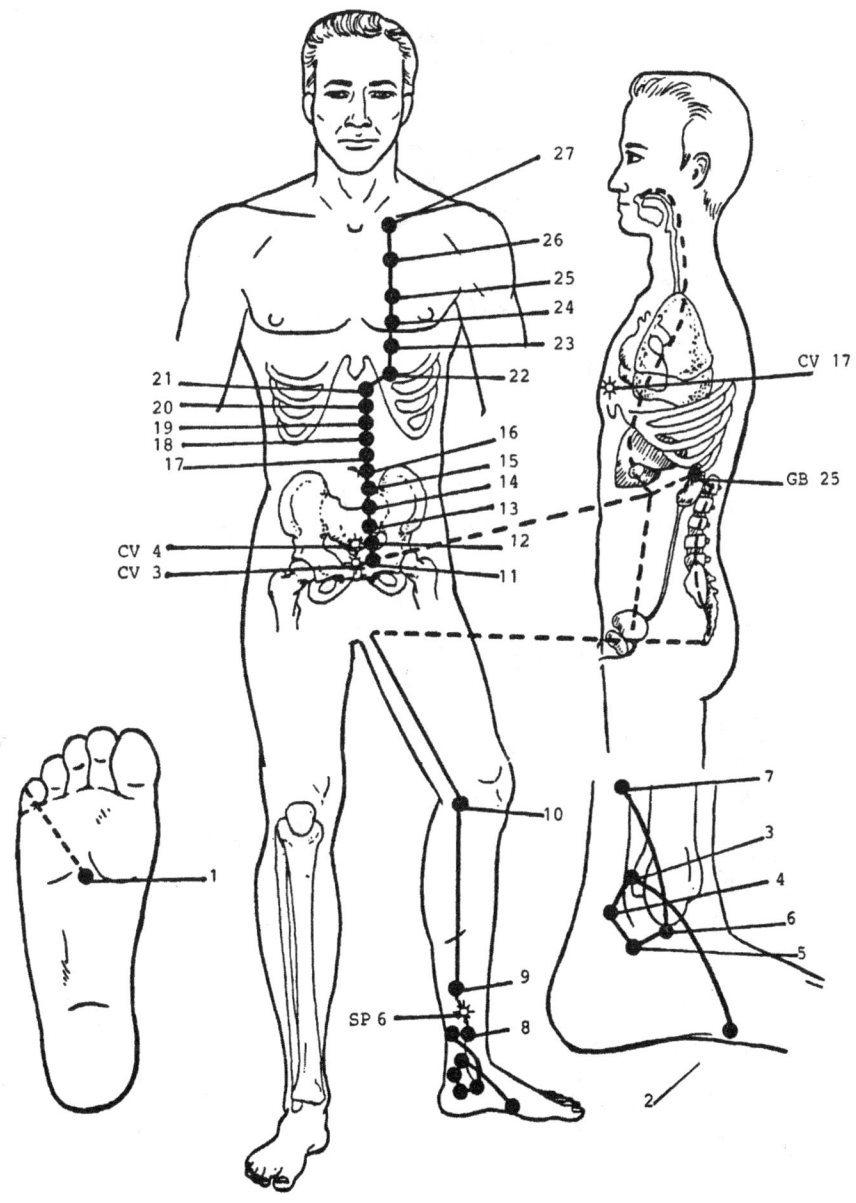

KIDNEY MERIDIAN
ILLUSTRATION COURTESY OF DR. JOHN AMARO,
INTERNATIONAL ACADEMY OF CLINICAL ACUPUNCTURE. COPYRIGHT © 1981.

heavy lifting. He has not reported further symptoms.

The Circulation/Sex or Pericardium Meridian 7-9 P.M.

Any hormonal imbalance in the body may be associated with the Circulation/Sex or Pericardium meridian. This meridian's deep inner energy radiates around the heart (the pericardium describes the fibrous protective sac surrounding the heart), extends down into the digestive organs and through the gonadal system or primary sex glands (the ovaries or testes).

The external part of the meridian runs from the lateral side of the breast or chest, around the arm and down to the middle of the palm of the hand. The Circulation/Sex Meridian also manifests a unique relationship with the pituitary gland, due

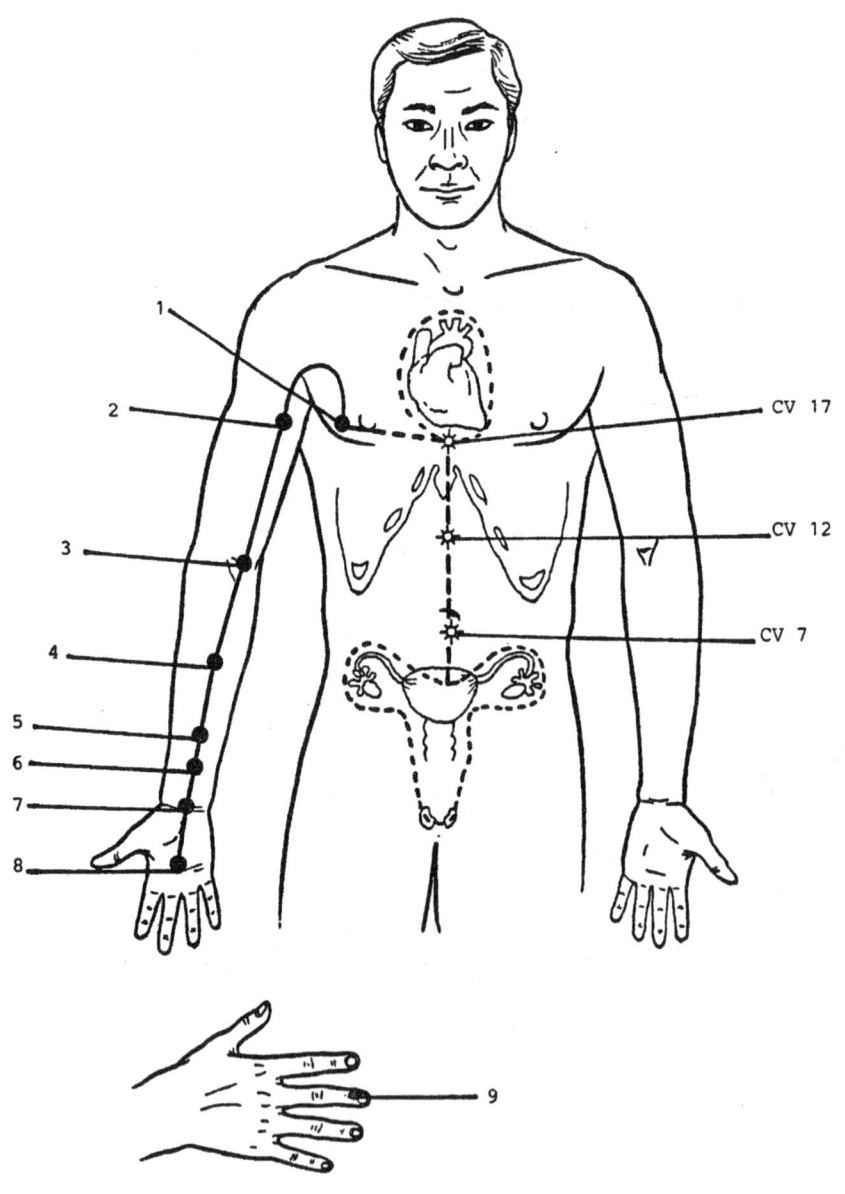

CIRCULATION/SEX-PERICARDIUM MERIDIAN
ILLUSTRATION COURTESY OF DR. JOHN AMARO,
INTERNATIONAL ACADEMY OF CLINICAL ACUPUNCTURE. COPYRIGHT © 1981.

to hormonal aspects, and with the hypothalamus, an "organ" of the brain which regulates many body functions.

The brain is infinitely involved in the energy of the Circulation/ Sex Meridian. The stimulation of various cerebral points, in addition to a whole subset of acupuncture stimulation, helps heal certain brain dysfunctions. Cerebral acupuncture also addresses other brain imbalances, including emotional problems such as depression.

As you might imagine, the Circulation/ Sex Meridian proves to be quite an overriding meridian. This meridian also contains a circulation point, located part of the way up the forearm, which may be tested for the presence of arteriosclerosis.

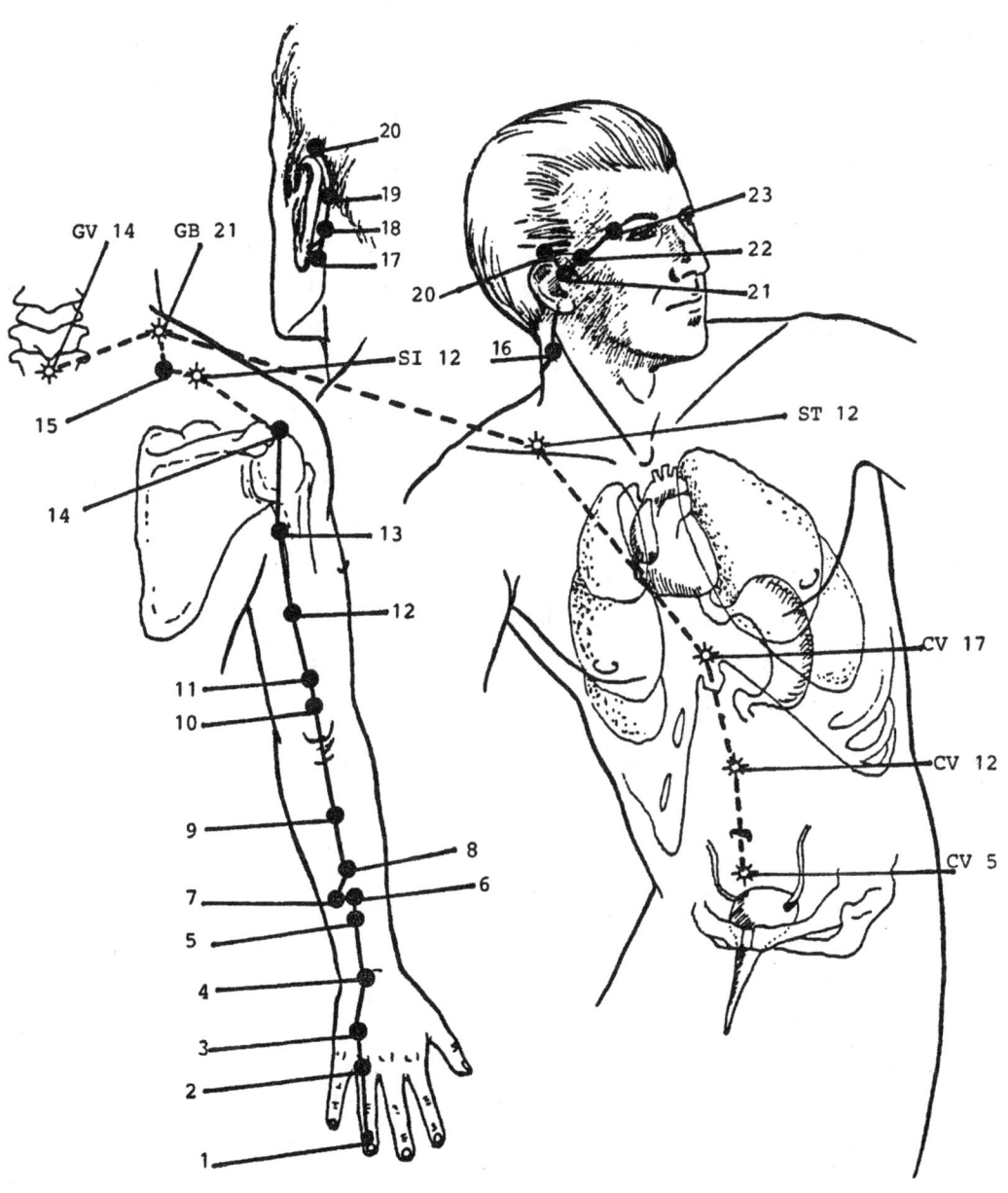

TRIPLE WARMER MERIDIAN
ILLUSTRATION COURTESY OF DR. JOHN AMARO,
INTERNATIONAL ACADEMY OF CLINICAL ACUPUNCTURE. COPYRIGHT © 1981.

Symptoms of Circulation/Sex Meridian Imbalance
- Eye problems
- Hormonal problems
- Hot flashes, sweaty palms, poor circulation
- Hunger, thirst, sleep disorders
- Rapid heartbeat, arteriosclerosis
- Swollen, painful underarm
- Depression, mood swings
- Poor memory, poor concentration
- Stroke

The Triple Warmer Meridian 9-11 P.M.

The Triple Warmer Meridian remains intimately tied to the function of the thyroid and, to a lesser degree, the adrenal glands. This pathway of energy emanates from the fourth finger, travels up the back of the arm, across the elbow, shoulder joint, and upper trapezius muscles. It winds around the back of the neck, around the ear, and flows to the edge of the eyebrow.

As its name implies, the Triple Warmer functions as the "silent regulator" of the three "fires" of the body. These include basic metabolism, digestive energy transference from food to cells, and body temperature regulation. People who complain of cold hands and feet, or get chilled easily, may experience a malfunction of the Triple Warmer Meridian and thyroid gland.

Symptoms of Triple Warmer Imbalance

Many aspects of the upper respiratory system may be influenced by the Triple Warmer Meridian/thyroid connection. These symptoms may indicate an imbalance:

- Colds
- Ear infection, tonsillitis, sore throat, swollen glands
- Eye problems, cataracts, pink eye
- Cold hands or feet, excessive sweating, hot flashes
- Jaw pain, shoulder, arm, wrist stiffness
- Thinning hair, dry skin
- Low energy, chronic fatigue immune deficiency syndrome
- Menstrual cycle irregularities

The Gallbladder Meridian 11 P.M.-1 A.M.

The second longest meridian, the Gallbladder Meridian, also contains the second largest number of acupuncture points. The energy channel begins at the edge of the eye, flows down the angle of the jaw, then shortcuts directly up to the hairline.

The meridian then zigzags across the head several times and down the back of the neck to an area around the armpit and lower front ribs. Angling across the pelvis to the hip joint, the energy laterals down the leg and knee to the calf, where it jogs all the way down to the lateral foot and ends near the nail of the fourth toe.

Symptoms of Gallbladder Meridian Imbalance

Additional problems which develop from low energy in the gallbladder meridian are:

- Headaches
- Muscle pain
- Gallbladder pain, stones
- Tightness in ribs, thorax
- Hip, joint stiffness
- Digestive problems, belching, gas
- Lower leg, ankle pain

Gallbladder Surgery

Surgeons routinely cut the Gallbladder Meridian during gallbladder surgery and energetic complications ensue. Any major surgery or scar surrounding the removal of an organ potentially disrupts the flow of acupuncture energy. Organ connections work the same as a sequential string of Christmas tree lights. If one little bulb goes out, the whole circuit is unable to function.

Surgery does not solve the imbalance that causes gallbladder problems. It simply removes the focus of the worst symptoms. The cause of the original imbalance still needs evaluation. In addition, once an operation has taken place, the surgical scar may further prohibit the Gallbladder Meridian from normal function. Two strikes against the gallbladder system inhibit further healing. A person missing the organ that connects to the meridian now has a scar cutting through the meridian—cutting off its energetic impulse.

Dr. Kiiko Matsumoto, author of *Five Elements and Ten Stems*, bases her entire acupuncture practice on treating surgical and injury scars.[2] In my own practice, I recommend the nutrient, superoxide dismutase or SOD for the liver, which revitalizes cells

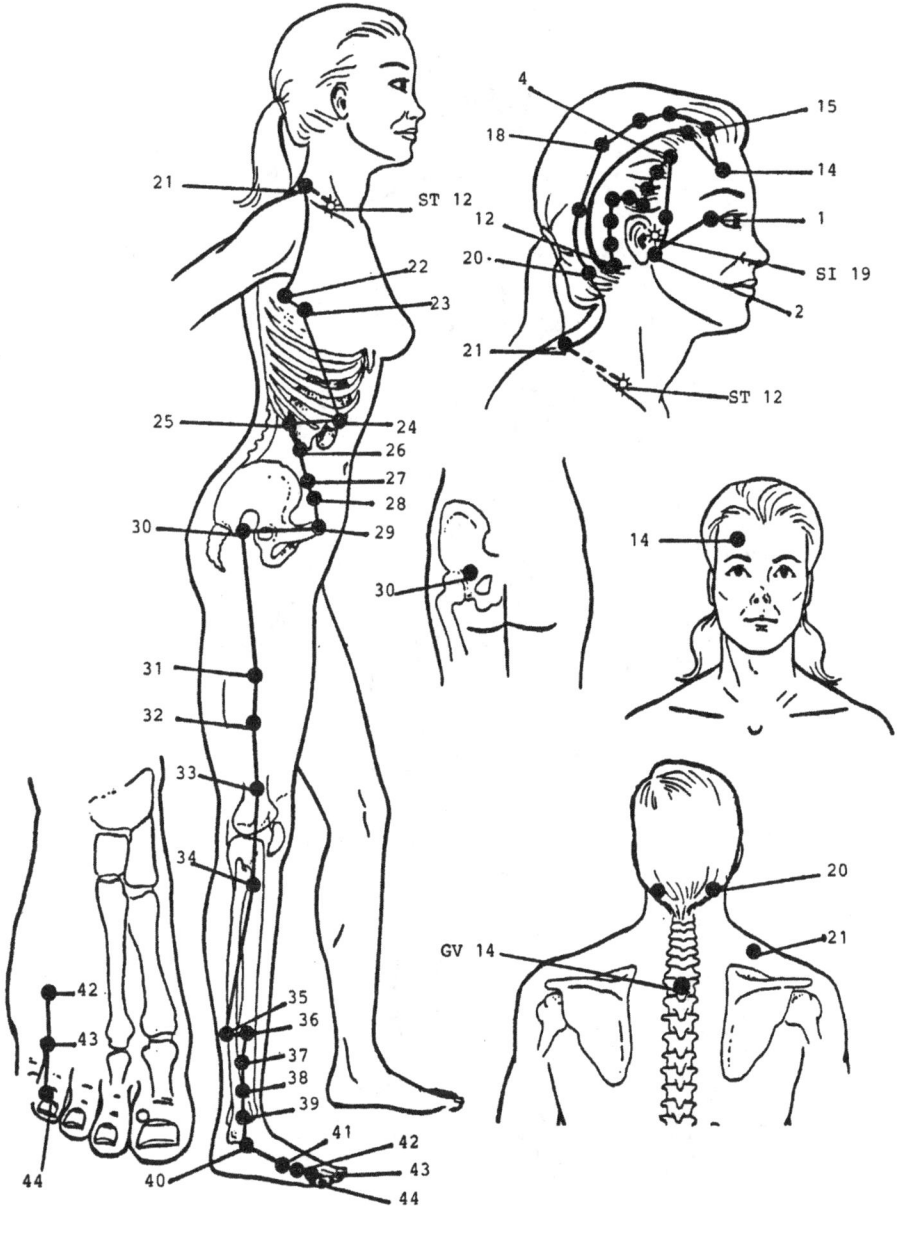

GALLBLADDER MERIDIAN
ILLUSTRATION COURTESY OF DR. JOHN AMARO,
INTERNATIONAL ACADEMY OF CLINICAL ACUPUNCTURE. COPYRIGHT © 1981.

and reduces excessive scar tissue, as well as treating the scar with acupuncture and/or laser.

For most people, gallbladder dysfunctions and remaining scars may be treated through acupuncture and diet changes. The primary factor involves regulating fat intake in the body. A diet containing processed or adulterated fat proves extremely irritating to the gallbladder, whether absent or present! In addition, a diet that is higher in processed fats may trigger heart problems later on.

The Liver Meridian 1-3 A.M.

The final energy pathway, the Liver Meridian, starts on the inner side of the big toe, travels upward and ends in the right lower ribs near the liver and on the left by the spleen.

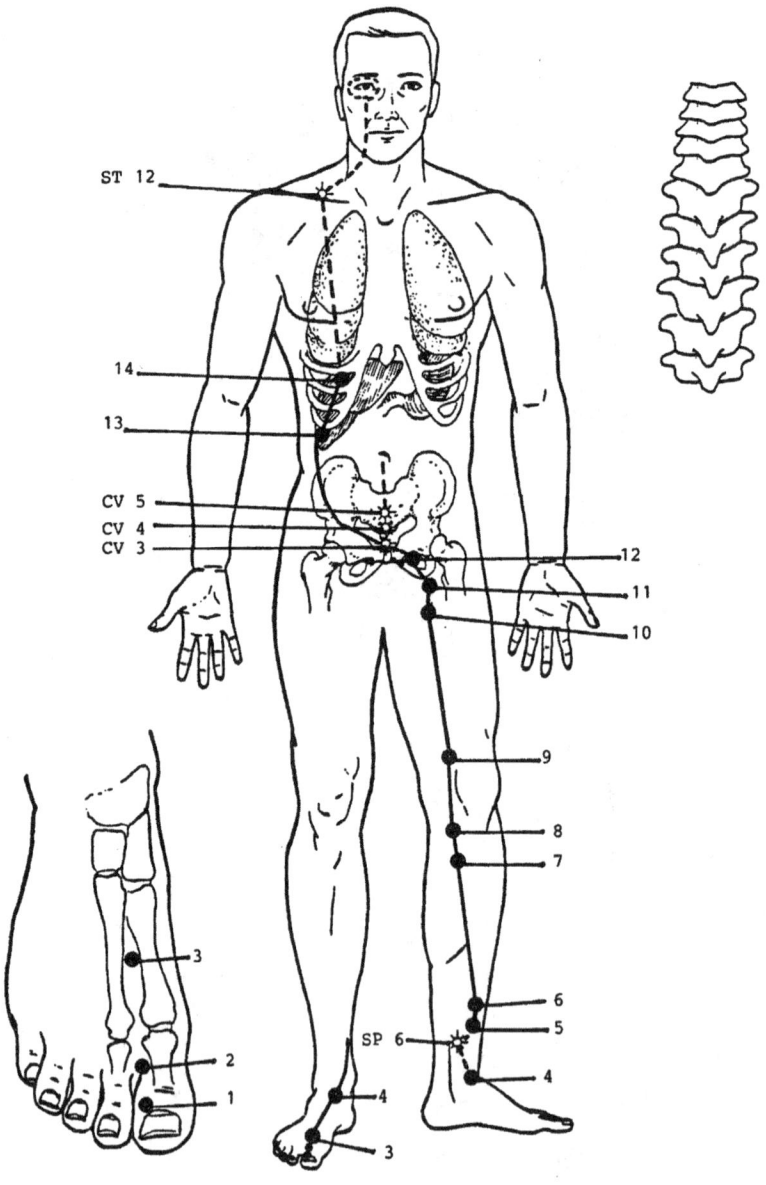

LIVER MERIDIAN
ILLUSTRATION COURTESY OF DR. JOHN AMARO,
INTERNATIONAL ACADEMY OF CLINICAL ACUPUNCTURE. COPYRIGHT © 1981.

44 YOUR BODY CAN TALK

Symptoms of Liver Meridian Imbalance

A Liver Meridian that is out of balance exhibits symptoms that may include:

- Eye irritation
- Lump in the throat
- Muscle, joint stiffness
- Back, rib pain
- Knee problems
- Uterus, ovary, or prostate complaints
- Arthritis
- Skin ailments: eczema, psoriasis, dermatitis

THE HEALING TOOL

Clinical Kinesiology helps practitioners to effectively use acupuncture in designing treatment programs to recover and maintain health. Once familiar with your energetic body and its acupuncture pathways, you can provide yourself the healing support needed to correct your body's functional imbalances.

Follow along as we cover the following treatment techniques:

- Acupuncture
- Acupressure/Teishin
- Lasers
- Therapeutic Magnets

Acupuncture Treatment

Acupuncture needles have been used for centuries in one form or another. Historians suspect pine needles and tiny bones from bird-legs served as the earliest methods for stimulating the points.

Acupuncture needles work much like tiny antennae. When inserted, almost painlessly, into an acupuncture point, the needle immediately begins drawing in the surrounding energy, which then shoots through the meridian and helps rebalance by removing blockages, adding or realigning energy.

Imagine shooting a high intensity blast of water through a corroded pipe. Immediately, you'd clear out most of the corrosion. A few more blasts and the pipe would be clean and functional once again. The acupuncture needles work much the same way.

Most acupuncturists use stainless steel, sterile, disposable acupuncture needles for optimum healing response. The narrow gauge, or diameter, of disposable needles makes them more comfortable and acceptable to most patients.

No matter what needle type, treatment requires direct stimulation of the acupuncture points for effective healing. Treatment relaxes the whole body and spirit and provides an extremely calming effect on inflammation or other active problems.

Initially, treatment of an active problem or inflammation requires longer needle-insertion time. The typical time varies from ten to fifteen minutes. Alternately, the shorter the length of time that the needles are in place, the less sedative effect.

Historically, older techniques required acupuncturists to manipulate the needles in and out, or up and down on the same point. Most manual stimulation involves twirling the needle between two fingers. Twirling the needles stimulates energy movement, or activates the *ch'i*. Today, most disposable needles contain a little handle on the end for such twirling purposes.

Brett's Story

Depending upon the imbalance, each individual body may require different treatment. Brett, a first-time male patient, pulled in so much of the energy being supplied from the acupuncture needle that his skin and tissue actually "tented." This acupuncture term describes skin that pooches up around an acupuncture needle just like a tent. Only after two hours and forty minutes did his body finally release the acupuncture needles.

Brett's body more or less held onto the needles "begging" for more input. Until his body reached a certain state of energy balance it refused to release the needles. Although difficult, it could have been possible for me to remove the needles, but traumatic for Brett's body. If the body says that it really wants that input, the wise thing to do is let the body decide its own pace and continue to allow it to absorb that energy balancing correction from the needle for the appropriate time.

Throughout the two hours and forty minutes, I checked on Brett periodically until his body said, "OK, I've had enough." Many times, there are emotional factors involved in such instances as we'll see in Chapter 3. In Brett's case, an upcoming move across the country may have been a big factor in the amount of energy his body needed during his acupuncture treatment.

The Needles

It's unnecessary to place an acupuncture needle extremely deep. This especially holds true when treating external meridian points. Treating external points affects internal points. So, one doesn't need to plunge the needles into the deepest recesses of the body to effect healing.

Acupuncture treatment is generally quite painless. Occasionally, depending on the particular imbalance, some points may prove noticeably tender. Patients who experience an active point in desperate need of treatment may find it quite tender upon needle insertion. Otherwise, there's absolutely no comparison to pain from an injection with a hypodermic needle more than six times as large. At worst, an acupuncture needle insertion feels more like a mild mosquito bite without any of the burning or inflammation.

When acupuncture needles are used, practitioners may gently "close the hole," by rubbing a finger over the open site where the acupuncture needle has been removed. The Chinese of old did this to stop any leakage of the person's *ch'i*—in essence—so they would not lose energy through the tiny opening.

Anyone who uses needle acupuncture must be trained. Appropriate concern for one's health and well-being includes choosing a health practitioner with sufficient training to understand how and where to apply the acupuncture with needles. It's important to remember that the effects of the acupuncture needles are quite dramatic. For example, inappropriate needle stimulation of specific points during early pregnancy can lead to miscarriage in some cases.

Acupressure and Teishein

I do encourage people to be involved in their own healthcare treatment which allows them to do many things for themselves. The *teishein*, or stainless steel acupressure tool may also be used to stimulate the same acupoint without needles. Spring-loaded with a retractable pressure applicator, the *teishein* resembles a ballpoint pen mechanism, and when tapped, applies pressure to an acupuncture point.

Energizing the meridian with the *teishein* comes first, followed by the small laser for additional stimulation. Such gentle tools enable treatment of tiny infants, small children, and other patients as needed.

I've helped several patients to purchase their own acupressure tool or *teishein* to use at home. While not easily available to the public, you may ask your acupuncturist to order a *teishein* for you and instruct you in its use. The best *teisheins* I have found are available through the International Academy of Clinical Acupuncture. (See Appendix for Product Guide and Associations.) Other acupressure point stimulators may be purchased through health-related magazines, catalogs and at tradeshows. In addition, Panasonic makes the Reach Easy Percussion Hand-Held Massager, which also stimulates acupressure points and can be ordered from specialty health stores or on the web.

Laser And Magnetic Therapy

Laser therapy provides another exciting field of energetic treatment recently opened to the West. Lasers involve treatment with a focused beam of light, called photon energy. Photon particles carry the force in an electromagnetic field.

Popular in Europe and China since the late 1960s, therapeutic lasers have been available in America since the 1990s. Growing in popularity, soft lasers are now being used successfully to augment acupuncture therapy. Acupuncture needles pick up and help direct needed energy into the body. A small laser may then be concentrated directly on the acupoint allowing its energy to penetrate along the course of the needle and into the meridian to help further the healing process.

Lasers project waves of light particles, or beams, into the body to a depth of a half-inch to an inch depending on tissue consistency. Some patients are sensitive enough to feel the beam of laser light as it connects with the energy from the meridian. When this happens, many times, the acupuncture needle itself begins to quiver from the added energy. Small soft lasers may also be purchased from specialty catalogs or through healthcare practitioners.

Joyce's Story

I treated Joyce, a female patient who lost a leg in a car accident. Initially, Joyce's complaint stemmed from continuing menopausal symptoms. Upon Clinical Kinesiology diagnosis, however, a liver imbalance pinpointed Joyce's true problem.

After locating specific acupuncture points on Joyce's leg that needed to be energized, I mentioned that it was my practice to stimulate both right and left sides in order to sufficiently treat an imbalance.

In addition to Joyce's acupuncture treatment, I added laser stimulation of the acupuncture point on her right side, even though no leg was present. Continued stimulation of Joyce's *etheric* body—her field of energy, or aura—and the existing current of uninterrupted energy for that area, proved extremely healing. Joyce's leg energy was not removed, even though her physical leg was no longer present.

Energy meridians remain intact. Proof of this may also be found in many situations of phantom leg pain. Joyce, too, described certain sensations in the area where her leg had been removed. What she felt energetically during the three years she'd lived with her amputation compared to reactions of a limb experiencing poor circulation or "falling asleep."

Following the laser stimulation Joyce experienced new energetic sensations much different from the phantom leg pain. She described a new, warm, tingling sensation, more aptly an awakening from "pins and needles." In Joyce's case, application of the laser stimulated her body to begin the necessary rebalancing.

The experienced effects of laser stimulation have proven an important therapeutic alternative for patients in similar situations. Once only considered to be a tool of the future, lasers now provide far-reaching cures in rebalancing the body and its energetic system.

Therapeutic Magnets

Therapeutic magnets supply yet another form of stimulation that may be applied to energize an acupuncture point. Clinical Kinesiology testing provides the means for discovering electromagnetic imbalances in the body. When such imbalances show up, effective treatment may require magnetic or polarity therapy.

Through Clinical Kinesiology muscle testing, a patient may be checked to determine if a "north pole" or a "south pole" magnet is required. Once a particular pole is indicated, the corresponding magnet, attached to a small, round adhesive strip, may be applied to the acupuncture point, where it remains for a few days to a week.

The individual power of therapeutic magnets are typically 800 gauss, (a measurement of magnetic field strength). Such a magnetic force doesn't overpower the body; however, it does help rebalance the electromagnetic system. I caution you against using any magnetic force on any generalized part of your body without specific testing by a trained healthcare practitioner.

Following acupuncture or related therapy, retesting with Clinical Kinesiology confirms the effectiveness of the treatment. Generally, acupoints

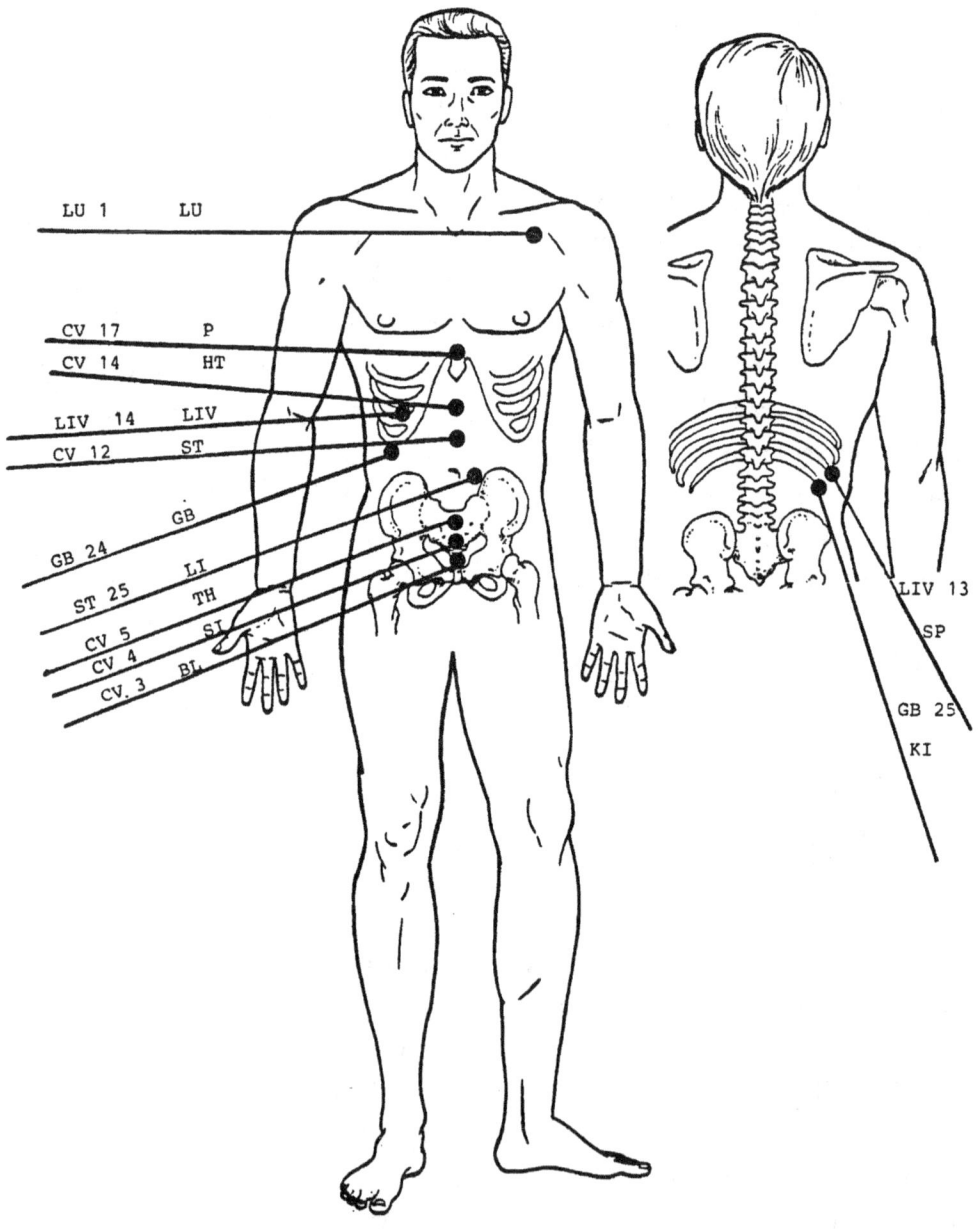

ALARM POINTS
ILLUSTRATION COURTESY OF DR. JOHN AMARO,
INTERNATIONAL ACADEMY OF CLINICAL ACUPUNCTURE. COPYRIGHT © 1981.

that registered weak prior to the application, now prove strong. If all is well, proceeding with further energetic testing determines any additional treatment needs, such as vitamin or nutritional supplementation.

ACUPUNCTURE ALARM POINT TESTS

When an organ/meridian system becomes out of balance, the body's innate wisdom is automatically programmed to set off an alarm, "Ah, there's a problem here!" You do not need to be "alarmed"... merely alerted. (A smoke detector goes off for many reasons other than simply for a fire.)

The acupuncture alarm point tests provide a series of "checkpoints" along your energetic system. If the body detects a problem, the alarm point is "set-off," and becomes active or often tender. If the alarm point is tender or responds weak to the Clinical Kinesiology muscle test, that alerts you that a particular organ/meridian system needs rebalancing.

The acupuncture alarm point muscle tests provide quick answers so that you do not need to check every individual point on each meridian. Do you need to be concerned about a specific organ or not? Testing the acupuncture alarm points may be the first step to uncovering an imbalance which may not yet be so advanced that it is noticeable through symptoms. Dr. John Amaro stresses the importance of the alarm points.

GO WITH YOUR ENERGY FLOW

If, during testing, you discover problems that indicate an energetic imbalance in your body, you have several choices. Deal with the most important priority first! Energetically treat the problem through acupuncture, diet, nutritional, homeopathic or herbal therapies—and change the imbalance. Treated now, your health may go in a whole new direction.

Left untreated, the imbalance, depending upon the direction the body takes—considering lifestyle factors and mindset—may lead to numerous different ailments. Generally, if you haven't been trained in acupuncture, it's best to seek guidance from an alternative health practitioner following your initial acupuncture alarm point tests.

How to Test Acu-Alarm Points

Most of the acupuncture alarm points may be located on the front of the torso, with a few points on the posterior or rear of the body. If you are right-handed, *therapy localize* or touch the Acu-Alarm point with your left hand, while the test is performed on your right arm indicator muscle by a test partner.

Lung Alarm Point Test

The alarm point for the lungs (LU 1) may be found on the front of the body, near the shoulder, just below the clavicle.

> Lung alarm point TL + Muscle test + Weak arm = Lung imbalance = Seek guidance from an alternative health practitioner.
>
> Lung alarm point TL + Muscle test + Strong arm = Lung balance.

Large Intestine Alarm Point Test

The large intestine alarm point (ST 25) may be located on the Stomach Meridian two thumb-widths lateral to the navel on both the right or left.

> Large Intestine alarm point TL + Muscle test + Weak arm = Large Intestine imbalance = Seek guidance from an alternative health practitioner.
>
> Large Intestine alarm point TL + Muscle test + Strong arm = Large Intestine balance.

Stomach Alarm Point Test

CV 12 indicates the point to therapy localize for testing the stomach alarm point. This point rests a couple of inches above the navel.

> Stomach alarm point TL + Muscle Test + Weak arm = Stomach imbalance = Seek guidance from an alternative health practitioner.
>
> Stomach alarm point TL + Muscle Test + Strong arm = Stomach balance.

Spleen Alarm Point Test

The spleen alarm point (LIV 13) may be located one rib above the kidney point or at the eleventh rib shown on the diagram. Rarely out of balance, the spleen, however, does have a relationship to the quality of the blood in the body. In addition, the female energetic system may be dramatically affected by spleen energy.

> Spleen alarm point TL + Muscle test + Weak arm = Spleen imbalance = Seek guidance from an alternative health practitioner.
>
> Spleen alarm point TL + Muscle test + Strong arm = Spleen balance.

HEART ALARM POINT TEST

On the mid-line of the Circulation Vessel Meridian lies the heart alarm point (CV 14). The heart point lies three or four inches below the pericardium point and even with the ninth or tenth rib inter space.

> Heart alarm point TL + Muscle test + Weak arm = Heart imbalance = Seek guidance from an alternative health practitioner.
>
> Heart alarm point TL + Muscle test + Strong arm = Heart balance.

Small Intestine Alarm Point Test

Another inch below the triple heater point, you may locate the small intestine alarm point (CV 4).

> Small Intestine alarm point + Muscle test + Weak arm = Small Intestine imbalance = Seek guidance from an alternative health practitioner.
>
> Small Intestine alarm point + Muscle test + Strong arm = Small Intestine balance.

Bladder Alarm Point Test

Directly above the pubic bone, (CV 3), the bladder alarm point may be located and tested fairly easily because the point corresponds closely to the physical organ.

> Bladder alarm point TL + Muscle test + Weak arm = Bladder imbalance = Seek guidance from an alternative health practitioner.
>
> Bladder alarm point TL + Muscle test + Strong arm = Bladder balance.

Kidney Alarm Point Test

The very bottom or shortest rib located on the posterior low back indicates the area of the kidney alarm point (GB 25). It's also helpful to locate the spine at the twelfth rib and follow it outward to the tip of the rib.

> Kidney alarm point + Muscle test + Weak arm = Kidney imbalance = Seek guidance from an alternative health practitioner.
>
> Kidney alarm point + Muscle test + Strong arm = Kidney balance.

Circulation/Sex or Pericardium Alarm Point Test

Locate the circulation/sex or pericardium alarm point (CV 17) directly above the inverted V between the ribs about an inch or two above the bony apex. This meridian provides the constant flow of energy that envelops the heart. Thus, it remains an important alarm point to test.

> Pericardium alarm point TL + Muscle test + Weak arm = Pericardium imbalance = Seek guidance from an alternative health practitioner.
>
> Pericardium alarm point TL + Muscle test + Strong arm = Pericardium balance.

Triple Heater/Thyroid Alarm Point Test

The immune system and thyroid share a strong relationship with the triple heater alarm point (CV 5). Because the navel is CV 8, to locate the triple heater point, you may drop down roughly 3 to 3 1/2 inches from the navel to reach the correct point.

> Triple Heater alarm point TL + Muscle test + Weak arm = Triple Heater imbalance = Seek guidance from an alternative health practitioner.
>
> Triple Heater alarm point TL + Muscle test + Strong arm = Triple Heater balance.

Gallbladder Alarm Point Test

The gallbladder alarm point (GB 24) lies at the lowest edge of the front side of the ribs. By therapy localizing the gallbladder alarm point you may also learn about an early gallbladder imbalance. Again, it's preferable to check the gallbladder point on the left rather than the right. Without the actual presence of the gallbladder organ beneath the point, you'll be guaranteed a much more accurate test.

> Gallbladder alarm point TL + Muscle test + Weak arm = Gallbladder imbalance = Seek guidance from an alternative health practitioner.
>
> Gallbladder alarm point TL + Muscle test + Strong arm = Gallbladder balance.

Liver Alarm Point Test

The liver alarm point rests on the lower right rib cage between the last two ribs that you can feel. The right liver point (LIV 14) is shown by the diagram; however, you may also test the corresponding point on the left. Often, I recommend the left point to avoid the confusion of therapy localizing over liver and gallbladder. For an accurate test, be sure to target the acupoint without allowing involvement of any nearby organ.

> Liver alarm point TL + Muscle test + Weak arm = Liver imbalance = Seek guidance from an alternative health practitioner.
>
> Liver alarm point TL + Muscle test + Strong arm = Liver balance.

Taking the time to treat an imbalance early, may create a new, happy and harmonious condition within your body. You, who were once ill, may soon be well! Will it be a miracle cure? I don't think so. All you will be doing is taking the time to "know" about yourself, your body, and the energetic flow of your meridians. It doesn't take many years, or a great deal of experience to get to know your body and to listen to what it has to say. All it takes is your time, attention, and willingness to be well.

This chapter has provided you with new information on the *physical* aspects of energetic imbalances and how Chinese acupuncture facilitates realignment and healing. In Chapter 3, *Energy and Your Emotions*, I'll help you understand the critical role that the *mental and emotional* body plays in maintaining physical health by presenting the Chinese Five Element theory, which interprets organ/emotion relationships through Clinical Kinesiology testing.

CHAPTER 2 SUGGESTED READING

Bauer, Matthew, L.Ac. *Healing Power of Acupressure and Acupuncture.* New York: Avery, published by the Penguin Group, 2005.

Beinfield, Harriet, L.Ac., and Korngold, Efrem, L.Ac., O.M.D. *Between Heaven and Earth: A Guide to Chinese Medicine.* New York: Ballantine Books, 1991.

Campbell, Anthony, MRCP (UK) FF Hom. *Acupuncture in Practice: Beyond Points and Meridians, 2nd edition.* Oxford, UK and Waltham, Mass.: Butterworth-Heinemann, 2001.

Campbell, Joan. *Acupuncture Channels and Points.* London: Churchill Livingstone, 2008.

Dougans, Inge with Ellis, Suzanne. *The Art of Reflexology, A Step-by-Step Guide: A Totally New Approach Using the Chinese Meridian Theory.* Rockport, Mass: Element, Inc., 1992.

Eisenberg, D., M.D. and T. Wright, *Encounters with Qi: Exploring Chinese Medicine.* New York: W.W. Norton and Company, Inc., 1995.

Fleischman, Gary F. *Acupuncture: Everything You Ever Wanted to Know.* Barrytown, New York: Barrytown/Station Hill Press, 1998.

Gach, Michael Reed, Ph.D. *Acupressure's Potent Points: A Guide to Self-Care for Common Ailments.* New York: Bantam Books, 1990.

Kaptchuk, Ted, O.M.D. *The Web that has No Weaver: Understanding Chinese Medicine.* New York: McGraw-Hill Books, 2000.

Kidson, Ruth Lever. *Is Acupuncture Right for You?: What It Is, Why It Works, and How It Can Help You.* Rochester, Vermont: Healing Arts Press, 2008.

Lee, Daniela. *Acupuncture for Cynics: Don't Be Scared To Be Healed.* CreateSpace Independent Publishing Platform (an Amazon company), 2012.

Levert, Suzanne and Glenn S. Rothfeld, M.D., M. Ac. *The Acupuncture Response: Balancing Energy and Restore Health—a Western Doctor Tells You How.* New York: Contemporary Books, 2002.

Liao, Waysun. *Chi: Discovering Your Life Energy.* Boston & London: Shambhala, 2009.

Mann, Felix, M.D. *Acupuncture: The Ancient Chinese Art of Healing and How It Works Scientifically.* New York: Random House Inc., 1972.

Matsumoto, Kiiko and Birch, Stephen. *Five Elements & Ten Stems: Nan-Ching Theory, Diagnosis, and Practice.* Brookline, Mass: Paradigm Publications, 1989.

Nambudripad, Devi S., M.D., D.C., L.Ac., Ph.D. (Acu.) *Living Pain Free With Acupressure: Acupressure Self Help.* Buena Park, Calif.: Delta Publishers, 1997.

———. *Say Good-Bye to Illness, Nambidripad's Allergy Elimination Techniques: A Revolutionary Treatment for Allergies & Allergy-Related Conditions, 3rd edition.* Buena Park, Calif.: Delta Publishers, 2002.

Willmont, Dennis. *The Five Phases of Acupuncture in the Classical Texts.* Marshfield, Mass: Willmountain Press, 2009.

Worsely, J.R. *Acupuncture: Is It for You?* Rockport, Mass: Element Books Ltd., 1985.

Yelland, Sharon, R.N., R.M., CAcC, MBAcC. *Acupuncture in Midwifery, 2nd edition.* Books for Midwives Press, 2005.

CHAPTER 3

Energy and Your Emotions

Several years ago, I attended a birthday party for my young nephew, Max. The entertainment featured a magician in top-hat and tails whose tricks held the crowd spellbound. At first, the magician's top hat appeared empty. He then magically reached into the hat and pulled out a beautiful red silk scarf. As he pulled, a blue scarf suddenly appeared, attached to the red. Then, a yellow scarf … and a green … and so on.

The magician pulled more hidden and varied scarves seemingly from deep within his hat. Watching these colorful scarves reminded me of another mysterious realm—human emotions. How deeply interconnected our emotions run and to what hidden depths they descend. When we can't "pull out" or express our emotions as readily as this magician pulled out the colored scarves, we suffer—physically, mentally, spiritually. Sometimes an inability to express deep thoughts or feelings of anger, sadness, or love causes emotions to become energetically congested in one or more organ/energy systems of the body. Clinical Kinesiology, then, becomes an invaluable tool in relief of symptoms associated with deep, underlying emotional imbalances.

THE MIND-BODY CONNECTION

In modern Western culture, science has separated mind and body. Other cultures in the world, however, have long held that mind and body are one. The ancient Chinese developed the Chinese Five Element Theory based on the belief that the energy of the mind and body exist as one with heaven and earth.

Dr. Alan Beardall incorporated the Chinese Five Element theory into Clinical Kinesiology testing to assess emotional states in the body. Since his death, several doctors, including Naturopath, Dr. Theresa Dale, and Neural Kinesiologist, Dr. Louisa Williams, have further explored diagnosis and treatment of the critical role emotions play in the well-being of the physical body.

Based on the Chinese Five Element Theory, this chapter focuses on the organ/meridian system as a storage site for deeply hidden negative emotions. In this chapter you will learn:

- How Clinical Kinesiology, through integration of different levels of mind-body energy, may be utilized to diagnose emotional imbalances.

- How homeopathic remedies can help eliminate emotional imbalances.
- How supplementation with amino acids, vitamins and minerals assists in brain metabolism.
- How words and attitudes augment healing through creative visualization and how self-testing the energetic body provides a deeper understanding of and access to underlying emotions.

Gaze into the sky on a starlit night and imagine the rotation of the moon around the earth. One evening, you might discover a beautiful full moon. Another night, only a quarter moon. The ever constant moon is always there, however, you may not always notice its quiet, dark side.

Just like the moon, the energy of your emotions is constantly expressed, whether noticed or not. Just as you cannot be separated from the environment, the effects of your feelings, thoughts, emotions, or preconceived ideas cannot be separated from body function, health, illness, or other life experiences.

CHINESE FIVE ELEMENT THEORY

Two to three thousand years ago, the earliest reference of the Chinese Five Element Theory was recorded in Shu Ching, a book of Chinese political philosophy.[1] Later, more in-depth theories appeared in the *Nan Ching*, an ancient medical classic.[2]

The book, *Five Elements and Ten Stems*, by Dr. Kiiko Matsumoto and Stephen Birch documents the development of the Chinese Five Element

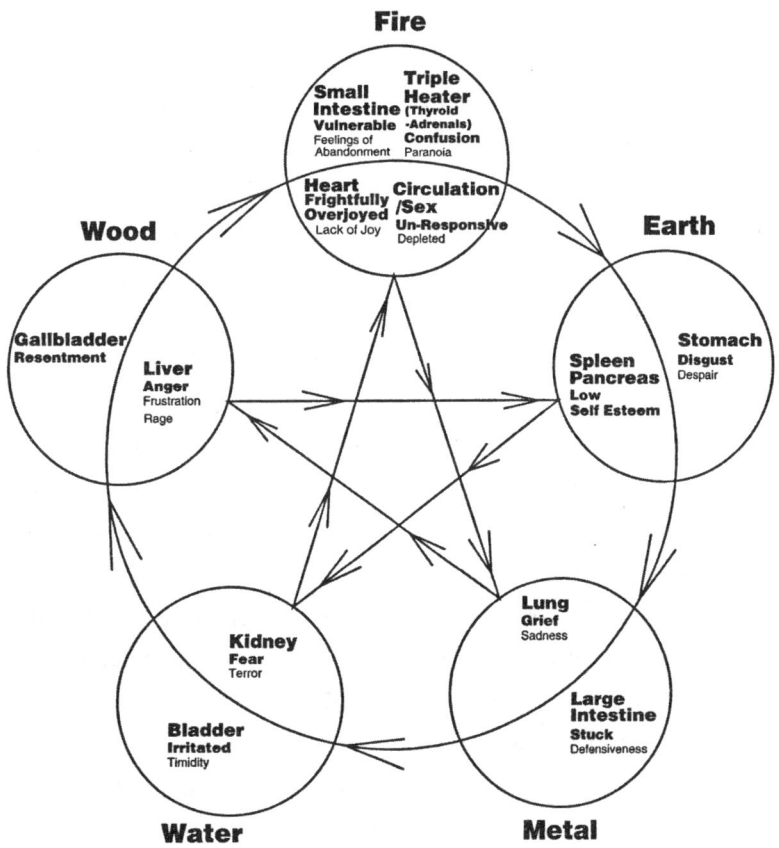

theory over many centuries.³ The concept of *yin* and *yang* best explain how the Chinese viewed the environment and its effect on human emotions. *Yang*, the energy of heaven, relates to each aspect of the five elements. *Yin*, the energy of earth, corresponds to the twelve main acupuncture meridians. This influence of heaven and earth on the body provides the basis for the Chinese Five Element Theory.

According to the Chinese Five Element Theory, every facet of health or illness may be governed by one of five elements ... wood, fire, earth, metal, and water. (Although emotions are the main focus of this chapter, the Chinese Five Elements also include aspects such as taste, color, odor, time of day, sound, and other distinct factors which indicate imbalances in the body.) Each of the five elements relate to a particular season of year, organ/meridian, and emotion.

According to naturopath Dr. Theresa Dale of The Wellness Center for Research and Education of Malibu, California, "... disease manifests as a result of resistance to feelings and emotions regarding an experience, idea or belief."⁴ This resistance may occur on a conscious or unconscious level. Take anger, for example. Most people encounter any number of anger-causing events throughout life. However, at the time, anger may go unexpressed for one reason or another. The vestiges of such unreleased anger are then stored inside the body.

New instances that trigger feelings of anger may not simply involve the current event or emotion. Rather, they may be connected to a chain of emotional events—all the way back to the earliest experiences of anger. Dr. Dale further believes, as the ancient Chinese, that such stagnant energy creates an "electromagnetic charge of energy" which may be stored in the corresponding organ/meridian system.

Plus Homeopathy

Dr. Dale, a former student of Dr. Alan Beardall, has expanded the application of Clinical Kinesiology adding the use of specific homeopathic remedies based on the *Materia medica*, and the Chinese Five Element Theory. Dr. Dale's Neuro-Emotional Remedies are specific formulations currently available only through healthcare professionals. (See Product Guide.) While they are used specifically by Clinical Kinesiology practitioners, other homeopathic remedies may be used as well.

Homeopathy, from the Greek words "homeo" and "pathos" means "similar suffering." Attributed to Samuel Hahnemann, homeopathy originated from the eighteenth century belief that real illness lies beneath the physical, mental and emotional levels at the energetic level, or level of *ch'i*.

Homeopathy is based on the premise that "like cures like," or as Hippocrates stated, "The same things which cause the disease cure it." Specific homeopathic remedies like Dale's allow release or drainage of "core" emotion/energy from an unbalanced organ or acupuncture meridian.

Furthering the energy/emotion balance may also require physical aspects of treatment including acupuncture, nutrition, gentle chiropractic adjustments, or other natural means. While prominent in most cases, emotional symptoms may be hidden by adaptations in others. As an organ responds to physical treatment, many times the underlying emotional aspect surfaces and requires treatment as well.

How Neuro Emotional Remedies Work

Clinical Kinesiology testing of emotions involves the location and testing of specific acupuncture points on the hands or feet. These reflex or "Jing-well" points were researched in the modern era by German doctors in the 1940s led by Dr. Reinhold

Voll, M.D. A weak muscle response in relation to a specific point can instantly diagnose underlying emotional imbalances for which a homeopathic remedy may provide rebalance.

Then, a number of homeopathic remedies may be evaluated by placing them directly on the patient's abdomen or in the energy field. The muscle testing is then performed to narrow down the correct treatment. Again, several other remedies are tested and arm muscle strength monitored until, by a process of elimination, the body "says" which remedy is best.

Discovering the Elements for Yourself

Follow along now as each element and its characteristics are identified. Since each element in the Chinese Five Element theory corresponds to a specific emotion in the body, use the data that follows to uncover your own "hidden" emotions. Challenge yourself to become aware of any emotions you may have been experiencing in the past weeks or months. Take as much time as needed to observe any emotions that may come to light. The suggestions that follow will help you in this process.

Many different techniques will help you to gain deeper insight into the energy of your emotions. For example:

- prepare a simple visualization that might allow you to transport yourself back in time and then allow yourself to quietly retrieve any past episodes of anger, grief or fear, etc.
- recall ways that you might comfortably intervene (verbal affirmations, crying, writing in a journal, pounding a pillow, etc.) at an emotional level to help your body overcome or cleanse any feelings that float to the surface.
- don't be afraid to speak about any unresolved, unfinished, or unexpressed emotions to a trusted friend or therapist.
- reward yourself for your efforts with something special: a walk, warm bath, visit to a friend, drive in the park, etc.

Wood Element: Liver and Gallbladder

Just as the earth experiences various "phases" or cycles, so does the body. The Chinese identified the seasonal elements through the Chinese Five Element Theory and further correlated it to the human experience.

The season of springtime awakens the wood element's predominant energy. Rebirth and renewal categorize the time of year for new grass, fresh shoots, tiny flowers, and budding trees. The whole world turns green.

The color green correlates significantly to the wood element's emotional relationship with its main organs, the liver and gallbladder. You may have heard people say, "He's 'green' with envy." Or, "She's 'green' with anger!"

In cases of jaundice, for example, the skin produces a yellow color, however, the actual hue represents more of a green-yellow shade than pure yellow. Diseases of the wood element often manifest such a skin tone.

Liver Emotions

In Chinese Five Element theory, the liver represents the seat of anger. When someone carries anger it often manifests physically as an imbalance in the liver. Gone unexpressed, the anger/emotion becomes trapped in the liver and problems may ensue.

According to Dr. Dale's research, other emotional aspects of liver imbalance may include:

- frustration
- rage

Caitlin's Story

Following her brother's suicide, Caitlin's liver problems manifested as bad headaches. At the time, Caitlin's parents refused to accept their son's death. Although she bore no responsibility for the suicide, her parents leveled their anger and blame in her direction.

Hurt and grief-stricken, Caitlin internalized her emotions, which included a great deal of anger. Eventually, the pent-up emotions stagnated her liver energy. Her Clinical Kinesiology test signaled that she needed a homeopathic liver remedy, along with acupuncture and other nutrients.

As Caitlin worked on releasing her anger with the remedy, I suggested she imagine her mind/body as a transparent balloon filled with grey smoke. The smoke symbolized her anger, along with other repressed emotions she'd stifled while defending herself against her parents blame.

As Caitlin took the remedy drops, she visualized the smoky grey anger slowly puffing up, up, and away. Her emotional cleansing continued through this visualization until she could "see" the true, clear color of her balloon.

Several months later, Caitlin scheduled a visit with her parents. Before leaving, she worked on her visualizations for about a month and a half. Then, with a great deal of trepidation, she made the journey. The trip went well, and turned out to be the best visit she'd ever had with her folks. While her parents' attitudes were much the same and Caitlin still experienced little jabs and negative comments, she was no longer paralyzed by them. She had vowed not to let her parents' accusations affect her. Caitlin couldn't change her parents' behavior, so she changed herself.

Gallbladder Emotions

The gallbladder is the body's physiological reservoir for bile, which flows from the liver. In emotional terms, the gallbladder serves as the reservoir for *resentment* which stems from stored anger. Other emotional factors of gallbladder imbalance involve:

- stubbornness
- emotional repression

You may hear the colloquial phrase, "I'm really galled!" Or, "That really galls me!" Most people don't realize that those words have a tremendous impact on the body. The gallbladder listens and hears. All emotions affect organ energy. The development of healthier strategies to deal with

---

A Balloon Meditation

You may want to try this simple balloon meditation as mentioned in Caitlan's story.

Start with imagining a clear balloon filled with grey smoke (representing your pain or emotional turmoil). Then, as you relax, breathing gently, or as you take a nutrient or remedy, "watch" the balloon color gradually change. (Pick a favorite color to brighten up the balloon, a color which makes you feel good.)

Watch as the balloon (your mind/body) becomes clearer and "floats" higher as negative emotions and excess anger leave your body. Cleansing trapped emotions helps release energy blockages on a cellular level and alleviates problems which interfere with body function and physiology.

We all experience emotions we need to feel and express. For Caitlin, taking the remedy drops wouldn't have been nearly as effective without including the mental processing, or visualization. This investment of herself—time, emotions and very soul—provided the true healing.

your anger situations and inner conflict today may strongly affect tomorrow's health.

Fire Element: Heart and Small Intestines

Imbalances of the fire element manifest in the height of summer through the change of leaves. The fire element encompasses four meridian systems: Heart, Small Intestine, Circulation/Sex and Triple Warmer.

The organs of the Heart and Small Intestine Meridian both comprise the fire element and relate to each other quite a bit. The fire organs provide the body with warmth, light and life.

Heart Emotions

An important emotion corresponding to a heart imbalance has been termed "frightfully overjoyed" by the Chinese. I also find lack of joy in many people. One example involves the pain of a broken heart. Another extreme heart emotion, which leans toward the opposite pole, may be termed "frightfully sad." According to Dr. Dale, other emotional aspects include abnormal or inappropriate laughter.

Physical heart problems may be easily pinpointed through Clinical Kinesiology energetic testing. Discerning whether any of the above emotions applies (especially if the person doesn't manifest these emotions) requires specific priority testing by a skilled practitioner. Once a remedy or treatment is administered, retesting confirms whether the heart strengthens with the remedy.

Small Intestine Emotions

The small intestine has been called the "sorter" of emotions. It processes those emotions of value to the mind/body and discards the rest.

The main emotional factor affecting the small intestine may be referred to as "vulnerable." Feeling vulnerable or lost in life may cause this imbalance to show up. Other related emotions involve feelings of abandonment.

Sandy's Story

Sandy came to me with a complaint of dizziness, which she attributed to an inner ear problem she'd been suffering from for over ten years. Treating the physical aspect of Sandy's problem pinpointed a relationship to her thyroid gland. Additionally, a blocked Eustachian tube and food sensitivities further contributed to the dizziness.

Simultaneously, Sandy suffered an emotional crisis. This immediately signified to me that something more serious might be going on. Through Clinical Kinesiology testing, Sandy's body indicated she needed three or four different remedies. *Vulnerable* proved to be the emotional imbalance that showed up most strongly. It made sense. If a person was feeling extremely vulnerable, his or her head would spin—he or she would feel dizzy.

Since several reflex points proved out of balance in Sandy's case, I suggested she read through a list of emotions and focus on two or three. She recounted abandonment as an issue she clearly related back to early childhood, and reported that she was currently addressing these issues with a psychotherapist. In addition, Sandy's heart proved out of balance. Several nutrients tested positive for strengthening her heart, and at one point testing also uncovered the need for a homeopathic remedy for female problems. Eventually, Sandy required treatment to rebalance every single organ/meridian system in the fire element.

Sandy acknowledged that for many years her emotions had gone unexpressed. Ultimately, they found an escape route through her illnesses—they rolled around in her head causing a great part of her dizziness.

Happily, with treatment, Sandy's ten-year span of dizziness came to an end after roughly four months. She made the transition from suppressed emotions and conflict regarding her career to a situation in which she'd created a three-day work week and a month's leave of absence to resolve her emotional issues, build up her strength, and closely evaluate her future.

Once blocked, both her emotional and physical illnesses were diagnosed and treated through Clinical Kinesiology, opening up for her the possibilities of a whole new life.

Fire Element Glands

The Thyroid and Adrenal glands of the Circulation/Sex and Triple Warmer meridian together are under the Fire element.

Research indicates that ninety percent of the imbalances affecting the thyroid and adrenal glands stem from emotions labeled "confusion." You may know someone who says, "I can't remember things," or "I can't put two and two together." Muddled instability reflects the main emotion along with the secondary emotion of paranoia.

The Pericardium

The Circulation/Sex or Pericardium meridian is named for the Pericardium, a tiny sac encircling the heart. A great deal of energy radiates around this sac. As a result, stagnation or energetic imbalances may, in turn, energetically block emotions from the heart. Someone who doesn't reach out or express emotions, who may not be thinking or emoting clearly, may indeed have a blockage around the heart.

When an individual suffers a shock or trauma it upsets positive thinking. You may be convinced you're a positive person and live life accordingly, however, when an emotional crisis arises, you may need to regroup and return that positive energy to the body as quickly as possible. Specific homeopathic remedies help clear up and release blocked emotions.

Male and Female Remedies

Emotional imbalances in the Circulation/Sex Meridian affect both males and females. According to Dr. Dale's research, the primary emotional factor involved with male and female problems is unresponsive. A number of homeopathic remedies address male and female problems.

Male/female imbalances affect unexpressive individuals or those who do not allow emotions out. An associated emotion has been categorized as "depleted" (from resisting responding).

Many people experience many problems in close relationships with the opposite sex. Most are unaware that emotions play a significant role in the success of those relationships. For example, with uterine or ovarian problems, prostate or testicular problems, the identifiable organ may be treated, however, without treatment of the corresponding emotion, physical response rarely comes as quickly as hoped. Severe problems call upon every factor in Clinical Kinesiology diagnosis to help rectify the situation.

Earth Element: Stomach and Spleen/Pancreas

The earth element predominates during late summer or "Indian summer," as the seasons change from green to yellow colors and plants withdraw into the earth for an early harvest. Imbalances of the earth element correspond to the stomach and spleen/pancreas. Although imbalances may occur at any time, a strong propensity remains for the earth element to flare up in the fall.

Stomach Emotion

The most relevant emotion assigned to the stomach relates to *disgust*. Many times, patients unknowingly feel disgusted about a situation, an experience, or something of that nature. The remaining ten percent of the impetus for stomach imbalance includes despair.

Spleen/Pancreas Emotions

The majority of the influence for spleen/pancreas emotional imbalance stems from *low self-esteem*.

Low self-esteem originates from feelings of rejection. According to the Chinese Five Element theory, any injury or damage suffered by the spleen or pancreas may also *trigger* low self-esteem.

The spleen manufacturers red blood cells and contains a great deal of lymphatic tissue. It's also a reservoir and recycling center for white blood cells. If the spleen becomes injured in a severe auto accident, it may rupture. Many times, removal of the spleen becomes necessary so an individual won't bleed to death.

Following spleen removal, people often develop immune system imbalances or other problems. Is there a correlation between low immune system functioning, or autoimmune diseases and self-esteem? Is sufficient self-esteem a common denominator in staying healthy? In the near future, these questions may be answered. Suffice it to say, the body and mind remain more interconnected than we ever thought imaginable.

Metal Element: Lungs and Large Intestine

Imbalances in the metal element occur most often in the late fall, its season of peak energy. The essence of metal symbolizes the power of molten rock and minerals which generate energy from deep within the earth's core.

The Chinese discovered imbalances in the metal element affect the lungs and large intestine.

Lung Emotion

Emotional imbalances of the lungs are bound up with *grief*, affecting more than ninety percent of people. The remaining emotion involves sadness.

Commonly, many people suffer a loss in the family and later come down with bronchitis, pneumonia or a cold. In addition, asthma cases often indicate a potential for grief that wasn't handled. Even childhood asthma makes one question what happened in the child's life (**even prenatally**) for which he or she carries grief. Refer to Grant's story on page 261 in Chapter 13.

Many times during evaluation, patients refer to grief issues or anger. They'll say, "Since my father died, I've never been well," or, "I felt breathless following my aunt's funeral." Such clues allow initial testing of a specific remedy. If a weak response occurs from the indicator muscle, further testing may be required to narrow down the type of homeopathic remedy which eventually strengthens the imbalance.

Stephen's Story

Sometimes, emotional problems manifest themselves severely. Stephen suffered from uncontrollable shivering each night after getting into bed. No matter how warm, or how bundled, Stephen couldn't stop shivering.

Dr. Burt Espy diagnosed Stephen's emotional imbalance through Clinical Kinesiology testing, and began treating his lungs and thyroid. However, not until well into treatment did Stephen begin to recall the trauma that led to his illness.

Ten years before, a ringing phone startled Stephen from a deep sleep in the middle of the night. Drowsily, he listened to a voice on the other end of the line inform him that both his mother and father had been killed in a car accident. Stunned, Stephen silenced his grief, carrying his pain around inside for the next ten years. Finally, the shivering—his physical manifestation of grief—became totally unbearable.

With Dr. Espy's help Stephen began to confront his unexpressed emotions. Through acupuncture, nutrition, treatment of his chakra energy centers (see Chapter 4), along with the appropriate homeopathic remedy, Stephen was able to peel away the negative emotions which literally "piled up" through body adaptations.

Large Intestine Emotions

Emotional imbalances related to the large intestine are best expressed by the term stuck. The colloquial term "intestinal fortitude," describes this immovable strength in the intestines.

Imbalances in the large intestine may affect one who requires a set of rules or principles (as in the dogma of a church, or political party) which may result in rigidity. This inflexible emotion may lead to intestinal problems at a later time. According to Dr. Dale, remaining emotional factors include *defensiveness*.

Although the energy of the large intestine projects a dogmatic or forceful aspect, some people with intestinal problems don't manifest these emotions, or, at least, not as obviously.

Water Element: Kidney and Bladder

In winter, everything which flows on earth slows to a standstill. Perhaps all that flows within the body may be affected in the same way. The time of year, winter, also provides a significant correlation to kidney and bladder imbalances of the water element.

Water comprises over seventy-five percent of the human body. Proper intake, balance, and release of water depends on two major organs, the kidneys and bladder. Together, they filter and excrete the body's wastewater and dissolved water products.

Kidney Emotions

Fear serves as the major emotion which affects the kidney meridian. Extreme fears such as phobias (including agoraphobia, panic attacks, fear of heights, water, or close quarters) fall into this category. Through Dr. Dale's research and my own clinical experience, as time goes on we may identify more. While the primary factor affecting the kidney relates to fear, the secondary emotion is *terror*.

Bladder Emotions

In psychological studies, fear and anger are closely involved. It is not surprising then, that the emotion associated with the bladder has been termed "irritated." Irritation may have more to do with feeling emotionally upset or slighted, rather than with full-blown anger. Another emotion classified with bladder involves *timidity*.

Considering fear in relation to the kidney and bladder, many people may recall experiencing an extremely fearful event actually causing incontinence. Although it is more joked about than probably occurs, incontinence remains a strong metaphor for how the emotion of fear is linked to imbalances of the kidney and bladder.

Brandon's Story

One of my patients scheduled treatment for her young son, Brandon, who had begun urinating more often than usual. At the onset, Brandon's medical doctor diagnosed the problem as a "neurogenic bladder." With no available treatment, the problem subsided for a short while, but later returned.

Still troubled, Brandon's mother questioned her son, who finally admitted he'd been kicked hard by one of the other children at school. Did his problem stem from the fear that he might be kicked again? What other fear issues were involved?

Due to his young age, Brandon's problem proved more likely to be emotional than physical. Further, Clinical Kinesiology testing was required to check that out. Brandon's test did prove positive for a homeopathic kidney remedy. After several months of treatment, Brandon experienced no further symptoms.

FIRST LINE OF EMOTIONAL DEFENSE

The Chinese Five Element Theory provides important answers to questions about how emotions interact with the total health of the physical body. In addition to the Chinese Five Elements, one of the most simple, "first line of defense" measures to ensure daily emotional health is to continually monitor your mental state and note how often you're experiencing negative thought patterns.

Pop by the mirror more often and take a look. Are you smiling, frowning, or looking frightened? Pay close attention to how your body reacts during stressful situations, after being presented with sad information or a stressful task to complete. Begin to "feel" and find out how you perceive and are affected by stressful events.

Negative Thoughts

It was King Solomon who said, "Death and life are in the power of the tongue."[5] And, it's true, words and emotions wield so much power. The subconscious mind takes everything literally. Listen to the daily thoughts that run through your head. They might provide important clues which affect your emotional well-being. Many people create unnecessary problems in their lives simply because of what they think and say.

Tonia, a young patient of mine, consistently entertained negative thoughts. Most mornings, as she left her house, she bombarded herself with several negative thoughts all at once: "I probably left the stove on … I hope I remembered to lower the garage door … Did I leave the water running"… and on and on.

I recommended to Tonia that she subjectively evaluate her thoughts and retrain her mind to create a more positive dialogue: "What a beautiful morning … I'm going to have a great day today … I just know I'm going to hear from a good friend!" I reminded Tonia that we "get" what we think about all day long.

In many ways life has become more intense and stressful than it's ever been before. Often, we don't take—or, can't take—the time to evaluate, sort out, cope or express the emotions we have. The quick solution? Unfortunately, seeking a chemical means for altering one's mood or perceptions has become second nature—almost a cultural norm.

The increased consumption of tranquilizers, sedatives, anti-anxiety drugs, anti-depressants, and other psychotropic drugs has reached epidemic proportions. Popping a pharmaceutical pill for these purposes **never** addresses the actual problem. Some individuals may seek prescriptions from one or more doctors to numb or void their emotional issues. This path is destined to fail since the underlying cause remains. Just like an annoying "pop up" ad on your computer screen, the actual issue will repeatedly pop up with various symptoms until you directly and effectively address it. Countless lives are damaged or lost to "self medicating" with alcohol, various street drugs, over-the-counter drugs, or hoarded prescription drugs. Of course, the worst damage comes from excessive dosing and combining incompatible substances. This cultural crisis is the precipitating factor pushing me to present my drug-free approach in my upcoming book concerning the downfalls of the "drug fix," which is ineffective and only offers a temporary "fix." This natural approach comes in many "flavors," yet typically requires one to be present with their feelings, emotions, motivations and reactions.

Most mind-numbing and tranquilizing drugs further suppress emotional problems and make coping with stress a nonissue. Tranquilized, we are still a sicker society today than we've ever been. However, it's something that each of us has the power to change. The first step means taking individual responsibility for our negative thoughts. Ronnie, another female patient, also played in her head a running commentary of terrible occurrences. During a lengthy span of treatment for kidney problems, she literally "wrote" her life with a succession of problems. It was one thing after another.

One day, Ronnie called in a state of panic and exclaimed, "I can't come to my appointment today. My apartment is on fire!" A chain-smoker, Ronnie had tried numerous times to quit smoking. This time, she accidentally caught her mattress on fire while smoking in bed.

Ronnie thrives on crises. She experiences crisis after crisis in her life because she's locked into a struggle. Why do people need to create such crisis situations? Unconsciously, they may create their problems from negative thought processes, which, in turn, create negative energy around them.

This negative mental processing, concentration, awareness, and expectation all add up to, "What's going to go wrong today?"

Recent studies speak volumes regarding how negative thoughts trigger physiological changes in the body. Research by Dr. Theresa Dale,[6] Dr. Joan Borysenko[7] and others in the field of psychoneuroimmunology, indicate an increase in lactic acid and adrenalin as the body reacts to negative word and thought.

Dr. Alan Beardall developed specific handmodes to delve into underlying emotional and psychological states using Clinical Kinesiology. Multiple personality, obsession, entrapment, personal vendetta and other conditions can be explored by using the handmodes documented in Dr. Beardall's handmode books.[8]

The Decision for Health

Many co-factors determine who gets sick and who doesn't according to Blair Justice, Ph.D., author of *Who Gets Sick*.[9] Beliefs, moods and thoughts affect the mind/body in many ways. Justice believes, "Whatever gives us an increased sense of control—whether it is love, faith, or cognitive coping—seems to mobilize our self-healing systems."[10] Successful recoveries through such mind/body control have allowed many to gain access to their inner self-healers throughout history and in the present day.

Author Norman Cousins led a personal crusade aimed at turning around negative states of mind. He championed the effects of positive thoughts and feelings in several books, including *Anatomy of an Illness as Perceived by the Patient* and *The Healing Heart* in which he documents his own conscious decision to fight the prognosis of a life-threatening collagen disease and subsequent heart attack.[11,12]

When doctors tell patients, "You will die," they risk giving them a death sentence. A terminal prognosis ... death in three, or six months—is a death sentence. When patients receive this kind of "programming" how can doctors expect them to live any longer? Health professionals should take into account a person's "fighting" spirit, commitment and will to overcome—to re-create his or her own reality!

In his book, *Who Gets Sick*, Blair Justice, Ph.D. reports, "... genetic or constitutional traits often determine which parts of our bodies are most vulnerable to dysfunction or disease."[13] Yes, however, even though genetic predisposition for diabetes runs in my family, I've made a conscious decision that I will not develop diabetes. I don't allow that negative mind-set to enter my thoughts. Protectively, I do take precautions, never eat sugar, and take numerous supplemental nutrients.

With any type of imbalance, problem, disorder, or dysfunction in the body, the first and strongest part of recovery is the decision, thought, inspiration, or "stick-to-it-ive-ness" to get well. When confronted with pain or illness, affirm with calm, positive self-statements, "I am getting well. My health grows stronger every day." And remember, you have the power and the ability to make yourself well.

Don't allow orthodox medical approaches ("Listen to what we say and do what we tell you...") to wrest power away from you, the patient. Instead of promoting dependency in their patients, health professionals should teach, and give options, accepting that the final outcome is not determined by them, but by you.

USING THE MIND FOR HEALING

You can learn to control your mind and thus relax and heal your body—through changing your brain waves.

Jose Silva, originator of The Silva Method Seminars, and many other researchers in human consciousness have developed simple methods of using mind and thought processes to control brainwave activity.

There are four different brainwaves, distinguished by their frequency or cycles per second: Beta (the highest frequency), Alpha, Theta and Delta (lowest frequency).

Beta waves characterize most of our thinking, conscious mind. Reading, writing, driving and focusing on many different activities may be done while in the Beta state. When we relax, the brainwaves slow down. It's now believed that this progression from Beta to Alpha (a slower brainwave frequency) becomes necessary to help the healing process. Different methods may be used to make this transition.

Sitting quietly, closing your eyes, listening to soft music or employing meditation, positive thinking or biofeedback can all help you to achieve a calm, relaxed state. Certain people with high levels of anxiety may benefit greatly by putting themselves in Alpha for a short period of time at least once a day.

This and other types of relaxation work were successfully used by Dr. O. Carl Simonton, (See Referral Guide.) Though Dr. Simonton (1942-2009) has passed, his revolutionary work remains successful and the Simonton Cancer Center continues to document remarkable victories with their cancer patients. One of their continued techniques is to have patients visualize or draw a cancerous tumor or mass. The patient is then guided to visualize scissors to the area and to cut the cancer away. Other visualizations involve the patient imagining armies of white blood cells attacking, gray, weak and confused cancer cells and ultimately killing them.

Whatever visualization you wish to create in your mind's eye may help trigger subtle changes. Practicing this type of concrete thinking initiates and expedites the process of healing in the body. As little as ten or twenty minutes, two or three times a day, should suffice.

In addition to visualizations, affirmations or mantras may be used to help heal your body. In her book *Heal Your Body*, Louise L. Hay gives a wide array of healing affirmations for literally hundreds of different maladies, as well as purposed causes for each of these dis-eases. These affirmations can be said aloud or repeated silently several times throughout the day in order for therapeutic benefit.

It's well known that humans only utilize between one and fourteen percent of their brain capacity. With that in mind, we've got a great deal of potential to use. By using our minds more positively, I believe we'll find more good things happening in our lives.

THE BRAIN AND EMOTIONS

The book, *The Amazing Brain*, by Robert Ornstein clearly describes the complexity of how the brain affects emotions.[14] The brain is relied on for important functioning of the physical body, emotions, and the stability of the psyche. Because of this, adequate neurotransmitter production remains paramount.

A healthy and adequate diet provides the foundation for supplying raw nutrients which enable the body to manufacture neurotransmitters in maintaining a healthy nervous system. Some individuals with poor absorption or genetic predispositions to brain disorders may need to take specific nutritional supplements to aid in neurotransmitter production.

Neurotransmitters consist of free floating chemicals which the body produces to enable messages to move among the nerves. Receptors represent physical spots or locations in the nervous system which receive and translate those messages. Each of us has explicit lock and key mechanisms which allow us to send and receive neurotransmitter communication.

To complete a myriad of nerve functions, the brain contains certain shaped neurotransmitters which connect with receptors for a perfect match. Such lock and key mechanisms maintain nervous system function at optimal levels. If the body cannot produce a neurotransmitter of the correct size and shape, the receptor won't receive its message—and cannot complete its job. That job function may entail producing a good mood, maintaining a calm body, avoiding depression, or other functions.

Neurotransmitters include both excitatory and inhibitory transmitters. Of the excitatory transmitters, acetylcholine regulates the autonomic nervous system, including all muscle movements. Other excitatory neurotransmitters include norepinephrine, dopamine, and serotonin.

Inhibitory transmitters, such as polypeptides, inhibit or slow nerve function. That function in itself can be extremely important because some messages may need to get through, while others must be held back. A lack of certain amino acids in the brain may result in anxiety, depression, phobias, and manic disorders.

Anxiety and Depression

The amino acid, Tyrosine proves to be an important neurotransmitter building block for treating depression. Tyrosine is composed of B_6, folic acid, niacin, copper and Vitamin C. These nutritional components are necessary in specific amounts, along with others, in order to help manufacture Tyrosine in the brain.

Other amino acids which facilitate brain and emotional function include: L-Glutamine, which has been used in treatment of alcoholism, L-Aspartate, GABA (gamma-aminobutyric acid), a well-researched, major inhibitory factor in treating anxiety and panic attacks when partnered with B_1, Taurine, and Glycine. Inositol is also an important brain supplement which aids other amino acids.

Deficiencies in the brain do alter thoughts. Therefore, many times emotional problems stem from nutritional deficiencies.

Christine's Story

Shortly after her sixteenth birthday, Christine was suddenly overcome with an inexplicable fear while driving her car. Heart pounding, blood rushing from her head—she felt as though she were about to faint. Forced to pull off to the side of the road, Christine sat flushed, shaking and weak.

The doctors at her medical clinic seemed puzzled: "We're not sure, but it's probably nerves," they told her parents. With no further tests, the doctors sent Christine home with her first bottle of tranquilizers.

Throughout her life, Christine continued to experience unexplained episodes of fearfulness. She learned to avoid crowds, to hover in safe corners of rooms. She even stopped going to restaurants in a vain attempt to mask the dreaded fear that could, at anytime, overtake her without warning.

Eventually, Christine fell in love with a caring young man and got married. Her first few months of marriage seemed blissful; then, something changed. Christine began noticing her husband's every move. He talked too loudly. He laughed too much. She felt so uncomfortable that she could barely sit in the same room with him. Slowly, Christine was developing a new phobia—one that could end her marriage.

Desperately, Christine searched for help, all the while taking more and more tranquilizers to cover her symptoms. She knew she had to find a real cure—and soon. Her panic attacks had progressed to serious phobias and she was now totally dependent on tranquilizing drugs.

With every ounce of energy, Christine began studying. She poured over hundreds of nutrition books and research studies. She became specifically interested in amino acid supplementation and their effects on neurotransmitter production in anxiety and panic attacks. Finally, the answer came.

Christine consulted a naturopathic physician who specialized in orthomolecular therapy. The physician helped her begin a program of supplementation with 500 mg. capsules each of the amino acids GABA, Taurine, and Glycine five times a day. She also supplemented her diet with B-Complex vitamins, and liquid Choline. In addition, Christine took a 1,000 mg. balanced complement of all the amino acids, extra magnesium, calcium, and vitamin C.

With faith, perseverance, and determination to heal, Christine found a cure. Today, her panic attacks and phobias are gone. She takes no tranquilizing drugs, her marriage has never been happier. Christine and her husband have three children and one grandchild. She remains free from her once crippling fear.

Amino Acids and Diet

Stunning research successes by Dr. Eric R. Braverman have propelled amino acid therapies into the forefront of nutritional healing and supplementation. Someday, these therapies may very well supplant the need for tranquilizing drugs. However, until more knowledge is gained, the search continues for long-awaited answers to emotional problems stemming from nutritional deficiencies.

The body requires twenty-two essential amino acids. Eating a well balanced, healthy diet, including a variety of whole grains, beans, legumes, and nuts, along with vegetables and some protein provide the best compilation of amino acids.

These foods supply complete and balanced nutrition and provide the major building blocks for neurotransmitters. If additional amino acid supplements are needed, you need to be aware of proper dosage and balance. Of course, Clinical Kinesiology evaluation remains the best method for determining the unique plan of supplementation for each person. To simply say, "Take so many milligrams of this or that," is merely a "cookbook" approach and doesn't address all people. Discerning how each individual body and physiology responds now remains crucial. The same test may prove different a month earlier, or a month later. Anyone who suffers a great deal of emotional stress, uses up more neurotransmitters. Precipitating factors—individual illness, lifestyle, diet and emotions—all affect testing results.

TESTING THE ENERGY OF EMOTIONS

Emotional aspects continue to affect many physical, as well as energetic health problems and conditions. Often, unexpressed emotions churning under the surface do not manifest obviously enough to be pinpointed except through energetic muscle testing. People in treatment for physical problems may admit emotional problems to others and themselves—or they may consciously or unconsciously hide that knowledge.

Just as Clinical Kinesiology muscle testing is used to evaluate physical imbalances such as a sore knee or ankle, it can also help the body-mind identify a "sore" emotional point which may be affecting health.

One simple method of using energetic muscle testing to uncover hidden emotional problems involves asking a test-subject a series of questions developed by Dr. Theresa Dale, based on the Chinese Five Element Theory.

The Organ-Emotion Questionnaire

This testing procedure is done on the mental level, thus, no verbal response is necessary. In this case, we're looking only for the muscle test response.

Before beginning any test of emotions, first ask the person being tested to lie down quietly and raise his or her indicator arm. Ask one initial question: *Is it appropriate to ask your mind/body the following questions at this time?*

> Question + Muscle test + Strong arm = yes, proceed with testing.
>
> Question + Muscle test + Weak arm = no, do not proceed at this time.

If the body of the person being tested "says" it's O.K. to proceed, begin asking the following set of questions calmly and clearly. Although the test questions are based on organ/emotion correlations, the test-subject should not therapy localize over any of the organs. Rather, the free hand should rest at his or her side.

As each consecutive test question is asked, the tester should simultaneously perform the muscle test and note either strong or weak muscle response. We're looking for the muscle test response. If asking a test question triggers a flow of thought, speech or verbalizing emotion, the person should be encouraged to talk about the feelings. That, in itself, may prove therapeutic.

The following Emotion Test Questions are listed along with the corresponding organ:

Small Intestine Question: *Do you feel vulnerable?*

> Question + Muscle test + Weak arm = Emotional imbalance affecting small intestine.
>
> Question + Muscle test + Strong arm = No emotional imbalance.

Thyroid/Adrenals Question: *Do you feel confused?*

> Question -f Muscle test + Weak arm = Emotional imbalance affecting thyroid/adrenals.
>
> Question + Muscle test 4- Strong arm = No emotional imbalance.

Heart Questions: *Do you feel sad? Do you feel frightfully overjoyed?*

> Question + Muscle test + Weak arm = Emotional imbalance affecting the heart.
>
> Question + Muscle test + Strong arm = No emotional imbalance.

Hypothalamus Question: *Do you express emotions easily?*

> Question + Muscle test 4- Weak arm = Emotional imbalance affecting the hypothalamus.
>
> Question + Muscle test + Strong arm = No emotional imbalance.

Stomach Question: *Do you feel disgust?*

> Question + Muscle test + Weak arm = Emotional imbalance affecting the stomach.
>
> Question + Muscle test + Strong arm = No emotional imbalance.

Spleen/Pancreas Question: *Do you have high self-esteem?*

> Question + Muscle test + Weak arm = Emotional imbalance affecting the spleen/pancreas.
>
> Question + Muscle test + Strong arm = No emotional imbalance.

Lung Question: *Are you grieving?*

> Question + Muscle test + Weak arm = Emotional imbalance affecting the lung.
>
> Question + Muscle test + Strong arm = No emotional imbalance.

Large Intestine Question: *Do you feel stuck? Are you tolerant of others?*

> Question + Muscle test + Weak arm = Emotional imbalance affecting the large intestine.
>
> Question + Muscle test + Strong arm = No emotional imbalance.

Bladder Question: *Are you irritated about something?*

> Question + Muscle test + Weak arm = Emotional imbalance affecting the bladder.
>
> Question + Muscle test + Strong arm = No emotional imbalance.

Kidney Question: *Do you feel fear?*

> Question + Muscle test + Weak arm = Emotional imbalance affecting the kidney.
>
> Question + Muscle test + Strong arm = No emotional imbalance.

Gallbladder Question: *Do you feel resentment?*

> Question -I- Muscle test + Weak arm = Emotional imbalance affecting the gallbladder.
>
> Question + Muscle test + Strong arm = No emotional imbalance.

Liver Question: *Do you feel anger?*

> Question + Muscle test + Weak arm = Emotional imbalance affecting the liver.
>
> Question + Muscle test + Strong arm = No emotional imbalance.

Male/Female Organ Question: *Do you express your emotions to loved ones?*

> Question + Muscle test + Weak arm = Emotional imbalance affecting the male or female organs.
>
> Question + Muscle test + Strong arm = No emotional imbalance.

This proves to be a simple method for delving below the surface emotions of an individual. If you are well acquainted with the person being tested, ask him or her to make a list of some emotional concerns he or she may have, or add to the list a few more which you may have observed.

Once an emotional imbalance is uncovered through a weak arm muscle response to the Clinical Kinesiology muscle test, seek guidance from a skilled practitioner who may follow up, test related reflex points and recommend appropriate treatment, Neuro-emotional or other homeopathic remedies. (See the Resource and Product Guide in the appendix of this book.)

ON TO WELLNESS

You can resolve the past, begin to create positive energy around you and reclaim the power over your miraculous mind-body. Begin your journey now with the recognition that sufficient self-esteem, along with the investment of your time, energy, and full range of emotions, may be the secret to maintaining good health on your mental and physical path to wellness.

Truly resolving physical and emotional problems also means addressing and understanding the *spiritual* aspect of health and healing. Often imbalances on the spiritual level have spontaneous effects on both emotional and physical well-being. In Chapter 4, we look at how *Divine Energy* affects and heals subtle energy centers in the body known as "the *chakras*."

CHAPTER 3 SUGGESTED READING

Barral, Jean-Pierre, D.O. *Understanding the Messages of Your Body: How to Interpret Physical and Emotional Signals to Achieve Optimal Health.* Berkeley, Calif.: North Atlantic Books and Palm Beach Gardens, Florida: Upledger Enterprises, 2007.

Boyd-Barrett, Leah. *Your Secret BodyMind Toolkit.* Ojai, Calif.: Earth Lotus Publishing, New Earth Books, 2012.

Borysenko, Joan, Ph.D., *Fire in the Soul: A New Psychology of Spiritual Optimism.* New York: Warner Books, 1993.

———, with a new Foreword by Andrew Weil, M.D. *Minding the Body, Mending the Mind.* Cambridge, Mass.: DaCapo Press; revised edition, 2007.

Braverman, Eric R., M.D. *The Healing Nutrients Within: Facts, Findings, and New Research on Amino Acids,* Laguna Beach, Calif: Basic Health Publications, Inc.; third edition, 2003.

———. *The Edge Effect: Achieve Total Health and Longevity with the Balanced Brain Advantage.* New York: Sterling Publishing CO, 2005.

Byrne, Rhonda. *The Secret.* New York: Atria Books, 2006.

———. *The Secret Gratitude Book.* New York: Atria Books, 2007.

Cousins, Norman. *The Healing Heart.* New York: Norton, 1983

———. *Anatomy of an Illness as Perceived by the Patient, Twentieth Anniversary Edition.* New York: Norton, 2005.

Goleman, Daniel. *The Meditative Mind: The Varieties of Meditative Experience.* Los Angeles: Jeremy Tarcher, Inc., 1988.

Hay, Louise L. *Heal Your Body: The Mental Causes for Physical Illness and the Metaphysical Way to Overcome Them Expanded/Revised Edition.* New York: Hay House. 1988.

Hunt, Douglas, M.D. *No More Fears.* New York: Warner Books, 1988

Justice, Blair, Ph.D. *Who Gets Sick.* Los Angeles: Jeremy Tarcher, Inc., 1988.

Matsumoto, Kiiko and Birch, Stephen. *Five Elements & Ten Stems: Nan-Ching Theory, Diagnosis, and Practice.* Brookline, Mass.: Paradigm Publications, 1989.

Nelson, Bradley. *The Emotion Code.* Mesquite, Nevada: Wellness Unmasked Publishing, 1st edition, 2007.

Ornstein, Robert. *The Amazing Brain.* Boston: Houghton-Mifflin, 1984.

Pelletier, Kenneth. *Mind as Healer, Mind as Slayer.* McHenry, Ill.: Delta, 1977.

Philpott, William., Dwight D Kalita, and Linus Pauling. *Brain Allergies: The Psychonutrient and Magnetic Connections, Updated 2nd Ed..* New Canaan, Conn.: Keats Publishing, 2000.

Sahley, Billie Jay, Ph.D. *The Anxiety Epidemic: A Wounded Healer Tells How to Use GABA and Other Amino Acids to Control Anxiety and Panic Attacks, 5th Ed.* San Antonio, Texas: Pain Stress Publications, 2002.

Steadman, Alice. *Who's the Matter with Me?, 13th Ed.* Marina Del Rey, Calif.: DeVorss, 1977.

Truman, Karol K. *Feelings Buried Alive Never Die: Revised and Expanded.* St. George, Utah: Olympus Distributing, 2003.

Weil, Andrew, M.D. *Natural Health, Natural Medicine: A Comprehensive Guide to Wellness and Self-Care, Revised Ed.* Boston: Houghton Mifflin, 2004.

Williams, Montel. *Living Well Emotionally: Break Through to a Life of Happiness.* New York: New American Library, 2009.

CHAPTER 4

Divine Energy: The Chakras

Displayed in the waiting area of my office is a macramé wall hanging which I designed. The intricately woven "landscape" symbolizes the flowing energy of life: As the snow melts from a mountain top, water flows down from the highest peaks, cascades into a waterfall and forms deep whirlpools of swirling energy. From there, the water of life plummets into a rushing stream that gushes down into a mountain lake. Trickling along, the water spills into a gentle pond rippling around a cluster of lily pads. Eventually the pond pours out into numerous streams—the dangling streamers that hang down from the piece. On its endless journey, the river of energy is always flowing and changing.

Like water, the energy in the body's subtle (spiritual) energetic centers known as the *chakras* flows downward from above. Some remains "on the peaks," to illumine the mind, "in the mountain lakes," to open the heart, some "in the pond" to balance the physical health of the whole body and some streams forever onward—to serve the Earth and her inhabitants.

HEALING CHAKRA IMBALANCES

The body is made up of "life energy centers" or chakras, which connect to all parts of the physical body. Although chakras cannot be seen in the physical realm, proof that they exist come from many-centuries-old religious, metaphysical, esoteric and long-standing spiritual traditions.

Varied approaches to explaining the chakras are found in ancient Eastern mysticism, Australian aboriginal lore, Native American stories, and Christian and Jewish esoteric doctrine. Although there are different outlooks, the common thread that links all approaches to the "spiritual body" involves a form of spiritual development that requires knowledge and practice to balance and create new healing through this channel of unseen Power or Divine energy from God.

When certain emotional problems, traumatic events, or lifestyle disturbances occur, energetic imbalances may begin to affect the physical body, manifesting in particular organs or meridian systems, through the chakras.

The practical goal of this chapter is to examine these deeper, ongoing emotional disturbances which can trigger imbalances in the spiritual body, or chakras. Deeply ingrained or long-lasting emotions, possibly stemming back to childhood, often lead to personality or behavior pattern changes that maintain or perpetuate disturbances in the chakras.

Returning balance and harmony to the body requires that one become an "instrument" or channel through which elimination of energy blockages in the chakras may be accomplished.

Different facets of the electromagnetic body respond to different therapies. Many therapies treat only the physical body, others heal the body of thoughts and emotions, while others treat the spiritual body. Some believe all states of health depend on this level.

Many people, including the late C.W Leadbeater, foremost author, clairvoyant and chakra researcher, consider that all disease originates only at deep spiritual levels. It is in this context that I will attempt to explain the importance of the spiritual role of the chakras in the total well-being of the body's energetic system.

"An energy center is very much like a flower bud. If it is properly cared for and receives the necessary sunshine, the bud opens and turns into a flower," say John Mann and Lar Short, authors of *The Body of Light*.[1]

In this chapter you will:

- Explore the body's spiritual garden, and begin to understand the basic characteristics of each chakra.
- Learn how the circulation of chakra energy or light helps open and heal chakra imbalances.
- Discover how Dr. Alan Beardall further developed Clinical Kinesiology by the introduction of Bach Flower Remedies to provide more accurate testing in locating deep spiritual imbalances.
- Determine through specific exercises and self-testing, how the revitalization and healing of the chakras—the body's spiritual flowers—may be attained through earthly flowers, The Bach Flower Remedies.

THE CHAKRAS

The word *chakra*, translated from ancient Indian Sanskrit, means "wheel." Although symbolic of a "wheel of fate" or life and death, in Clinical Kinesiology diagnosis the chakras relate to a series of wheel-like energy vortices. The Chinese liken the chakras to spiritual or Divine flowers with many petals.

Chakras represent subtle energy centers in the etheric or spiritual body. Unconfined to the physical body, they channel psychic and healing energy from the glandular and nervous systems. This vital force comprises the conscience, "aura" or etheric body, and links physical, psychic, and superphysical or clairvoyant states of consciousness.

The body's seven major chakras consist of an energetic force localized in the physical body but extending beyond the physical body. The chakras coincide with different levels of the spine, (usually in conjunction with an organ). Chakra energy projects several inches from the front of the body, envelopes and flows out the back of the body.

Identifying Chakras

Chakras, seen only by clairvoyant sight, appear as colorful wheels of light whose centers vary in brightness and hue. Active chakras each contain a corresponding color closely aligned with the type of *vitality* sent to it through other chakras and from the sun.

Similar to the Chinese Five Element Theory, each chakra corresponds with a specific element: earth, water, fire, air, or ether (mind). These elements manifest as solid, liquid, fiery or gaseous, airy, and etheric. Each element also represents rising levels of consciousness. For example, the earth element chakra represents the lowest levels of consciousness, while the "ether" elements represent the higher, more developed levels.

C.W Leadbeater, expert in chakra energy research, suggests that people "... imagine themselves to be looking straight down into the bell of a flower," such as a morning glory, in order to grasp the general appearance of a chakra.[2]

Perpetually rotating, chakra energy centers may be likened to a vortex or whirl of energy spinning at seven distinct centers of the body. Leadbeater further describes chakras as "... the hub or open mouth in which a force from the higher world is always flowing."[3] He states, "Without this inrush of energy, the physical body could not exist."[4]

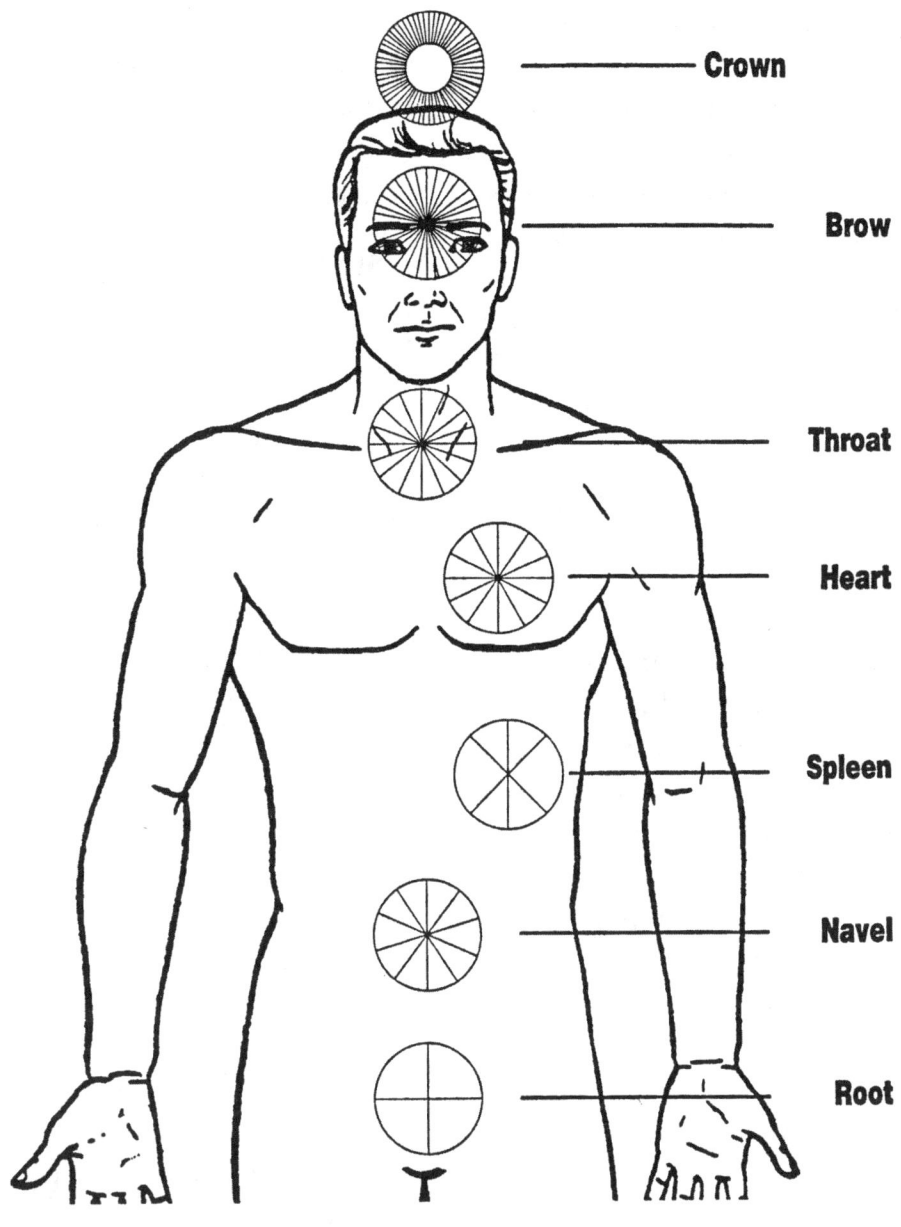

THE CHAKRAS
ILLUSTRATION COURTESY OF DR. JOHN AMARO,
INTERNATIONAL ACADEMY OF CLINICAL ACUPUNCTURE. COPYRIGHT © 1981.

Kundalini Energy

The Root or Base Chakra represents the seat of energy, the basic force that infuses life. The Hindu religion refers to this base as the reservoir of *Kundalini* energy. Kundalini is believed to emanate from a central core of the body, physically related to the spine. Through a channel called the *Sushumna*, the energy rises through a cavity in the bony canal of the spinal cord. This physical canal also provides a central connecting electrical system from which the peripheral spinal nerves of the body communicate with the brain.

Kundalini energy rises like a snake along two coiled paths of the Sushumna channel: the *Ida* or female, and *Pingala* or male. The Kundalini base energy then combines with incoming streams of Divine energy from the Power of the Divine Spirit or God. This current sets up a pressure which causes the mingled forces of energy to form a whirl. As the energies in the Ida and Pingala cross over on their rise up the body, each positive and negative crossing point creates a chakra "flower."

The Silver Cord

Sanskrit teachings detail a "silver cord" connecting the human spirit with God, a Higher Power or an overriding Spiritual Principle. This Divine energy flows down through the top of the head, or Crown Chakra. An extension of Sushumna energy, the "silver cord," connects the spirit and body together.

Kundalini yoga or meditation practitioners often teach techniques which implement the movement of Kundalini energy from the Root Chakra at the base of the spine, all the way up the Kundalini Path of energy to the Crown Chakra—and on to connection with the Divine spirit and spiritual reality.

How Do Chakras Work?

According to most spiritual traditions, chakras operate similarly in everyone. However, in Leadbeater's view, in a spiritually undeveloped person, chakras may whirl in a comparatively sluggish motion, merely forming the necessary vortex for the force and no more. Comparatively, in a more spiritually-evolved individual, enormously greater amounts of energy pass through the "flowers," opening additional faculties and possibilities.

Naturally divided into three groups, chakras represent the lower, middle and higher—or respectively, the physiological, personal, and spiritual—aspects of life. Some believe each petal of the force-centers also represent a moral quality. The development of that quality brings each center into activity.

YOUR SPIRITUAL GARDEN

In order to experience chakra energy, you might imagine taking a stroll through your own body's spiritual garden. To assist in this visualization, picture your favorite type of garden—an English Country garden, or a simple meadow filled with wildflowers.

Ask a friend to read you the descriptions of the seven chakras which follow. Lie down peacefully and imagine yourself sensing the fragrance of each "flower." As you "walk" serenely along your garden pathway:

- Locate each spiritual flower or chakra energy center within your body.
- Hold your hand approximately an inch or two above your body at the location of the chakra.
- Inhale and exhale deeply as you picture each whirling "flower."
- Note any correlations between your spiritual energy and symptoms you may be experiencing.
- Focus briefly on any energy sensations (feelings of warmth or coldness), as you sense each "flower" along the way.

The Root Chakra

The Root Chakra or *Muladhara*, centered at the base of the spine, is the lowest or base chakra. It also represents the least highly developed area of the spiritual self: the embodiment of the flesh, regeneration, and physical reproductive functions.

The Root Chakra became the focus for ancient yogic meditation rituals. With certain breathing techniques and other practices, the Kundalini energy was encouraged to rise up the spine, thereby raising the level of consciousness of the practitioner. This same spiritual quest also marked the tradition for monks to remain celibate. Such solidarity trials allowed them to focus on the subtle essence of their spiritual nature and further understand the connection between their spiritual beliefs (or Creator) and themselves.

Physically, the Root Chakra may be found in close proximity to the anus or rectum and connected to the sacrum and coccyx.

Symptoms corresponding to Root Chakra imbalance include glandular problems with the gonads manifesting as:

- Ovarian problems in women, or
- Testicular problems in men.

Other Root Chakra associations include:

- Root Chakra color: fiery orange/red
- Element: earth
- Negative emotion: fear
- Spiritual Petals: four

The Spleen Chakra

An especially radiant, glowing and sun-like chakra, the Spleen Chakra, *Swadisthana*, may be located slightly left of the body midline over the spleen. From Leadbeater's own clairvoyant research, the Spleen Chakra characterizes devotion "... to the specialization, subdivision, and dispersion of the vitality which comes from the sun."[5] Physically, the Spleen Chakra corresponds with the First Lumbar vertebrae, or the area surrounding the ribs. Energetic imbalances in the Spleen Chakra affect:

- Adrenal glands
- Intestines

Other associations include:

- Spleen Chakra color: rose red
- Element: water
- Negative emotion: excessive desire, lust, attachment
- Spiritual Petals: six

Because of the Spleen Chakra's relationship with the water element, chakra imbalances often trigger abnormalities of thirst centers resulting in excessive thirst or dryness. In addition, the adrenal glands and kidneys relate closely, which predisposes Spleen Chakra imbalances to the kidneys.

The Navel Chakra

The Navel Chakra or *Manipura* may be located two to three inches above the navel in the area commonly known as the solar plexus. The term solar plexus originates from the word "sun," which *defines* the center of our solar system.

Rays of the sun are often depicted as concentric circles radiating wider and wider throughout the entire body. Many energy reflex points contain both a solar and a subsidiary plexus. Likewise, the solar plexus represents the gravitational center of the body. Someone who is said to be "centered" or grounded possesses a balanced solar plexus, in harmonious relationship with the earth.

A *plexus* describes a gathering place of tiny nerves that come together in a cluster to communicate messages. Additional nerves also intersect at a plexus and branch off in different directions, similar to the activity of a bustling train station.

Many, many "trains"/nerve impulses arrive from various directions and convene at one spot. Energetic messages ride in on one train, get off and transfer to another train for the final destination. From one central point, or solar plexus, many nerves take off or send their messages in many different directions.

Navel Chakra imbalances associate with:
- pancreas problems
- liver problems
- stomach problems stemming from self-pity

Other Navel Chakra associations include:
- Navel Chakra color: green
- Element: fire
- Negative emotions: anger
- Spiritual Petals: ten

The Heart Chakra

The Heart Chakra, or *Anahata*, centers over the heart, or physically correlates to the sternum. The Heart Chakra may also be referred to as the Thymus Chakra, because of its connection with the Thymus gland.

Other classifications of the Heart Chakra include:
- Heart Chakra color: yellow/gold
- Element: air
- Negative emotion: greed
- Spiritual Petals: twelve

Chest pains often stem from physical reasons. Initially, however, a Heart Chakra imbalance may have precipitated the physical heart to become out of balance. Emotional trauma and shock are among the main reasons why Chakras become imbalanced.

The Throat Chakra

The fifth, or Throat Chakra, also known as *Vishuddha*, corresponds physically to the neck and throat. The endocrine gland involved is the thyroid, which suggests the name Thyroid Chakra in some instances.

Other traits include:
- Throat Chakra color: silvery, gleaming blue (like moonlight rippling on water)
- Element: ether or mind
- Negative emotion: pride, egotism, grief
- Spiritual Petals: sixteen

The Throat Chakra evolves from a center of self-expression—the voice. Many times this chakra becomes out of balance when an inability to work through negative emotions, such as pride, ego, or grief exists. Some people then manifest a sore throat, laryngitis or some type of thyroid problem. They may wish to speak and express something, however, suddenly the words don't come.

The Brow Chakra

The Brow Chakra, or *Ajna* in Sanskrit, classifies the sixth chakra, located between, or possibly an inch or two above, the eyebrows. Due to its nerve plexus relationship with the carotid sinuses, the Brow Chakra often affects blood pressure.

The Pineal gland, which may be reactive to light, is affected by the Brow Chakra. Imbalances in the Brow Chakra may cause Seasonal Affective Disorder in some individuals.

Other classifications include:
- Brow Chakra color: deep, vibrant or Indigo blue
- Spiritual Petals: ninety-six

A vivid blue color signifies mental awareness, while shades of violet to purple suggest spiritual awareness.

The sudden leap in the number of petals from sixteen in the Throat Chakra to ninety-six in the Brow Chakra suggests that this energy center represents an altogether different order from the lower level chakras of the etheric body. More complex and higher principles of life exist in this realm. An increasingly greater modification of

> ### Third Eye Experience
>
> - In a relaxed state, focus on The Third Eye point, slightly above the point where the eyebrows converge. Allow your awareness to penetrate slowly beneath the surface of the skin.
> - Note any sensations or experiences. Repeat the phrase, "This is the center of my experience." Make gentle contact with the point by lifting your forefinger to the area. After ten seconds, remove your finger and notice any new sensations.
> - Continue focusing, breathe in and draw new energy to the area, hold your breath for a few moments, allowing that energy to expand.
> - Breathe out any emotional tension.
>
> Repeat this exercise as often as you wish.
>
> From: *The Body of Light* by John Mann and Lar Short Published by: Charles E. Tuttle Co., Inc. Copyright 1990 John Mann and Lar Short All Rights Reserved

energy is required to create the psychic and spiritual expression which this chakra represents.

The Brow Chakra has often been referred to as the Third Eye. The ancients spoke of spiritual enlightenment as the opening of the Third Eye. Austerity practices such as fasting and meditation were attempts by Tibetan or Aurveydic (Hindu) monks to lessen input to the physical senses and thereby open the Third Eye.

When the Third Eye opens, spiritual vision opens. At once, one gains the ability to focus, learn, perceive, and impart knowledge on a new spiritual level. A simple method for experiencing the Third Eye is reported in *The Body of Light*, by John Mann and Lar Short.[6] This practice involves using conscious breathing to focus on the Third Eye.

The Crown Chakra

The Crown Chakra or *Sahasrara*, most resplendent of all, displays two "flowers." In full expression, it radiates 960 outer petals of violet, and twelve inner petals of gold. The Crown usually remains the last chakra to be opened or "awakened." As one gains the optimal in spiritual enlightenment, this magnificent spiritual flower blooms.

Clairvoyant C.W. Leadbeater characterized the Crown Chakra as "... full of indescribable chromatic effects and vibrating with almost inconceivable rapidity."[7] Containing properties unmatched by any other chakra, the Crown Chakra emanates a "... subsidiary central whirlpool of gleaming white flushed with gold in its heart"—through which the divine force flows in from without.

Leadbeater contends, "Only when one realizes a position of divine light ... this chakra reverses itself, turning as it were inside out; it is no longer a channel of reception but of radiation ... standing out from the head as a dome, a veritable crown of glory."[8]

Ancient Sanskrit drawings often depict individuals with a closed flower bud at the top of the head. Symbolically, this person has yet to reach enlightenment. In great men or women of high spiritual development, however, the Crown Chakra displays a fully open, nearly thousand-petaled flower, historically depicted as a golden glow or halo around the head. This is the basis for the appearance of a halo in many early Christian paintings and figures.

The hypothalamus represents the nerve plexus associated with the Crown Chakra. Endocrine glands affected by Crown Chakra imbalance include the pituitary and pineal.

DR. BACH'S DISCOVERIES

At the same time C.W. Leadbeater (1847–1934) described his clairvoyant research into the nature and functions of the chakras, Dr. Edward Bach (1886–1936), an English microbiologist, made a remarkable discovery of his own. Bach determined that energetic imbalances in the body's "spiritual flowers" could be remedied by earthly flowers.

In the early 1920s, Bach noted that certain patients exhibited differing symptoms and illnesses, although laboratory tests proved all had been infected with the same bacteria. As he puzzled over the different manifestations of the individual "dis-ease" processes, he correlated the inconsistencies with the scientific understanding of the day and developed a new theory, a new explanation for the inconsistency. Bach recognized a link between emotional states (which correlated to personality types) and physical illness.

Seven Personality Types

Soon, Bach began categorizing individuals according to seven basic personality types, finding that patients invariably fell into a certain category or personality type *according to their response to illness*. In essence, the disease-causing bacteria became less important than the underlying personality type which would inherently deal with it.

The seven types which Bach identified included people who manifested: fear, loneliness, uncertainty, overcare for the welfare of others, oversensitivity to ideas and influences, despondency and despair and insufficient interest in present circumstances.[9]

Bach's theory not only documented how the seven personality types responded to illness, but how they responded to or coped with life!

Wandering in the English countryside one day, Bach was struck with a spark of Divine revelation. Magnified around him, he suddenly noticed beautiful flowers carpeting the meadows. Bach instinctively knew that these flowers held the answers to healing his seven personality types.

This Divine inspiration allowed him to identify a system of picking and categorizing each flower. He placed each one in a crystal bowl of spring water, the universal solvent, and left them to bask in the sunlight. Slowly, the essence of each flower absorbed into the water. He then bottled and used each essence as a concentrate to cure the seven personality types.

All homeopathic remedies, including Bach Flower Remedies, heal on a vibrational level. If the remedy were tested in a lab, its composition would mainly contain a mixture of spring water, diluted by a concentrated essence of flower-soaked water.

As time went on, Bach formulated thirty-nine remedies (currently available at most health food stores), including one special mixture of flowers which he named "Rescue Remedy." Rescue Remedy was specifically formulated to be used for urgent or imminent danger, and crisis situations. The remedy includes essences of Rock Rose, Clematis, Impatiens, Cherry Plum, and Star of Bethlehem flowers.

Averi's Story

On one occasion, a young woman and her baby, Averi, arrived at my office. The child was feverish, restless and pulling at her ear. She and her mother had just flown into town from another state. Little Averi had been fighting a small cold before take-off; however, due to cabin pressure changes, she quickly developed an ear infection. By the time I saw her she was extremely irritable, and cried at every attempt at treatment.

Because Averi suffered from so much pain in the Eustachian tube from her throat, she'd stopped taking fluids and proved to be slightly dehydrated. At once, I administered Bach Flower Rescue Remedy to her in a glass of water: the first time she'd successfully drank any quantity of any liquid. Within minutes, Averi calmed down and allowed me to proceed. I was then able to diagnose and treat her ear infection, which resolved a few days later.

Marjie's Story

Crying uncontrollably, Marjie, a distraught patient had just discovered that her beloved cat, Butterscotch, had been killed. An immediate dose of Rescue Remedy enabled her to regain composure. Within a few minutes, Marjie became calm and settled into a quiet state of peace.

Healing Chakra Imbalances

The Bach Flower remedies have many effective applications. The originator of Clinical Kinesiology, Dr. Alan Beardall, studied Dr. Edward Bach's theories and remedies and developed them as a successful adjunct to Clinical Kinesiology diagnosis. Dr. Alan Beardall correlated Bach's seven personality types to the chakras as follows:

- Root Chakra: "for those who have fear."
- Spleen Chakra: "... loneliness"
- Navel Chakra: "... uncertainty"
- Heart Chakra: "… overcare for the welfare of others"
- Throat Chakra: "... oversensitive to ideas and influences"
- Brow Chakra: "... despondency and despair"
- Crown Chakra: "... insufficient interest in present circumstances"

According to Bach, it didn't matter if a person had a cold, an injury or an ailment as serious as kidney failure—depending upon their personality type, they basically responded with fear, loneliness, uncertainty—even despondency and despair. The actual illness or irritating factor was secondary to the response.

Through testing, Beardall discovered that negative emotions may be pinpointed and released to heal energetic imbalances in the chakras.

Bach had classified the Flower Remedies according to their application to each of the seven personality types. Beardall applied this classification to the chakra system beginning with the lowest or Root Chakra, up through the Crown Chakra. Once again, the way in which the appropriate remedy was chosen depended upon the testing of the body's sensitive energetic system.

During initial evaluations of new patients, Clinical Kinesiology may be used to test for chakra imbalances. At first, emotional imbalances may be hidden in body adaptations. However, many times, hidden chakra imbalances appear once other energetic imbalances have been corrected.

Especially difficult cases involve organ problems which remain static; not responding to treatment as they should. That, in itself, may be a signal to dig a little deeper to discover chakra imbalances formerly gone unseen. Any chakra imbalance, once identified, provides a major turning point. As rebalancing begins, formerly static organ conditions often progress dramatically.

Lindsey's Story

During one seminar, I tested a young woman, Lindsey, for chakra imbalance. Lindsey assumed the chakra handmode position, which is four fingers straight, with the thumb bent at the last or distal joint, the tip of the thumb touching the large knuckle of the index finger. The test of Lindsey's indicator arm muscle proved weak, indicating a chakra imbalance. Once an imbalance was indicated, we were able to move up and test Lindsey's other points to see which one triggered a weak muscle response.

Lindsey assumed the correct handmode position and resisted as I performed the muscle test. Her arm went weak in relation the Root Chakra, indicating *an imbalance of that chakra*.

Experience tells me that a strong muscle test on the lowest or Root Chakra automatically guarantees blockage of all successive chakras. With testing, this proved to be the case for Lindsey.

Initially, the first step in healing Lindsey's blocked chakras concentrated on rebalancing her lowest or Root Chakra. *Again, testing and healing evolves from bottom to top.* When more than one chakra tests out of balance, the lower one must be treated first due to the tendency for the energy to move from the Root Chakra upwards.

As noted earlier, according to Dr. Beardall the lowest or Root Chakra relates to the negative emotion, fear. Often, people who experience a great deal of fear and anxiety manifest imbalances in the Root Chakra. Through Clinical Kinesiology testing, the appropriate Bach Flower Remedy may be identified to successfully alleviate fear and anxiety, allowing it to dissipate and become a less common occurrence.

Since several Bach Flower remedies correlate to the Root Chakra, the question was finding the correct remedy compatible with rebalancing Lindsey's Root Chakra. The possible remedies include Aspen, Cherry Plum, Mimulus, Red Chestnut, and Rock Rose. I tested each bottle of remedy in the energy field of Lindsey's body, while monitoring the strength of her indicator muscle.

Lindsey resisted as each remedy was put to the test. Her etheric body responded and was not quite balanced with Rock Rose, so I tried the next remedy, Aspen. Ah, good muscle strength! Lindsey pushed and resisted again. She did not respond well to the Cherry Plum remedy. Mimulus? Again, not encouraging. Red Chestnut? What does Lindsey's body say? "OK, but not great."

How Much and for How Long?
Aspen proved the most effective Bach Flower Remedy to rebalance Lindsey's Root Chakra. With the correct remedy determined, I needed to find the correct dosage. Using Clinical Kinesiology testing, Lindsey's body communicated to me how many drops of the Aspen remedy would be required, and for how long.

Testing for dosage required filling a cup with fresh spring water and then adding several drops of the Aspen Remedy. Lindsey held the water container directly on her abdomen in the energy field of her body. One drop ... two ... three ... four ... five! I test after each drop until Lindsey's indicator muscle proves strong. Generally, dosages range between three and seven drops.

In Lindsey's case, Clinical Kinesiology testing determined that five drops, twice per day for a period of three months was the appropriate dosage. The new remedy is poured into Lindsey's personal remedy bottle. Many alternative practitioners have been taught to *succuss* or tap the water bottle containing the new remedy several times on the palm of the hand to set up a vibration which activates the energy.

Patients who use Bach Flower or other remedies often benefit from doing a bit of positive visualization or meditation at least twice a day, along with taking the drops. Allowing the physical body to come into play along with emotional and spiritual aspects of the chakra rebalancing often speeds recovery.

The Bach Flower Remedies may be found in most health food stores. You may request that a store employee assist you in muscle testing various remedies, or seek help from a qualified practitioner who utilizes the remedies.

Once the correct remedy is found, dosage may be calculated as explained in Lindsey's case. Merely test the drops from one up to seven until a strong Clinical Kinesiology muscle test responds to the correct dosage.

ENERGY THERAPY

An adjunct treatment that helps rebalance chakras involves light energy therapy, similar to therapeutic touch. As patients relax, practitioners may place one hand under the body and the other directly over the body at the level of the unbalanced chakra.

Energy focused by moving the hands in a circular motion helps stimulate circulation of chakra energy centers. The energy sets up a flow which continually moves between hands—hooks up to the unbalanced chakra—and moves through the etheric body.

Treatment entails working about three inches above the body, allowing the energy flow to vibrate back and forth. The subtle energy may be felt by the patient in many cases. Treatment continues in a clockwise motion in an attempt to move, normalize and rebalance energy.

Many people actually feel added energy if they stop, sit quietly for a couple of minutes, focus and perceive. Often patients describe the sensation as one of "warm light" or of a "pulsating feeling or vibration."

Energy treatment does not drain practitioners of their own energy. They're not taking energy from within. This underlines the whole idea of subtle energy or the spiritual side of healing. The person doing the healing work cannot give away his or her own energy or he/she will weaken his/her own body.

Healing energy is drawn in through the top of the head and allowed to flow out through the hands. Practitioners simply open themselves to a Higher Awareness, meditate a bit, and allow God's Divine healing energy to infuse their own bodies. The practitioner's awareness of the Sushumna pathway, the Crown Chakra and his or her own soul connection to the unseen healing Power facilitates the healing of others.

The Energy Exercise

Have you ever suffered a bug bite, stubbed toe, or accidentally run your knee into a desk drawer? What happens? If you are like most people, you probably automatically grab the area, hold it…and rub. Without knowing it, you're using your inherent healing energy to help the wounded area. It's an automatic response.

The following exercise provides an effective method for gaining awareness of the powerful energy in your body.

1. First, place both hands opposite one another, palm facing palm approximately an inch apart. For a moment, simply begin to perceive the energy between your hands. You may "feel" something between them … then again, you may feel nothing.
2. Now, rub your palms together as if you were trying to warm them from the cold. Notice the friction created after practicing this exercise for at least a minute.
3. Let your hands separate and feel the sensation within each hand. Slowly move your palms toward one another again, and hold them steady allowing your fingertips to barely touch. Notice any energy sensations between the palms.
4. Next, hold the fingertips of one hand over the palm of the other. Again, observe the different energy sensations. With both hands bouncing energy off one another, many people report that the radiation becomes much more noticeable.

5. Once you've activated the energy built up in your hands, place them over one or more of your chakra energy centers. The practice provides a nice way to wake up the subtle energy in your hands—and body.

The same principle has been used in "palming." Dr. William Bates, who wrote *The Bates Method For Better Eyesight Without Glasses,* originated the treatment of laying the palms over the eyes, without physically touching them, merely to release energy from the hands to help the eyes.[10]

VITALITY: THE COLOR OF ENERGY

According to C.W Leadbeater, "Just as the sun floods the system with light and heat, so does it perpetually pour out—a force to which has been given the name, 'vitality.'"[11] The color of the chakras corresponds closely with the type of vitality radiated from the sun.

Vitality radiates on all levels and manifests itself physically, emotionally, and mentally. Upon entering the physical atoms of humans it increases their energy, and renders them animated and glowing. Unlike electricity in the atoms, the force of vitality infuses the atom from without, not from within.

Through Clinical Kinesiology testing, imbalances of color may be tested to help rebalance chakras. For example, imbalances in the Root Chakra, whose color is red and orange, may respond more strongly to one shade than another. Sometimes, people don't experience enough of a healing color. Sometimes they experience too much.

On the whole, it's a good sign if you feel comfortable with a certain color, gravitate toward that color—or, just "love it!" However, one should never dictate, "For Root Chakra imbalances, wear orange or red." On the contrary, that becomes a blanket recommendation. Instead, appropriate colors may be tested for each individual through Clinical Kinesiology testing.

The Color Purple

The color monitor on my computer in the office provided a reason for testing recently. During set-up, the computer programmer asked me, "What's your favorite color?" I immediately told him, "Purple." He then proceeded to format the computer monitor screen in a computer version of "purple."

Unfortunately, "computer purple" wasn't the right color, shade or intensity for my office assistants, and caused fatigue for both my receptionist and therapy assistant. To solve the problem, I had them each sit in front of the computer, without looking at the screen, and administered the Clinical Kinesiology muscle test. Both responded with a strong indicator muscle. Then, I instructed them both to stare at the purple screen for approximately one minute. When I retested, their indicator muscles proved weak.

I immediately called the computer programmer back to the office, told him the background looked beautiful, however, the shade and intensity of the computer purple wasn't healthful for us.

With the programmer's help, I tested all of the remaining screen colors until we found a truly healthy, balanced color for everyone involved. In the end, my favorite color was not the best for everyone—and, the computer purple wasn't even compatible with me.

CHAKRA STRESSORS

Along with color, mental states and emotional stressors negatively affect chakra energy. Experiencing constant irritation on a mental, emotional, environmental or spiritual level, provides continual negative input, which may throw the chakras out of balance.

Deanna's Story

Deanna, a woman in an abusive relationship, manifested a definite chakra imbalance. During initial treatments she didn't tell me about her physically abusive relationship. However, each time she left my office and returned to her threatening situation, fear enveloped her.

Although treatment continued, a powerful degree of mental anguish continually disrupted the energy flow in her Root Chakra. Each time we met, Deanna was back to ground zero, never gaining any improvement.

I reevaluated Deanna's treatment and suggested a different remedy for fear, along with some therapeutic touch over her Root Chakra. Again, Deanna went home and suffered threats and abuse. Her emotional state and abusive situation negated the benefit of her treatment because the causative factor remained.

Protecting Chakras

To the degree that one is open to outside influences, the people we are closest to may affect our chakra energy. That can be either beneficial or problematic. Meeting an individual whose Heart Chakra or Navel Chakra is quite open or strong, may cause us to be affected in the same chakra area.

Many times, individuals energize or draw energy from one another without being aware of what is happening. Acknowledging that our inner state may be negatively or positively affected by others provides opportunities to further discover chakras and how they affect and harmonize our lives.

The following are some simple ways of protecting the chakras.

- Visualize your chakra centers as being "pulled in" closer to your body allowing them more protection than being out in your "aura" or "etheric" body.
- Place a hand over a chakra that may need protection. Especially in cases involving the Heart Chakra or solar plexus you will notice that during a frightful situation, the hand automatically is drawn over the Heart Chakra or solar plexus. Use the hand to protect that chakra and not allow vital energy to leave through that area.
- A four-step tradition known to Catholics and others as "making the sign of the cross" on the body also helps protect the Heart Chakra, Third Eye and the shoulders (which are major joints known as minor chakras). The "making the sign of the cross" procedure begins with touching the right hand to the Third Eye ... to the heart ... left shoulder and right shoulder.

ELECTROMAGNETIC IMBALANCES

Outside forces, such as environmental electromagnetic fields, also adversely affect chakra imbalances in a myriad of ways on a physical level. The dangers of overexposure to high-voltage power lines, electrical appliances, and microwave ovens may require a closer inspection of your environment in order to minimize electromagnetic pollution. (These issues will be discussed in-depth later in Chapter 9: *Unfriendly Energy: Electromagnetic Pollution.*)

SELF-TESTING FOR CHAKRA IMBALANCES

Self-diagnosing imbalances in the energy chakras proves helpful for both energetic and emotional well-being. Because the chakras are so closely associated with various mental and emotional states, unlocking the key to chakra imbalances also leads to recommendations for various Bach Flower Remedies, which can rebalance the chakras.

Chakra energy testing begins as any other Clinical Kinesiology muscle test, with verification of the strength of the test-subject's Indicator muscle. (See Chapter 1 for instructions.)

The most expedient test for identifying an unbalanced chakra is to simply use the chakra point test. Each chakra corresponds to a specific acupoint and specific emotional imbalance.

Dr. Alan Beardall developed handmodes which may be used to access specific information regarding the chakras, much like the files in a typical office cabinet. The use of handmodes begins a diagnostic process of delving into the underlying secrets of the body. This establishes a priority, order or sequence in resolving an underlying problem. Assume the handmode position on one hand *while the Clinical Kinesiology muscle test is performed on the opposite arm.*

When testing for chakra imbalance, always begin testing with the lowest or Root Chakra. Should an energy block be found in the Root Chakra—all other chakras will be blocked.

Step 1: First, the individual being tested should assume the Chakra handmode position for the Diagnostic test of chakra imbalance.

> Chakra Handmode/Diagnostic Point + Muscle test + Weak arm = chakra imbalance. Proceed with further testing.
> or
> Chakra Handmode/Diagnostic Point + Muscle test + Strong arm = No chakra imbalance. No further testing is needed.

Step 2: Use the thumb to touch each specific point. As you proceed through each test, keep in mind that a weak muscle test on a particular point identifies which chakra may be out of balance.

> Chakra Handmode/Root Point + Muscle test + Weak arm
> = Root Chakra imbalance.
> or
> Chakra Handmode/Spleen + Muscle test + Weak arm = Spleen Chakra imbalance and so on.

Once identified, a chakra imbalance may be remedied by the corresponding Bach Flower Remedy, which may be tested as follows:

Step 3: Place each recommended remedy in the energetic field of the body (usually on torso).

Step 4: Perform the muscle test again while the subject remains in the chakra handmode position which tested weak.

Specific, helpful remedies may be narrowed down by observing which sample remedy triggers the strong muscle response during testing. Refer to the Bach Flower Remedy chart on the following page for more information.

> Weak Root Chakra Handmode Point + Rock Rose + Muscle test + Weak arm = Check another remedy.
> or
> Weak Root Chakra Handmode Point + Aspen + Muscle test + Strong arm = Use remedy to rebalance Chakra.

BACH FLOWER REMEDIES

Root Chakra
Aspen, Cherry Plum, Mimulus, Red Chestnut, Rock Rose

Spleen Chakra
Heather, Impatiens, Water Violet

Navel Chakra
Cerato, Gentian, Gorse, Hornbeam, Scleranthus, Wild Oat

Heart Chakra
Beech, Chicory, Rock Water, Vervain, Vine

Throat Chakra
Agrimony, Centaury, Holly, Walnut

Brow Chakra
Crabapple, Elm, Larch, Oak, Pine, Star of Bethlehem, Sweet Chestnut, Willow

Crown Chakra
Chestnut Bud, Clematis, Honeysuckle, Mustard, Olive, Wild Rose, White Chestnut

Note: If all chakras are blocked, use Bach's Rescue Remedy.

Helpful Hint

It's best to treat only one chakra at a time. When a weak muscle response indicates a problem with one of the lower chakras, start with that chakra, figure out the remedy and take only that remedy. Do not treat another chakra immediately because it takes some time to rebalance the first chakra. Helping any unbalanced lower chakra will have a positive effect on the higher chakras. This allows the progression of healing energy to move from lower to higher chakras, more easily "clearing" the energy channel.

Only slight variances of arm strength may be discerned between each tested remedy. However, as you become more proficient at testing, the correct remedy may be easily found.

Most health food and nutrition stores are open to clients for purposes of in-store testing of Bach Flower Remedies. You may want to contact the store in advance or take a friend with you to enable quick testing of the remedies.

HEALTHY CHAKRAS

For the most part, leading a healthy lifestyle helps everyone maintain healthier chakra energy centers in the body. Part of that healthy lifestyle includes providing the body and spirit with clean sources of vital energy, as well as additional ways of increasing vital energy.

On the most basic level, evaluate diet. Take only pure foods and liquids into the body, and avoid cigarette smoking, alcohol, prescription or recreational drugs. Introducing such impurities only weighs down and deadens the enlightenment you wish to obtain.

Provide the body with daily, gentle and reasonable exercise, avoid chemical and environmental pollutants, and always try to remain vitalized. When you are not at risk from these negative forces, you may focus on bringing more natural energy into your life.

Revitalize your chakra energy centers with prayer, meditation, yoga, spiritual or breathing exercises, *tai ch'i*, or other forms of mental awareness. Maintain a positive state of mind, and seek out a natural balance of sun, air and water. Develop your marvelous mind-body through the energy centers known as the chakras and experience a whole new world of energy and healing in your life.

From food for the spirit, we now move to food for the body. In exploring the body's multileveled energetic system, we've seen how The Bach Flower Remedies provide higher levels of emotional and spiritual nurturance. Now, we return to the physical body to illustrate how Clinical Kinesiology diagnoses energy sensitivities to food.

CHAPTER FOUR
SUGGESTED READING

Bach, Edward, M.D. and F.J. Wheeler. *The Bach Flower Remedies, Revised Ed.* New Canaan, Conn.: Keats Publishing, Inc., 1997.

Barnett, Larkin. *Practical Centering: Exercises to Energize Your Chakras for Relaxation, Vitality, and Health.* Wheaton, Ill.: Quest Books, Theosophical Publishing House, 2012.

Craydon, Deborah, C.F.E.P; Bellows, Warren, Lic.Ac. *Floral Acupuncture: Applying the Flower Essences of Dr. Bach to Acupuncture Sites.* Berkeley, Calif.: Crossing Press, 2005.

Dale, Cyndi. *The Complete Book of Chakra Healing: Activate the Transformative Power of Your Energy Centers, 2nd edition.* Woodbury, Minn.: Llewellyn Publications, 2009.

Davies, Brenda, M.D. *The 7 Healing Chakras: Unlocking Your Body's Energy Centers.* Berkeley, Calif.: Ulysses Press, 2000.

Dossey, Larry M.D. *Healing Words: The Power of Prayer and the Practice of Medicine.* San Francisco: HarperCollins Publishers, San Francisco, 1994

Gerber, Richard, M.D. *Vibrational Medicine: The #1 Handbook of Subtle-Energy Therapies.* Santa Fe, New Mexico: Bear & Company, 2001.

Kaslof, Leslie, J. *Traditional Flower Remedies of Edward Bach: A Self-Help Guide.* New Canaan, Conn.: Keats Publishing, Inc., 1988.

Krieger, D. *Accepting Your Power to Heal: The Personal Practice of Therapeutic Touch.* Santa Fe, New Mexico: Bear and Co., 1993.

Leadbeater, C.W. *The Chakras, Second Ed.* Wheaton, Ill.: Theosophical Publishing House, 2013.

Liberman, Jacob, O.D., Ph.D. *Light: Medicine of the Future.* Santa Fe, New Mexico: Bear and Co., 1991

Mann, John and Lar Short. *The Body of Light: History and Practical Techniques for Awakening Your Subtle Body.* Boston: Charles E. Tuttle Company, 1993.

Minich, Deanna M., Ph.D., C.N. *Chakra Foods for Optimum Health: A Guide to the Foods That Can Improve Your Energy, Inspire Creative Changes, Open Your Heart, and Heal Body, Mind, and Spirit.* San Francisco: Conari Press, an imprint of Red Wheel/Weiser, LLC, 2009.

Moore, Thomas. *Care of the Soul: A Guide for Cultivating Depth and Sacredness in Everyday Life.* New York: Harper Perennial, 1994

Pond, David. *Chakras for Beginners: A Guide to Balancing Your Chakra Energies.* St. Paul, Minn.: Llewellyn Publications, 2003.

Simpson, Liz with Foreword by Teresa Hale. *The Book of Chakra Healing.* New York: Sterling Publishing Co., Inc., 1999.

Wood, Betty. *The Healing Power of Color: Using Color to Improve Your Mental, Physical, and Spiritual Well-being.* Rochester, Vt.: Inner Traditions, 1998.

PART II

ENERGY AND THE IMMUNE SYSTEM

CHAPTER 5

Energy Sensitivities to Food

Warm sunlight flooded the tiny playroom strewn with colorful toys and stuffed animals. In his happy, well-behaved state, Justin, a young child with severe food sensitivities, sat on the floor eating a snack of white bread and jelly. After a few moments, researchers added a dollop of peanut butter to his bread.

Suddenly, the pleasant world erupted in chaos, as Justin began to writhe, scream, throw toys and tear the playroom apart. For the next several hours he experienced a continuous state of agitation until, near exhaustion, he finally fell asleep on the playroom floor.

Justin had experienced a severe allergic reaction, not simply to one food, rather to a combination of food items. His behavior presented startling and clear proof of the far-reaching dimensions of food sensitivity problems. Like Justin, millions of people are similarly affected by food sensitivities—perhaps on a lesser, but nonetheless serious, scale.

This chapter provides a new perspective on the myriad ways food can be toxic to the body and its energetic system. Today, more than ever, diet affects the immune system, either supporting or negatively impacting the body's major line of defense against disease.

Determining healthier food choices includes the ability to interpret the warning signals or symptoms of immune system malfunction stemming from food sensitivity. It isn't enough to eat well. *The ability to differentiate between compatible and incompatible foods serves as the basis for diagnosing, treating and healing food sensitivities.*

With Clinical Kinesiology testing, discover how easy it is to rely on the body's inner knowingness to access firsthand information on the foods your body can and cannot tolerate. Instant feedback from this indispensable tool provides the vital link to deterring incompatible food patterns, halting the downward spiral of disease.

This chapter will help you familiarize yourself with foods that create imbalances in current states of body physiology, immune, and digestive systems; it will address poor digestion, digestive disorders, and liver toxicity, as well as examine common high-sensitivity foods that contribute to organ imbalances of the liver and thyroid. It will discuss the dangers of hybridization and microwaving.

You will discover simple methods for breaking the patterns of food sensitivities, finding energetically compatible alternatives which restore the body and immune system. Finally, you will be encouraged to examine symptoms and determine addictions, through self-testing your own foods, vitamins, and pharmaceutical prescriptions. After reading and digesting the information in this chapter, you will have a strong foundation for further study of Chapter 7, *Candida Causes and Treatment*, and Chapter 8, *Leaky Gut and Your Digestion*.

Take the important first steps to developing a new attitude toward food. As you begin to conquer food sensitivities, discover renewed health and energy, and a more loving relationship toward food and yourself.

WHY LOOK AT FOOD?

Food provides nurturance to life, satisfying not only physical, but emotional, psychological, spiritual, social and cultural needs. In many cultures, an expected sign of hospitality includes offering food or drink to guests, thus solidifying friendship or other bonds.

Throughout the world, age-old religious mores—even taboos— still exist surrounding certain foods. Different religions designate specific foods as clean and unclean, blessed and unblessed, appropriate for certain occasions ... while prohibiting other foods from being eaten at all. Throughout history, fasting served as a spiritual cleansing of the body and soul. (Although today, many consider fasting or abstention from eating food to be merely a physical cleansing technique.) Those who practiced fasting used it to renounce or detach from the physical or secular world.

Psychologically, food has long been used as a reward and a comfort. From early ages, children (quite inappropriately) are told, "If you behave yourself you'll be rewarded with cookie ... an ice cream ... a candy bar." Unfortunately, this type of behavior modification reinforces good behavior or good feelings directly associated with sweet or unhealthy food. Nurturance of the physical body remains closely tied to nurturance of the emotional self. Unfortunately, for many people, the urgent need to provide emotional nurturing often includes unhealthy food choices or unneeded quantities.

Often, obese individuals "comfort eat" to provide nurturance and love to themselves. On the other hand, people with the illness *anorexia nervosa* feel completely unworthy, unable to receive praise, undeserving of rewards, refuse to be rewarded, and therefore stop eating entirely.

Such early patterning often leads to food sensitivity, addictions and eating disorders. Emotional and psychological problems, nutritional deficiencies, family dietary patterns, and cultural conditioning drive many people to eat solely for taste and enjoyment rather than health and well-being.

Of course, it's appropriate to enjoy food! It is not necessary to eat only sprouts for the rest of your life. However, people who continually go beyond healthy dietary parameters may begin to develop problems.

Food is fuel. Eating the correct foods in the correct amounts adds to body energy and health. That's why it's so important to learn what foods to eat, including how each body reacts to different foods, in order to avoid food sensitivities and addictions.

Clinical Kinesiology food sensitivity testing provides a simple method for assessing the appropriate foods for each individual body. By using this tool, you will begin to develop a new relationship to food, as you examine its positive and negative effects on your energetic body.

THE IMMUNE SYSTEM AND FOOD

Diet affects the immune system, white blood cell count, muscles, joints—even thoughts and moods. Medical, environmental, and physiologically induced factors diminish immune system function.

One thing is clear: If symptoms of food sensitivities exist, such as cravings, dark circles under the eyes, sinus problems, joint and muscle dysfunction, emotional behavior problems, mood swings, headaches, rashes, coughing or other respiratory problems—even hay fever—*the immune system isn't functioning at its best.*

Hay fever and other allergies do not often exist in people with optimum physical health. These other allergies often stem from the immune system being weakened by food allergies. Clinical Kinesiology food-sensitivity testing can identify sensitivity to offending items, including common ones.

In the case of my patient Priscilla, for instance, her rash clearly stemmed from a food allergy, but I also suspected other underlying problems. Physically, much more was going on to cause it. Priscilla's immune system had become overburdened and had stopped working at optimum capacity.

The Oaken Bucket

Dr. Steve Olson, a holistic dentist who removes mercury fillings to strengthen the immune system, describes the immune system as a wonderful, solid, oaken bucket that faithfully collects everything dumped into it.

Everyone starts out with perfect health, Olson explains. As reactions to many external and internal irritants occur, the oaken bucket fills up with everything the immune system must handle, from environmental problems, such as chemical and electromagnetic pollution, to germs, viruses, stress, and now, food sensitivities.

The immune system copes only to the current level of the body's health. Ultimately, the bucket becomes full, its maximum load achieved! That's when many people suddenly begin noticing a number of different symptoms. For some, this "last straw" constitutes a serious crisis.

Instead of filling the oaken bucket to the brim, I suggest you begin to incorporate healthy habits with which to "bail out" your bucket. In doing this, you greatly diminish the chance for illness in the body.

Instead of compromising the immune system, find ways of rebuilding it. Look at the contributing factors for food sensitivity, evaluate the dysfunction, and seek treatment which will ultimately return you on the road to health. Clinical Kinesiology will assist you in doing all of this.

THE ENERGETIC BODY

Every substance known on earth possesses a specific energetic quality. Every person exhibits a different compatibility with different foods and the energetic qualities they possess. The same holds true in cases of specific organ imbalances, or genetic patterns.

Food sensitivities occur when pre-existing energetic weaknesses in the current state of physiology, immune system or digestive function inhibit certain food items from matching the current energy pattern of the body. In short, the body's energetic system proves incompatible with certain foods.

Like an automobile, the body runs on a specific type of fuel. Only that fuel contains the correct components, enabling the "engine" to perform at optimum efficiency or health. We all know that certain cars require regular gasoline, others need unleaded or diesel. For a fuel to be appropriate for one car (or body), it must contain a certain energetic balance and chemical composition. Evaluation of the molecular structure of a particular fuel may find it compatible for one type of "engine." Substitute a different fuel, and the engine may not perform appropriately.

Because the body proves much more sensitive than any human-made instrument (such as a car), it's important to use a custom diagnostic tool. Clinical Kinesiology testing quickly and easily indicates the compatibility of any substance with the energy pattern of the body. Once that energy pattern is identified, changed and strengthened, food sensitivities may dissipate.

You can learn to listen carefully to the information that your body imparts about what foods it needs and what foods it doesn't. Then, you can combine that knowledge with Clinical Kinesiology testing in determining wiser, healthier and more *energetically compatible* food choices.

HEALTHY AND UNHEALTHY CHOICES

One study involving kindergarten students shed new light on children's natural understanding of healthy food sources; i.e., the children intuitively knew the connection between food, exercise, health and body fat and were attuned to what foods could be potential health hazards. The study proved that even young children can make correct food choices although such knowledge is not always translated into daily practice.[1]

Adults also make correct food choices, but the majority place heavy emotional connotations on certain foods. Adults also maintain preconceived ideas about foods that they want or don't want to eat.

Busy working adults, such as Karen, one food sensitive individual, more often take the path of least resistance when it comes to food. "I just don't have time to stop and prepare foods myself," Karen complains. The results become habitual dependence on fast or processed foods. In this way, the conscious mind often overshadows the correct decision.

Research indicates that the average American consumes a total of only twenty different food items. Although the items may be prepared in different ways, *twenty items* still constitute a limited diet. This practice alone proves to be a main contributor to food sensitivities.

Continually bombarding the body with the same food items, (especially if proven slightly energetically incompatible) becomes an open invitation to food sensitivities. Time after time, antigens or toxins from that energetically incompatible food cause the body to become more sensitive.

This practice tends to be a problem in the elderly population. Many older people hold long-ingrained habit patterns concerning the choice of food items. Some use the same grocery list every week.

Myra and Roland, two of my elderly and underweight patients, actually began to lose a great deal of weight because they routinely bought and ate the same items over and over. For some, the weight loss may have been healthy and welcomed, but neither Myra nor Roland were overweight to begin with, so it was unhealthy. Following Clinical Kinesiology food sensitivity evaluation and treatment, they regained most of the lost weight and developed a "healthier" and more diverse shopping list.

If You See GMO "Foods" ... Run!

Educating yourself about genetically modified organisms (GMOs) could save your life, your health, and your children's well-being. The creation of GMO "foods" is ominous, and threatens the entire ecosystem, biodiversity, and our individual health.

Genetically modified organisms were modified by humans attempting to "improve" upon nature. Genetic material from one organism is artificially placed into the chromosomes of other organisms for calculated, desired effects. The end result is boosting the profit margin of the industry, yet leaving the consumer with a less nutritional, potentially harmful, often allergenic,

"Franken-food." Serious cases of gastroenteritis (inflammation of stomach and intestines) in people who have consumed these foods are on record. Even some deaths are recorded. The industry that creates these has manipulated to have these products classified as "natural," and have no labeling requirements in America.

Monsanto is the GMO-industry leader. They produce the well known pesticide Round Up® (2, 4-D). Now they have engineered corn with the genetically entrenched quality of resisting Round Up® so that more and more applications of the potentially carcinogenic toxin can be sprayed on cornfields, killing all other plants, except the "Round-Up-Ready Corn." Besides polluting the air, soil and water, this chemical gives your intestinal tract and liver a good dose of poison if you eat this corn. Monsanto has already concocted the "next generation." That would be corn plants that exude pesticides to their immediate environment while growing. What do you think happens when you eat this corn and your digestive enzymes begin to break it down?

My patient Charlie can tell you. He was hospitalized for severe gastroenteritis and diverticulitis that he knows was caused by eating a small serving of corn hours prior to experiencing debilitating pain in his abdomen. Charlie was incapacitated for weeks. After a several day hospitalization, receiving intravenous feedings, and virtually no food, he required several weeks at a rehab facility to regain strength. After he was discharged, I went to his home and administered several home treatments before he felt strong and steady enough to drive again. One small serving of corn effectively took two months out of his life, and cost thousands upon thousands of dollars in medical bills. Charlie has no interest in consuming GMO corn again.

What can we do? Educate ourselves about GMO products and agricultural practices. Keep your children away from GMO crops. Avoid eating these foods and products, and also stay away from their growing areas. Particles from these crops get into the wind and dust and can wreak havoc. The good news is that the Non-GMO project exists, educates, has a website (http://www.nongmoproject.org/) and performs DNA testing on produce. The Non-GMO-project *verified seal* is your new best friend.

The following is a list of highly suspect foods. Avoid them unless they are Non-GMO verified.

- Alfalfa (often fed to livestock), so eggs, milk and meat are high-risk for GMO contamination
- Canola—as a grain or oil
- Corn, corn oil, cornstarch, corn sweeteners, fructose (corn is also fed to livestock)
- Cotton-clothing, sheets, towels, etc.
- Flax
- Papaya
- Rice
- Soy, tofu, edamame, soy sauce, soy protein, etc.
- Sugar beets—refined sugar, molasses
- Wheat, flour and products made with wheat or wheat flour
- Yellow summer squash
- Zucchini

Remember to refer to the Non-GMO shopping guide that is easily accessible through the Non-GMO website. Routinely request Non-GMO produce and products at your grocery store and your health food store. Simple grass-roots efforts like these will save lives. Boycotting these destructive and potentially poisonous "Franken foods" may diminish their production due to slow sales.

This thumb-nail description about natural, unadulterated food sourcing probably seems overwhelming. My intention is to generally educate and warn you of dangers inherent in our food supply. Many countries have been ravaged by GMO practices and the roughshod coercion of farmers by Monsanto. A deplorable condition exists in Venezuela, where many children are dying due to GMO toxicity and pollution. Be sure to read the sidebar from Dr. James Mercola's website.

Here's the bottom line regarding healthy food choices:

> IF NATURE MADE IT, AND NO HUMANS TAMPERED WITH IT, CONSIDER EATING IT AND FEEDING IT TO YOUR PRECIOUS CHILDREN.

Let this principle be your starting point for dietary choice making. You will thereby eliminate many detrimental epigenetic factors, and promote your family's health. You can further refine your dietary selections based on taste preferences, as well as other parameters. Examples of other parameters may be food sensitivities, actual food allergies (refer to Chapter 5), dental or oral cavity issues, dietary style preferences, digestive system tolerances, religious or belief system dietary choices.

INDICATORS OF FOOD SENSITIVITIES

A weakened immune system that stems from food allergies leaves the body susceptible to a wide

---

Monsanto Above the Law?

Dr. Medardo Vasquez, the neonatal specialist who heads up the Children's Hospital in Cordoba [Venequala]. Dr. Vasquez tells him [Joseph Mercola]: "I see new-born infants, many of whom are malformed. I have to tell parents that their children are dying because of these agricultural methods. In some areas in Argentina the primary cause of death for children less than one year old is malformations."

Argentina's population is being sickened by massive spraying of herbicides on its genetically engineered soya fields. Glyphosate, the main ingredient in Roundup, is blamed for the dramatic increase in devastating birth defects as well as cancer. Sterility and miscarriages are also increasing.

A 2012 nutritional analysis of GMO versus non-GMO corn shows shocking differences in nutritional content. Non-GMO corn contains 437 times more calcium, 56 times more magnesium, and 7 times more manganese than GMO corn.

GMO corn was also found to contain 13 ppm of glyphosate, compared to zero in non-GMO corn. The EPA standard for glyphosate in American water supplies is 0.7 ppm, and organ damage in animals has occurred at levels as low as 0.1 ppm.

GMO corn contains extremely high levels of formaldehyde—about 200 times the amount found toxic to animals.

Unfortunately, President Obama recently signed into law a spending bill that included a devastating provision that puts Monsanto above the law. The provision limits the ability of judges to stop Monsanto and/or farmers from growing or harvesting genetically engineered crops, even if courts find evidence of potential health risks.

http://articles.mercola.com/sites/articles/archive/2013/04/09/argentina-gmo-crops.aspx array of infections and illnesses. Many seemingly unrelated maladies can be attributed ultimately to an intolerance or an allergy to a specific food, or a combination of specific foods.

Disorders attributed to food sensitivity include inflammation of all types such as:

- arthritis
- bursitis
- gastritis
- irritable bowel syndrome

Also, people who suffer from seasonal hay fever usually have inflamed respiratory tracts which leave less room for proper airflow.

People with bodies that tend to swell or inflame usually exhibit a number of food sensitivities due to water retention. In addition to swelling, other signs of food sensitivities include:

- red, blotchy skin
- musculoskeletal soreness or stiffness
- muscle cramping, spasm or other weakness

Pinpointing and eliminating specific food sensitivities automatically calms the system.

Other common disorders stemming from food sensitivities include:

- conjunctivitis or "pink eye"

Extremely infectious, "pink eye" stems from food sensitivities and immune systems in turmoil. Usually, in the spring, a little pollen floats by and it's the last straw for the immune system. The problem results in inflammation, excessive tearing, sensitivity to light, and blurred vision.

Along with the eyes, come the ears. Any type of disorder with the ears may be related to food sensitivities:

- ear noises, ringing, infections
- Meniere's Disease

In my clinical experience, ear infections often correlate with milk allergies. In addition, the beginnings of joint dysfunction or arthritis, liver and intestinal dysfunction and elimination problems all begin before usual means of diagnosis have discovered food sensitivities.

Progression from joint pain—to stiffness—to swelling or dysfunction—to arthritis, signals that food sensitivities have been causing trouble in the body for a long time.

The beginnings of sinus problems or repeated sinus infections also indicate food sensitivities. As soon as suspected symptoms occur, food sensitivity testing using Clinical Kinesiology and appropriate treatment should be undertaken to arrest or reverse the process.

DIGESTION AND FOOD ALLERGIES

If everyone ate the correct diet for their bodies, they would experience good digestive function and most or their health problems would be eliminated. Unknowingly, in many cases, the digestive process has been "over-AMPed" by food incompatible to the body's energetic system.

When food is not digested properly it leads to further problems such as:

- constipation
- indigestion
- nervous stomach, pains and cramps
- spastic colon
- excess gas, bloating
- nausea, vomiting
- gastric ulcers and other gastrointestinal disorders
- hemorrhoids

Bedwetting in children or young adults is also a symptom. With frequent or burning urination, food sensitivities cause the urine to be more irritating. As a result, the body excretes more frequently to try and rid itself of the problem. Again, my own clinical tests show that the inability to digest milk is the most common link to bedwetting.

Gallbladder attacks may also stem from food sensitivities, or ingesting too much fat from fried food.

Biochemist, Jeffrey Bland, Ph.D., the Chief Science Officer of Metagenics (2000-2012), and the President of Metaproteomics explains the seriousness of improper digestion: "Food fragments cross from the intestines into your bloodstream, and cause tissue damage."[2] The condition, known as Leaky Gut Syndrome, occurs when insufficiently broken down pieces of food enter the bloodstream as oversized particles. Leaky Gut will be discussed in greater length in Chapter 8, *Leaky Gut and Your Digestion*. This happens from a lack of digestive enzymes and/or hydrochloric acid in the body. Without sufficient digestive enzymes the body cannot absorb the nutrients it needs to create more digestive enzymes leading to the downward spiral of digestive malfunction. Because these large undigested particles cannot be utilized at a cellular level, they end up triggering allergic reactions in the body.

What becomes of toxic residue left floating around in the blood-stream? It travels to the liver to be broken down, reconjugated or recycled. Already taxed with reprocessing and detoxifying unrecognizable food molecules, the liver must then cope with a large number of antigen/antibody reactions, eventually becoming overburdened itself.

These macro molecules of undigested food exact an even greater toll on the already energy-stressed liver, whose own dysfunction goes hand-in-hand with resulting joint dysfunction stemming from food sensitivities. Initially, many people mistake this condition as arthritis; however, it is actually a biochemical reaction in the body to food.

People who unknowingly spend their whole lives battling food sensitivities will have a low tolerance to the insufficiently broken down chemicals which freely enter the bloodstream from the liver. From age thirty-five to fifty, these people may notice a variety of major symptoms.

Their complaints: "My joints feel stiff," "My knees are so swollen that I can barely walk," stem from advanced metabolic poisoning.

The build-up of toxic residue in the joints begins the process of inflammation of those joints. As Gary Null reports in *Gary Null's Complete Guide to Healing Your Body Naturally*, "Because of the specific physiology of the joints, they are especially susceptible to the buildup of toxic materials …"[3] Over time, this metabolic dysfunction truly forms the basis for disorders and imbalances in the body previously mislabeled as "arthritis."

Fifteen or twenty years from now, a set of X-rays may confirm that food sensitivities have progressed to "true" arthritis. However, it's not too late to change eating habits that may prevent that diagnosis from occurring in the future.

Thyroid Imbalance

Along with the liver, the thyroid, a regulator of metabolism in the body, may become overly stressed due to food sensitivity. The ancient Chinese never referred to the thyroid gland, only its functions, or "three fires," which they called the *Triple Warmer*.

In Chinese theory, the thyroid controls the energetic aspect which extracts heat and energy from food and converts it to energy. This metabolic and energetic process of digestion and assimilation (not to be confused with the chemical process) became known as "cellular respiration."

Food sensitivities indicate that the body's energy has become out of balance. The thyroid may then become overworked in trying to assist in converting improper foods into usable energy. In this way, food sensitivities and the consumption of energetically incompatible foods adversely affect the liver and thyroid.

Marlene's Story

Shortly after her fiftieth birthday, Marlene developed terribly painful joints, which her doctor labeled as "rheumatoid arthritis." She experienced stiff knees, ankles, shoulders, wrists, and fingers. During her Clinical Kinesiology food sensitivity evaluation, Marlene tested weak to the entire group of Nightshades. (The Nightshades refer to a fleshy family of foods, which include the white potato, all peppers, paprika, eggplant, and tomatoes. Several edible ornamental plants such as the petunia, chalice vine and angel trumpet also belong to the Nightshade family.) Immediately, Marlene was encouraged to discontinue eating the Nightshades for a period of three months. (Generally speaking, anyone who experiences muscle or joint stiffness may benefit from avoiding the Nightshades, pending food sensitivity testing.)

One evening Marlene attended a county fair where, due to a complete lack of good food choices, she decided to eat a baked potato. Instantly, she suffered a severe exacerbation of her symptoms.

During Marlene's treatment, the Nightshades were retested and the potato remained the only item to which she tested weak. Because Marlene hadn't been eating the others for nearly three months, they no longer tested as irritating to her energetic system. However, it only took one potato to trigger stiffness and soreness in Marlene's body.

Until her metabolism and digestion become fully rebalanced, I recommended that Marlene avoid the Nightshade family of foods. Low tolerance for one Nightshade automatically sheds suspicion on all the others, as far as I'm concerned. Of course, the true test lies in Clinical Kinesiology food sensitivity testing.

Reaction time to sensitive foods may often be confusing because, unlike Marlene's case, for many people hours or days may pass before symptoms occur. Again, every individual experiences food differently. Without testing, it is difficult to pinpoint food sensitivities.

OVERVIEW OF ALLERGENIC FOODS

The most commonly allergenic foods are milk and dairy, corn, wheat or other grains, citrus and meats. In order to further understand why these particular foods trigger so many instances of food sensitivities let's look at each now.

The most difficult food sensitivities to overcome involve milk and dairy products and usually, during Clinical Kinesiology testing, if someone indicates a dairy sensitivity, he or she should restrict all dairy for several months (at least three) to reduce reactivity.

Milk: Not So Perfect Food

For decades, advertisers have "sold" Americans on milk—nature's perfect food! If that's true, why does an intolerance for dairy products show up most often during food sensitivity testing?

Today's milk is no longer consumed in its natural state. Milk's extreme homogenization and pasteurization process kills natural enzymes which normally help people digest milk. In addition, heating destroys the protein and vitamins. To a degree, it also alters the milk's chemical and energetic quality.

Other problems occur as the homogenization process breaks down the milk's large fat molecules. In many cases, homogenization renders the fat molecules so small that the body cannot recognize them. The result? They go undigested through the bloodstream, coating blood vessels with arterial plaque. This process ultimately leads to arteriosclerosis.

Additionally, many people are introduced to milk at too early an age. In my opinion, milk is "the perfect food" *to grow tiny calves into great big heifers*. That's what milk was naturally designed to do. The consistency of cow's milk is much different from mother's breast milk. The amount of fat is much higher. It takes just one year for a baby calf to mature. By the age of two, it's completely full-sized. Obviously, human babies don't develop at the same rate of growth as a cow. That's why human infants require a much gentler approach with nutrient intake. Breast milk is their intended food.

Most commercial milk contains a number of additional chemical additives and preservatives (many of which we are uninformed about). These additives are one reason some milk retains such an unnaturally long shelf life. Some processors have even been known to add preservatives to the wax coating on the inside of the carton. In this way, they avoid identifying such toxic substances on the label.

Other additives in commercial milk include synthetic Vitamins A and D. All these factors cause people who may have been milk intolerant from an early age to experience more food sensitivities than normal.

People who say, "Oh yes, I'm lactose intolerant, but I take lactase tablets or a lactic acid enzyme," perhaps won't experience as much gas, however, *they're still sensitive to milk* and the way it's processed. Once someone proves milk intolerant, that intolerance usually applies to all forms of milk—yogurt, cheese, regular and skim milk. However, the fermented forms may be better tolerated by many. And, as long as this person continues to drink milk, his or her body will continue to experience symptoms.

Lactase persistence (lactose tolerance) is seen predominantly in individuals with northern European ancestry, especially Scandinavian, and in certain other populations, including some of the nomadic peoples of the middle east and Africa. Lactase non-persistence (lactose intolerance) is observed in a majority of the world's populations, including most of those with Asian or African forebearers.[4]

More discussion about milk and milk products can be found in Chapter 7, *Candida: Causes and Treatments* and Chapter 13, *Optimizing Your Children's Health*.

Mary Lou's and Faye's Stories

I treated two adults for ear infections, and both had severe food sensitivities and weak thyroid glands. One woman, Mary Lou, really toyed with, "Can I give up my milk?" She went off milk for awhile, then back on milk, resulting in another ear infection.

The other patient, Faye, also complained of a sinus problem. Following food sensitivity testing, I recommended, "The simplest thing to do is try a two-week stint without milk and see how you feel."

She did it and reported, "I feel great ... never felt better. I can actually breathe when I lie down at night!" Within a month, Faye was back on milk. She explained, "I decided it was more important for me to have my milk."

What happened? Both Mary Lou and Faye keyed into their desire for milk ... and the addiction. It's a personal choice, ultimately.

Grain Sensitivity

Grains rank third among the most common food sensitivities, with wheat predominating. Many people test positive to four or five different grains and one of them is usually wheat. (Should they eventually recover from all the grain sensitivities save wheat—that particular food sensitivity may prove lifelong.)

Corn

Corn also ranks as one of the most common allergenic foods. Anyone who tests sensitive to corn should be wary of corn in all forms—popcorn, corn syrup, cornmeal, cornstarch, even fructose. The vast majority of all corn in America is not heirloom. It is Genetically Modified, indigestible, and downright harmful. You will find more discussion of this in Chapter 8, *Leaky Gut and Your Digestion*. No matter what form of corn is eaten, the energy pattern remains discordant. Only the physical form has been changed. If you test energetically sensitive to it, watch out!

Hybridization: The First Step to Changing the Genetic Structure

Extreme hybridization is my theory as to why corn, wheat, and citrus (another high-sensitivity food) render so many people weak during food sensitivity testing. *Hybridized foods retain little of the natural properties of the foods they once were.* Indian corn, for example, is an original heirloom and unadulterated corn. Look at an ear—no straight rows and no perfect kernels; and the ears themselves are a natural hodgepodge of variable sizes. It's difficult to harvest that type of corn with modern farm machinery. The genetics of Indian corn plants were altered solely because of machines.

Corn must be a certain size, the ears a certain proportion, to be harvested by standard machines used today. Scientists also designed ears of certain length and rows of straight kernels to please customers.

The same genetic alterations apply to wheat, and other grains, although wheat remains the most hybridized. Again, because the farmer's combine is only so tall, the wheat is hybridized to match. Certain varieties of wheat require less water, while others have been developed to last longer in storage before being ground.

In citrus fruits, today's "orange" originated as the much smaller mandarin orange. Easily broken and torn, the mandarin orange peel itself is obviously different from hybridized "oranges." In addition, the tiny segments appear more crescent-shaped than today's genetically altered oranges; the seeds more firmly attached to the membranes.

In my teens, during employment at a small produce store, I learned that oranges were named by the size and number that fit into a carton. The smaller Valencia oranges came seventy-two to a box. So, the only identifying factor was the number 72 stamped on the side of the box. The store owner would often instruct me to bring out a box of 72s or 48s (which were navel oranges).

Many reasons exist why our food has been genetically altered— not all of them compatible with health. Scientists create new (and increasingly unnatural) life forms every day. Down-sized lettuce, the "super tomato," and apple-flavored carrots are only a few of the other "foods" being crossbred in laboratories. Hybridization, genetic mutating, and inoculation of genes of one species into another is confusing the whole food system—not to mention the human body. The altering of DNA in various foods is done for a multitude of reasons, generally financially driven, and is known as "<u>G</u>enetic <u>M</u>odification." These "Franken-foods" are often devitalized and, in many cases, carcinogenic (cancer causing). Refer back to pages 96–98, where we discussed the use of GMO foods; this trend alone provides a good impetus for growing your own food, thereby maintaining quality control.

Meat

Meat sensitivities also prove hard to overcome due to the difficulty in digesting heavy protein content. Clinical Kinesiology food sensitivity testing includes the testing of standard grown, versus naturally grown meat.

With commercially grown beef, pork and poultry, a high likelihood exists of numerous drugs being ingested throughout an animal's life. Chemical additives and pesticide residue may also be traced to the animal's feed. So, in addition to the meat allergy, there may be a chemical sensitivity. During testing, a person may prove sensitive to conventionally grown meat but not have a significant reaction to the organic meat. It's helpful to test both in order to know whether to restrict all conventionally grown meats or recommend organic meats for that person.

Eggs

Animals do have emotions, and many lead desperately unhappy lives. Today's chickens are treated terribly. Penned up their entire lives, they never see sunlight, never scratch. Imagine, chicken on top of chicken—each one catching the droppings of the ones above. In addition, today's chickens ingest antibiotics and synthetic hormones in incredible numbers. Once those drugs enter the food chain, they pose an even bigger hazard—food sensitivities in humans.

A big difference exists between the egg of one-hundred years ago and the egg today. It's also the reason eggs often prove highly allergenic to many people. As with meat, it's appropriate to test both regular commercial eggs and organic free-range eggs.

Transdermal Lambchops with a Side of Pharmaceuticals

It's frightening to learn about hybridization and its effects on food sensitivities, especially in light of the latest bioengineering experiments now being conducted on animals.

In the last decades of the twentieth century, Tufts Veterinary School spearheaded a biotechnology research program involving sheep and cows in England and Scotland. Geneticists inject sheep with human DNA in order to produce certain clotbuster, or heart drugs, which can be obtained cheaper through the animals' milk. (Early experimental animals already produce thirty grams per liter of drugs in their milk. In addition, these "transdermal sheep" are worth over $100,000 each to the pharmaceutical companies that back the research.)

At issue here is that drugs are being introduced in a high concentration into the food supply. Many people have reactions to prescription drugs which they are *knowingly* taking. Imagine the reactions we may see with drug-sensitive people who had no clear idea they were eating a food biotechnologically laced with pharmaceutical drugs.

Why *are* drug companies so interested in this type of genetic alteration? Mainly, because it's cheaper to produce drugs in sheep, goats and cows than in the laboratory. The pharmaceutical industry is simply further commercializing the production of drugs at the expense of innocent animals and, quite possibly, the entire human race. This biotechnological research that began late in the 20th century is still in practice at an even greater degree in today's world. The far reaching grasp that the pharmaceutical industry has obtained is disturbing and will be discussed in my up-coming book concerning the downside of drugs. You will learn about countless safe alternatives to discuss with your trusted healthcare practitioner.

Coffee and Sugar

Another mass-marketed product, caffeine, also remains highly addictive and allergenic to most people. Symptoms of caffeine sensitivity include headaches, flushing, nervous jitters, even diarrhea. Many times, caffeine and sugar go hand in hand because sugar is often used to mask the bitter taste of both coffee and chocolate, two widely used foods containing caffeine.

The sugar cane and sugar beet represent whole foods that contain a natural complement of nutrients which help metabolize the carbohydrate. In sugar processing, those natural nutrients are fractioned out. What's left behind is a toxic chemical to which many adults have become addicted. So addicted, that the average American consumes between 150-170 pounds of sugar each year.

Sugar also triggers a food sensitivity reaction that directly affects the immune system. One research study found that sucrose, fructose, honey and orange juice all decreased the capability of neutrophils (a type of white blood cell) to kill bacteria. The decrease in effectiveness of the white blood cell to kill bacteria lasted up to five hours after consuming sugar.[5]

The body's white blood cells maintain a continuous search for foreign particles, chemicals, dead tissue debris, or suspect cells in the body. As tiny garbage collectors, their job entails cleaning up dead cells in the body.

Because the white blood cells complete such a relentless and detailed search, they often find sugar to be a toxic, foreign chemical in the body and immediately go on the attack. The white blood cells then sacrifice themselves by engulfing that sugar toxin. It poisons them instantly, and they die. That's why less white blood cells can be found in the body following sugar consumption.

Additives and Preservatives

Other chemical toxins which annihilate white blood cells include additives and preservatives unnaturally added to preserve certain foods.

Used in a myriad of ways, additives and preservatives never test compatible with the body's physiological or energetic system. These and other environmental toxins simply add to the propensity for food sensitivity problems—and fill up that "oaken bucket," overtaxing your immune system.

Along with hybridization, pesticides and herbicides pose additional threats to the food chain. Pesticides are commonly used in both wheat and citrus farming, and leave residues in grain and other produce.

In testing sensitivity to both organic and regular wheat, most people react to the contaminated wheat, but not the organic wheat. For this reason, it's recommended that everyone buy organic food and produce whenever possible from reputable health food supermarkets.

Railie's Story

Railie suffered a great many headaches stemming from food sensitivities. Her exam indicated she was allergic to the MSG or monosodium glutamate in many Chinese dishes, among other items. Her particular sensitivity also added to a great deal of heart-related stress. Following treatment, Railie went for days with no headaches. Then, the bottom fell out.

"What happened?" I asked.

"Well, I went out for Chinese food again," she admitted.

"Did you remember to tell the waitress 'No MSG.'"

"No, I forgot." she sighed. Unfortunately, her headache didn't forget.

ARE YOU ADDICTED TO FOOD?

Food sensitivity and addiction go hand in hand. People who wake up each morning and find they simply must have their milk or coffee, may be suffering from a food addiction. Extreme compulsiveness about any food usually signals food sensitivity or an allergy to that item. As we pointed out earlier, with food eaten too frequently the likelihood of developing a sensitivity or addiction increases. Finding ways to break those patterns of food addiction involves exploring other choices.

There's no need for complicated rotation diets, systems, gimmicks or color codes. Simply eat a variety of foods. This one important change stops the perpetuation of habits leading to food sensitivity.

FOOD SENSITIVITIES MAY BE INHERITED

Other addictions also compound food sensitivity susceptibility. An individual whose mother experienced significant food sensitivities and consumed those foods during pregnancy (while the child was *in utero*) often develops the same sensitivities. Particularly, mothers who use drugs (pharmaceutical or otherwise), alcohol or cigarettes, risk causing their children to become addicted. Such factors compromise the baby's immune system resulting in significant problems. This topic is explored further in Chapter 13, *Optimizing Your Children's Health*.

Leon's Story

Unquestionable proof that addictions are passed on to children is seen in fetal alcohol syndrome. I evaluated and helped formulate treatment for a fourteen-year-old boy, Leon, who appeared to be borderline mentally retarded.

While *in utero*, Leon's mother was an active, heavy drinker. Thus, Leon was born addicted—and severely allergic to sugar. As a result, he was extremely hyperactive ... moving every minute! Leon also exhibited various kinds of choroid movements: flicking fingers, moving hands, shaking his head, and twitching his body continuously.

When I first met Leon, he was in detention at a boy's ranch for having attempted to set his mother on fire. Each day, Leon was expected to help with the ranch duties. Instead, he refused to cooperate, picked fights with the other boys and continually found himself in trouble.

Leon begged, borrowed, or stole money for soda pop. Prior to being taken into custody it was routine for him to drink at least a case of pop a day. Because of his inherited addiction, Leon's body had been severely damaged at birth. The resulting antibody reaction to alcohol set up his sugar addiction, which he liked to placate in liquid form.

Leon's case points out how food sensitivity developed in utero can seriously affect mental and emotional behavior. I recommended the elimination of soda pop from the entire ranch and suggested that the pop machines be filled with canned juices, especially for Leon.

Unfortunately, Leon was unable to recover from his addiction and subsequent destructive behavior. He was eventually sent back into the penal system.

CLINICAL KINESIOLOGY FOOD TESTING

Clinical Kinesiology food sensitivity testing bypasses the conscious mind, including one's preconceived ideas about food. Testing "asks" the energetic system of the body which foods prove compatible. In turn, the body talks, relaying information regarding the appropriate "fit" of the energy pattern of a particular food with the energy pattern of the whole body *at the current time*. (With treatment, that answer may change over time.)

In my office, Clinical Kinesiology food sensitivity testing utilizes a battery of approximately 244 food items. The food groups normally tested include seeds and grains, red meat and poultry, nuts, dairy products, herbs and spices, seafood, vegetables, legumes, fruits and other miscellaneous items such as chewing gum, coffee, and soda pop. A grouping of natural and artificial sweeteners, salts, and seaweed items are also included.

Clinical testing requires the placement of each food item directly in the energy field of the body, or on the abdomen. During testing, food items should be concealed from the patient, so as not to bias the test. Otherwise, the patient might be thinking, "Oh, I hate alfalfa sprouts!" Or, "I just love sugar or coffee," and thereby change the energetic field of the body.

Food items may be tested directly in their plastic containers, just as blood samples are evaluated by a Chromo Spectrophotometer in a laboratory. These sample test-food containers prove basically inert, which means they don't interact energetically. Additionally, dried food proves most stable for testing purposes.

How Testing Works

I tested a thirty-five-year-old man, Clyde, for food sensitivities. As instructed, Clyde lay down comfortably on the examining table and I performed a preliminary test to check the strength of his indicator muscle. As I pushed, I asked Clyde to resist. His arm proved strong.

The first test items represented the seeds and grains group. Clyde resisted and his muscle responded strong to alfalfa seeds. In this way, his body indicated through the Clinical Kinesiology muscle test, that it was safe for him to eat the alfalfa as sprouts or ground up as an alfalfa supplement.

The next item tested, amaranth, often thought of as a grain, is truly a little seed. Amaranth provides a good alternative for anyone sensitive to wheat or other grains. The amaranth test? Again, Clyde's indicator muscle reacted strongly.

The testing continued with artichoke semolina. I pushed, Clyde resisted—and proved strong.

Barley? A big push and the indicator muscle suddenly fell weak. At this point in time, Clyde's body proved energetically incompatible with barley. Why? I speculated to myself: Had Clyde eaten too much barley too commonly in his life? Could barley have been introduced in a cereal before his infant digestive tract was mature enough to accept it? Or, was barley simply inappropriate for Clyde's system due to organ imbalance, genetics, individual body chemistry or current digestive process?

Therapy Localizing for Food Sensitivity

Food that tests incompatible with the energy of the central abdomen or whole body may be "therapy localized" over each organ (see Chapter 1). An indicator muscle may react weakly to a food placed over the liver, yet hold strong in the energetic field of the thyroid. In this way, organs most sensitive to the item may be pinpointed and treated.

Testing over the liver provides the best indication of food sensitivities. The liver functions as the "workhorse" that breaks down chemicals in the body. Treating the liver or other organs that may contribute to food sensitivity (such as the digestive organs) quickly strengthens the whole body.

Once the affected organs become restrengthened, retesting and reintroduction of foods once sensitive to the body may occur after ninety days. Foods which prove inappropriate during initial tests may now test fine. One caveat? Avoid eating any formerly offending food on a daily basis.

Clyde's Test Continues ...

... Clyde resisted and proved strong with couscous. What about flaxseed? Again, strong. Kamut, a grain only slightly longer than the wheat grain came next. (Many times when a person indicates a food sensitivity to wheat it's advisable to substitute kamut for a period of time.) Oats? Once again, Clyde tested strong. Wild rice, pumpkin seed, quinoa, soy flour, and sesame seeds all tested strongly in Clyde's energetic field.

Clyde tested through wheat and wheat products—such as wheat germ, wheat bran and wheat macaroni—with flying colors. Often patients indicate a sensitivity to all four, or at least to one.

Following completion of the 244-item food sensitivity evaluation, Clyde studied his exam sheet on which each food sensitive item had been circled.

Half-Full Not Half-Empty

I compiled a list of food items for Clyde to avoid for ninety days. (During that time, evaluation and further treatment of organ imbalances, or digestive function might be necessary.) In addition, I recommended nutrients and supplements to help rebuild and re-strengthen liver and thyroid function, the organs most affected by food sensitivity.

As Clyde scanned the data from his exam, I encouraged him to concentrate on new food items he'd never eaten before. "Wow, I can eat cucumbers, endive, and kale—but I never eat them," he said. On further investigation he discovered many more new and appealing items to choose. I recommended interesting recipes for organic quinoa and couscous dishes he'd previously never tried.

Following food sensitivity testing, Clyde began experimenting with new-found foods and further varying his diet. As with so many aspects of life, we always have the choice of whether to see the glass as "half-empty" ("Oh no, look at all the foods I can't eat") or "half-full" ("Look at how many healthy new food choices I have to increase my energy and well-being").

Clyde continued with treatment of specific organ imbalances that helped restrengthen his digestive process. He also added vitamin, glandular and enzyme supplements to his diet. After three months, I performed a follow-up food sensitivity test which indicated that Clyde was no longer sensitive to many of the originally unacceptable food items. In this way, his body "told" me that his immune system had sufficiently strengthened and Clyde was well on the way to recovery from food sensitivities.

Nambudripad Allergy Elimination Technique (NAET)

California acupuncturist Devi S. Nambudripad, D.C, O.M.D., Ph.D., has developed the Nambudripad Allergy Elimination Technique (NAET) to work with hidden allergies. Dr. Nambudripad uses Kinesiology and acupuncture at her Buena Park clinic to change the energetic body's unbalanced response to food items and other substances. Dr. Nambudripad's technique, described in her book, *Say Goodbye To Illness*, allows the food sensitive person to again co-exist with food sensitive items or environments. As a result of her technique, eighty to ninety percent of Dr. Nambudripad's patients have now become allergy free. Thousands of doctors across the country have now been trained in NAET.[6] For more in-depth testing, and allergy elimination techniques such as Dr. Nambudripad's, see the Appendix of this book or consult your local alternative or natural healthcare practitioner who can provide follow-up guidance specifically pertaining to food sensitivities.

FOOD SENSITIVITY SELF-TESTING

Meanwhile, you can learn to do some simple self-testing for food sensitivities, instantly identifying foods as compatible or incompatible with your own particular energetic system. This knowledge and practice can be helpful in discovering underlying effects of specific foods on your body. The following steps will help you and a partner/ tester quickly discover a particular food substance to which you may be sensitive.

Step 1: Always begin any series of Clinical Kinesiology testing by first performing the Indicator muscle test. This test determines the base-line strength of the arm the test-subject will be using. (See Chapter One for instructions.) Once Indicator arm muscle strength is determined proceed with further testing.

Step 2: Have the person being tested select a food item to which he or she suspects a sensitivity. Instruct him or her to lie down comfortably and place that food item in the energy field (on the central abdomen) of the body. Perform the test as follows:

> Food + Muscle test + Weak arm = Food sensitivity.
> or
> Food + Muscle test + Strong arm = Energetic compatibility with body.

To simplify food sensitivity testing, be sure to test only with organic food first, thereby leaving out any influences from modern processing. Negative reactions to an organic product provides a good indication of food sensitivity to the food itself and not to other factors.

Microwaved and Genetically Engineered Food

Along with muscle testing for the energetic compatibility of natural foods, you may also want to test the human-made varieties. Microwaved food sends up another red flag for anyone with known food sensitivities. It's radiated, chemically altered and incompatible with the body. To check sensitivity to microwaved foods, do a sample test.

Step 1: First, check for food sensitivity to a potato.

Step 2: If the muscle test proves strong, cut the potato in half. Microwave one half and bake the other half in a conventional oven.

Step 3: Retest the microwaved potato versus the baked potato and note any difference in the sensitivity tests to each potato.

I strongly recommend consulting with a natural health practitioner to assist in strengthening the digestive system and organs over a ninety-day period following food sensitivity testing. Perhaps after a time, as in Clyde's case, the food that tested energetically incompatible may be acceptable.

Following initial self-testing, should any food remain questionable in your mind, retest the food a second time held over the liver, and a third time over the kidney. Sometimes a food item that may irritate the liver or kidney will not irritate the body as a whole.

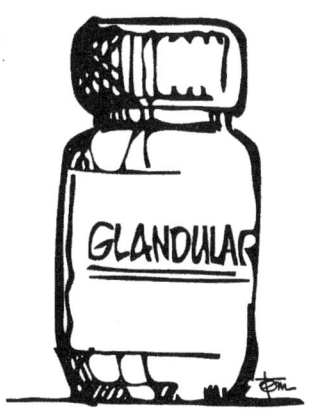

Testing Vitamins, Herbs, and Prescription Medicine

The same principles used in testing foods may also be used for Clinical Kinesiology testing of vitamin supplements, herbs, homeopathic remedies—even prescription medications.

Muscle testing can determine if almost any natural or chemical substance is energetically compatible with your specific body energy. Many times, people think, "Vitamins are always good for us." I say, *it always depends on the energetic quality of the substance.*

In the case of vitamins, many questions should be raised. What are the raw ingredients? How is the processing done? How careful was the manufacturer in not adding chemicals? (You may not be aware that some vitamins are made by the same pharmaceutical laboratories that manufacture chemical drugs.) Discount brand vitamins that appear bright purple or green or contain a hard, shiny yellow coat are not natural! As a result, they may irritate the body. The irritation may not show up during the general test, however, during therapy localization over the liver, the muscle test may render the arm weak.

When testing supplements, herbs, homeopathic remedies or medications, test them while in their labeled containers—whether unleaded glass or plastic. This will maintain cleanliness of the substance, and avoid confusing one item with another.

Remember, muscle tests may change with time, based upon current body balance, the season of the year, or what may be occurring in each individual system. The tests do initially confirm substances energetically compatible with the body. However, self-testing should become a life-long practice to meet the varying needs of each body.

When self-testing prescription drugs, most people find that, typically, the drugs render the arm muscle weak—especially during therapy localization over the kidney, liver, or both. Be aware of this. Find ways of strengthening the liver and kidney such as periodic cleansing (See Chapter 10 for various liver and kidney flushes), vitamin, herbal or glandular supplementation. Do what you can to strengthen the body so that it no longer exhibits the weakness for which the drug was prescribed. Chapter 14, about how drugs interact with your body, offers many natural alternatives for you to discuss with your trusted healthcare practitioner.

CONQUERING FOOD SENSITIVITIES

As you begin to feel good about the food you eat, you'll also feel good about yourself. Clearing up suspected problems with food sensitivities or addictions, following specific recommendations and indicating to others new dietary commitments and restrictions are the keys to renewed health.

As you gain new perspective, be encouraged to consider food as physical, emotional and spiritual nourishment. With each bite, lovingly chew your food, and let go of any former mental blocks about that food that may affect your current and future health.

Enjoy foods in their natural forms, along with the energy, vitality and bounty they bring to life. Eat simply to live. As you begin to supply nutrients to help body function you'll not only satisfy your hunger, you'll also be rewarded with

---

Supplement + Muscle test + Weak arm = Energetically incompatible. Purchase only natural supplements from a reputable alternative healthcare provider or health food store and retest.

Supplement + Muscle test + Strong arm = Energetically compatible.

or

Prescription Medication + Muscle test + Weak arm = Energetically incompatible. Consult your natural healthcare practitioner for alternative treatment in strengthening the organ or condition which required the prescription drug.

"high performance" health for an optimal length of time.

As we've seen, the incompatibility that develops between food and the body's energetic system stems from a malfunction of the immune system. Just as the immune system protects the body from its own poorly digested foods or natural by-products of metabolizing that food—it also protects from other unrecognized chemicals and foreign invaders. Chapter 6, *Energizing Your Immune System*, offers specific methods of fighting disease through a healthy and functioning immune system along with protecting it from unnecessary drugs, antibiotics and immunizations, which further undermine immune function.

CHAPTER 5 SUGGESTED READING

Anderson, A. *Flourishing with Food Allergies: Social, Emotional and Practical Guidance for Families with Young Children.* Southbury, Conn.: Papoose Publishing, 2008.

Aronson, Dina, M.S., R.D., Vesanto Melina, M.S., R.D. and Jo Stepaniak, M.S. Ed. *Food Allergy Survival Guide: Surviving and Thriving with Food Allergies and Sensitivities.* Summertown, Tenn.: Healthy Living Publications, 2004.

Balch, Phyllis A. C.N.C. *Prescription for Dietary Wellness: Using Foods to Heal, 2nd Ed.* New York: Penguin. 2003.

Brostoff, Johnathan and Linda Gamlin. *Food Allergies and Food Intolerance: A Complete Guide to Their Identification and Treatment.* Rochester, Vt.: Healing Press, 2000.

Crook, William M.D. *Tracking Down Hidden Food Allergy.* Jackson, Tenn.: Professional Books, 1980.

Fenster, Carol. *Cooking Free: 200 Flavorful Recipes for People with Food Allergies and Multiple Food Sensitivities.* New York: Avery. 2005.

Joneja, Janice Vickerstaff, Ph.D., R.D.N. *Dealing with Food Allergies: A Practical Guide to Detecting Culprit Foods and Eating a Healthy, Enjoyable Diet.* Boulder, Colo.: Bull Publishing Company. 2003.

Katzinger, Jennifer. *Flying Apron's Gluten-free & Vegan Baking Book.* Seattle: Sasquatch Books, 2009.

Koeller, Kim and Robert La France. *Let's Eat Out: Your Passport to Living Gluten and Allergy Free.* R & R Publishing, 2005.

Marienhoff Coss, Linda. *How to Manage Your Child's Life-Threatening Food Allergies.* Lake Forest, Calif.: Plumtree Press, 2004.

Mosely, Cindy. *Great Foods without Worry.* Aventine Press, 2003.

Nambudripad, Devi S. *Say Goodby to Illness: A Revolutionary Treatment for Allergies and Allergy-Related Conditions, 3rd Ed.* Buena Park, Calif.: Delta Publishing, 2002.

Orenstein, Neil S. Ph.D. and Sarah Bingham, M.S. *Food Allergies: How to Tell If You Have Them, What to do about Them If You Do.* New York: Perigee Books, 1988

Pascal, Cybele. *The Whole Foods Allergy Cookbook: Two Hundred Gourmet & Homestyle Recipes for the Food Allergic Family.* Ridgefield, Conn.: Vital Health Publishing, 2006.

Philpott, William, Dwight D. Kalita, and Linus Pauling. *Brain Allergies: The Psychonutrient and Magnetic Connections, Updated 2nd Ed.* New Canaan, Conn.: Keats Publishing, 2000.

Santillo, Humbart, B.S., M.H. *Food Enzymes, The Missing Link to Radiant Health.* Prescott, Arizona: Hohm Press, 1993.

Sicherer, Scott H., *Understanding and Managing Your Child's Food Allergies.* Baltimore: The Johns Hopkins University Press, 2006.

Twogood, Daniele A., D.C. *No Milk: A Revolutionary Solution to Back Pain and Headaches.* Victorville, Calif.: Wilhelmina Books, 1992.

CHAPTER 6
Energizing Your Immune System

Amy nervously paced the halls of the hospital children's ward as her three-year-old daughter, Kaycee, underwent surgery to implant Myringotomy ear-draining tubes.

In the preceding months, Kaycee had been prescribed dose after dose of antibiotics. The little girl always seemed better for a short while, then suddenly developed another ear infection. Each visit to the medical clinic resulted in still more prescriptions of antibiotics.

Eventually, the few remaining strong bacteria in Kaycee's intestinal system multiplied and mutated, forcing the doctor to pull out his strongest arsenal of antibiotics—to no avail. Surgery became the doctor's final solution to months and months of repeated ear infections for which he could find no other cure.

Every day, children like Kaycee literally experience a merry-go-round of drugs that ultimately destroy their young immune systems. As a result, their bodies are left open to a downward cycle of illnesses for which they have no immune system "army" left to fight.

A HEALTHY IMMUNE SYSTEM

Although a strong immune system is capable of fighting off any disease, its function remains a mystery to most people—*including most medical doctors*. The body relies so much on the integrity of the immune system that, often, until the immune system stops working, most people are unaware of it.

This chapter introduces you to the complex components of the immune system—the network of cell fighters and immune organs. Monitoring that system which provides optimal health requires knowledge of its strongest foundation—diet and nutrition.

Daily care and maintenance of a healthy and functioning immune system also involves individual evaluation of immune function, available for the first time through Clinical Kinesiology energetic testing.

Armed with new knowledge, you will be encouraged to find ways to avoid or change factors which suppress or compromise immune function, including genetic pre-dispositions, overuse of antibiotics, stress, and medical and governmental immunization programs based on money and politics, rather than health.

This chapter will further discuss *informed consent*, your right to choose to protect the health of your immune system, and that of each member of your family, from yearly "flu shots" and other mass advertised vaccination programs.

You can learn to re-establish and maintain natural immunity through self-testing, education, natural diet changes, detoxification, and alternative therapies.

How The Immune System Works

Many people today are increasingly faced with immune system problems. AIDS, chronic fatigue immune deficiency syndrome, lupus, rheumatoid arthritis, multiple sclerosis, scleroderma and cancer all occur mainly because immune systems have become weak. In most of these auto-immune diseases the body mistakes normal tissues for invading substances, triggering full-blown attacks on itself. In this mass state of confusion, the weakened body no longer has any resources with which to fight.

The role of a strong immune system in warding off cancer has become central to most treatment. Immune system cells are continually on the lookout for problem areas in the body. Everyone harbors a certain number of cells which, from time to time, begin to divide in crazy patterns. Every year, cancer cells develop in everyone's body. Luckily, a strong immune system takes care of them.

A network of killer T- and B-cells, lymphocytes and suppressor cells comprise the many types of cells throughout the immune system. Fighters that provide natural immunity, these cells remain continuously on patrol and searching—**if** the immune system is strong and healthy.

Several organs and tissues also defend the body from infectious disease, external chemical irritants and internal imbalances. That defense includes protecting the body from bacteria, viruses, chemicals, and many other foreign invaders. Anytime an individual develops an auto-immune disease, the critical element is a malfunctioning immune system.

T-Cells

The soldiers of the immune system army constitute several different types of white blood cells called lymphocytes. The most active and most daring are the killer T-cells.

Produced in the thymus gland, located directly under the sternum, the killer T-cells seek out and destroy cells in the body which have been invaded by foreign organisms, as well as cells which have become cancerous. A simple self help method to stimulate your immune system is tapping over your thymus in the area of your sternum. This can easily be made into a playful and healthful activity for parents and children.

When an individual develops the AIDS virus, the killer T-cells are most affected. Dangerous viruses, such as HIV, contain some DNA, although not the complete molecule. Viruses typically invade a cell, parasitize it and use the DNA of the host cell to propagate and increase in number.

The host cell may be a blood cell, or any other cell in the body. Ultimately, the host cell becomes "bleached out." With its nutrients expended by the virus, it explodes and spews many viruses throughout the body.

Another set of cells, the helper T-cells, serve as "directors" of the immune system. Helper T-cells identify invaders and stimulate the production of other immunity cells located in the spleen and lymph nodes. Through chemical means, the helper T-cells call up the masses to the problem area.

The macrophage cells, another of the lymphocytes, take on the role of "housekeepers," and function primarily as the front line of defense. Macrophages are readily available throughout the body. Chemically programmed to be attractive to various bacteria and viruses, macrophages engulf and digest any particles left behind as the result of an initial attack.

Electron micrograph enhanced images beautifully portray the activity of a macrophage cell shooting out a killer substance through its own protoplasm, encircling a bacteria and neutralizing it. Most often, macrophages engulf debris in the body left over from wound healing; in effect, preventing decaying matter from lying around, becoming available for bacteria to feed on.

B-Cells

The B-cells, or beta cells of the immune system, lie dormant in the spleen and lymph nodes. They act as tiny "guards" in guard-posts scattered throughout the body, awaiting the call to duty. The B-cells wait silently in strategic locations and may be activated quickly.

Stimulated by helper T-cells, the beta cells produce potent chemical weapons called antibodies. Antibodies attach themselves to foreign substances in order to neutralize them, allowing other white blood cells to seek out and destroy the dangerous substances.

Once danger passes, the suppressor T-cells play a vital role in calling off the attack after an infection has been conquered. To enable the body to maintain immunity for future invasions, memory cells are also produced during the initial infection. These cells may circulate in the blood or lymph for years, allowing the body to respond more quickly to a repeated attack or infection.

White and Red Blood Cells

White blood cells comprise the fighters, while red blood cells provide the nutrients, or reinforcements, when a problem develops. The red cells carry oxygen and take on carbon dioxide, helping to move it out of the area.

As cells die or are destroyed the body must recreate most of its one hundred trillion cells. Certain nutritional supplements may be used to help create many of the different immune system cells.

Varying ideas exist on how long it takes to replenish the entire body with new cells; however, a common estimate is seven years. But, most red blood cells live only 120 days. So, if an anemic person is provided with a good diet and adequate supplements, within a short time, his or her red blood cell count improves.

Toxicity in Immunity

Every antigen/antibody reaction works like a lock and key mechanism. The shape of the antigen and antibody molecules are specific and must fit together. When this doesn't happen, immune cells must gobble up offending organisms. Chemicals, pollutants, and toxins in the blood are eradicated in this way too.

Obviously, the less extra chemicals, toxins, and pollutants from food additives, preservatives, and unnatural items in the blood stream, the more efficiently white blood cells can work to fight off the organism. So, toxicity also becomes an issue in immunity. The more toxic the body, the lower the immunity.

The importance of diet and nutrition as the healthy foundation of the immune system cannot be stressed enough. You are what you eat! Maintaining healthy immune cells and rebuilding lymphatic tissue depend on diet. It alone may be the change that positively affects the immune system for the rest of your life.

The Immune Organs

The dynamic, movable parts of the immune system consist of the white blood cells, while the stationary parts include the thymus gland, located under the sternum or breastbone; the thyroid gland, a butterfly shaped gland in the front region of the throat; and the lymph nodes, located on both sides of the neck and groin, and in each armpit.

Other important areas of lymph tissue strategically placed in the body include the tonsils, appendix, and throughout the intestinal tract. All of these glands and organs support immune system function.

Through the years, myself and many of my colleagues have noticed a high incidence of dental cavities in people who have had their tonsils removed. The tonsils exist as a tiny reservoir for white blood cells. When bacteria reaches the mouth, if the tonsils are doing their job the immune system holds strong.

The tonsils also help stave off upper respiratory infections and kill off bacteria in food that enters the stomach. The appendix provides another important reservoir for the immune system. Contrary to some beliefs, neither the tonsils nor appendix are simply worthless organs that should be eliminated without thought. Reasons exist for the presence of the tonsils and appendix!

A primary organ imbalance which almost always accompanies a weak immune system involves the thymus gland, the main producer of killer T-cells. The thyroid gland often proves to be the weakest secondary organ most affected.

EVALUATING IMMUNE SYSTEM FUNCTION

Immune system function can be evaluated through Clinical Kinesiology energetic muscle testing. A complete exam also involves investigating past health history and current concerns.

Copper metal is a well-known conductor of electricity. Dr. Burt Espy, a colleague of Dr. Alan Beardall, discovered that utilizing a copper plate placed on the body in conjunction with Clinical Kinesiology energetic muscle testing, lends specific information as to the functioning of the immune system, particularly in determining immune organ dysfunction. The copper "works" by ascertaining the body's currents as either strong or weak through the muscle test.

Following placement of the copper plate on the body, the Clinical Kinesiology muscle test may be performed. If the indicator muscle registers weak, the response determines a lack of proper energetic function of the immune system.

In order to further evaluate if an unbalanced organ is primarily thymus or thyroid, the copper plate may be touched over each of these organs to see if the weak muscle strengthens. The self-testing section at the end of this chapter provides specific instructions for evaluating the current status of individual immune system organ response.

A second method of Clinical Kinesiology evaluation may be used to test thymus- or thyroid-strengthening glandular supplements. Following the initial indicator muscle test, hold the supplement *along with the copper in place*, directly in the energy field of the body. Perform the muscle test. The correct remedy will render the formerly weak muscle strong. Such supplements strengthen the energy balance of a weak organ or gland along with further balancing the immune system. (See the product guide in the Appendix of this book for supplement distributor information.)

FACTORS WHICH SUPPRESS IMMUNITY

Stress and Toxicity

Anyone subjected to extraordinary stress calls upon the immune system to fight needless battles. The immune "soldiers" become over-worked and worn out. The results? They may not be as alert, available or ready in adequate numbers to fight off an invasion. Emotional stress, depression, and mental fatigue are all factors which compromise a healthy immune system.

The field of psychoneuroimmunology has developed in the last few years to research this problem. It studies the relationship between emotional states of mind and the immune system. Candace Pert, Ph.D. (1946-2013) was a leading neuroscientist. She had been affiliated with Johns Hopkins, Georgetown University and Rutgers University. Dr. Pert discovered neuropeptides—neurochemical substances that cause alterations in mood, and brought this information to the world in her book, *Molecules of Emotion: the Scientific Basis behind Mind-Body Medicine.*

Most significantly, neuropeptides have been discovered not only in the brain, but in the spinal cord, glands, organs and other body tissues. Neuropeptides found throughout the body also affect the functioning of the "whole" body, including the immune system.

Quantification of various types of white blood cells and their activity have been performed and correlated to various states of mind. In other words, we can think ourselves sick! Dr. George F. Solomon, a longtime researcher in psychoneuroimmunology, suggests that an "immunosuppression-prone" personality type often uses hostility or simply gives up when illness strikes.[1] Such depression and lack of interest in one's own well-being affects some people to the point that they become sick from suppressing their immune systems. Other factors which suppress the immune system include: toxicity due to overload of chemical residues from pollution, food preservatives and additives or medications. In addition, toxicity stems from the end-products of poor digestion (rendering food material into metabolic waste). Such end-products continue to reside in body tissues until a cleansing, a major illness, or purging takes place.

Stress, poor diet, toxicity and other lifestyle factors often work together to diminish the effectiveness of the immune system.

If we provide the immune system with the proper conditions, or strengthen a slightly weakened immune system through natural means, we have a greater likelihood of preventing future infections or other illness in the body.

Antibiotics

Contrary to negative reports in various media, bacterial and viral illnesses do not lurk behind every corner waiting to jump out and inundate the human race with sudden illness. It's true, microbes thrive all around us. However, maintaining the strength of the immune system remains the key to warding off disease.

Louis Pasteur himself developed a theory of immunity that has been largely forgotten by medicine. He suggested that the microbe proliferates only when the host has become too hospitable due to preexisting illness.[2] Today, pre-existing illness, which characterizes the ability of the immune system to function correctly, stems from the lifestyle and basic level of health of an individual. As Pasteur suggests, maintaining a healthy and functioning immune system is the only proven way to fight disease.

Today when humans or animals contract a type of bacterial infection they are most frequently prescribed an antibiotic. The drug, however, kills off only the weakest of the bacteria. The strongest live, begin reproducing, and eventually may genetically alter the bacterial gene-pool so that the infection flares up again! Then, another antibiotic is administered that kills off a few more bacteria. Once again, the strongest survive and recreate a new generation of even stronger bacteria. The bacteria mutate and constantly change to meet different conditions in the body and environment, especially to escape the effect of antibiotic drugs.

Much of the standard medical treatment since the middle of the twentieth century has been destructive to the immune system. Many individual doctors have unknowingly prescribed drugs that brought terribly destructive results.

Antibiotic drugs suppress immune cell production. Anytime the body is given a "substitute" (typically, a chemical substitute) for a natural function, the body automatically slows down or halts that function. For example, if the thyroid gland proves slightly under-productive for thyroxin, and a prescription for synthetic thyroxin is taken, the normal function of the thyroid falls off. That's why most patients given synthetic drugs are commonly told, "You must take this for the rest of your life." The reason? The individual's thyroid function diminishes and deteriorates once the medication is taken.

Antibiotic usage diminishes the strength of the immune system in much the same way. Pharmaceutical companies have developed what they call "broad-spectrum" antibiotics. Imagine going to target practice and aiming to shoot a bull's eye. Instead, the resulting effect of these powerful broad-spectrum drugs becomes more like a machine gun cleaning out the entire area.

NATURAL IMMUNIZATIONS

Remember Kaycee, the three-year-old who underwent surgery to insert ear-draining tubes? Who hasn't known a small child who's been prescribed antibiotics? And it's never one dose that is prescribed. On the contrary, it's *repeat … repeat … repeat*, and all the while, the child's immune system becomes weaker.

Experiencing childhood illnesses remains the only natural way to stimulate and strengthen the immune system. Such illnesses actually serve as a way of exercising the immune system. In effect, "use it or lose it." That's not to say that children need to contract pertussis or polio, but the milder childhood diseases including the mumps, measles, and chicken pox provide the building blocks in establishing a workout and development program for the immune system. These natural illnesses stimulate the immune system to work at a higher functioning level so children may easily ward off other, more serious, illnesses.

At best, life is a growing and learning process. A little baby learns to crawl first, then walk. The immune system must be trained in the same way. First, a child experiences a little cold, or roseola. Later it's a virus such as measles or chicken pox. Typically, all these childhood diseases are extremely gentle.

Throughout the centuries, the immune system has handled various exposures and diseases. Obviously, some individuals are weaker than others and people have died. We'll never stop that. Vaccines have never stopped that either!

Dangers of Immunizations

Immunizations constitute a great concern because the public has not been informed of the short and long-term side effects, traumas, neurological damage, and deaths which are part and parcel of the artificial immunization or vaccination of children.

In the last century, the medical profession, along with government authorities, have instituted public immunization programs and issued blanket prescriptions of antibiotics to countless people. Ethical, medical and social edicts regarding "blanket" immunization decisions are more often based on money and politics—and not health.

The immunization issue involves decisions that have been made at the highest levels—for the benefit of a few at the expense of many.[3] Each succeeding generation's immune systems have been weakened as a result.

Initially, scientists who studied immunizations may have thought they represented a valid, plausible idea. However, shortly before Louis Pasteur's death, he rejected the whole idea of immunizations. Pasteur proclaimed that he wished for the world to understand that the only way to fight disease was to maintain a healthy and functioning immune system.

Immunization or vaccination involves a process of exposing an individual to a mild form of a disease in hopes that an antigen/antibody reaction will be stimulated. In truth, it takes a stretch of the imagination to believe that injecting a virulent bacteria or virus (even in a weakened state) into the body, would be good for health. The whole idea that the body must begin fighting this deadly invader is frightening.

When an individual sustains a huge gash or wound (a dogbite, for example), bacteria is injected directly into the bloodstream. (Does someone have a better chance of fighting bacteria that way or by using the respiratory system as a filter, along with the immune system army? How many times have you been exposed to someone with a cold ... *and not gotten the cold*?)

Once bitten by a dog, the body must work extremely hard to avoid infection. However, the skin provides the first line of immune defense, while the white blood cells, including the entire immune reserves, wait in the wings.

What defense do you have from an injection of a virus into your bloodstream? By the time an immunization or particular vaccination is produced, the strain of that bacteria or virus may have changed or mutated significantly enough that the vaccine's effectiveness is lessened.

Most major diseases are cyclical, just as everything in life—day and night, summer and winter, hot and cold, birth and death. As diseases evolve, the rate of infection may rise; however, it also always drops. Many of the serious diseases—ones we presently immunize against—were most prevalent in the twentieth century. The danger of contracting them is much less than it was historically.

Many diseases have naturally diminished due to the attrition of one illness and occurrence of other new illnesses. Therefore, when building up and protecting the immune system, the significant risks of immunization mistakes and immunization-caused illnesses must be weighed.

Richard Moskowitz, in "The Case Against Immunizations," states that immunizations promote certain types of chronic diseases. "Far from providing a genuine immunity... vaccines may act by actually interfering with or suppressing the immune response ..."[4] Moskowitz soon discovered "... I could no longer bring myself to give the injections even when the parents wished me to."[5]

Dr. Moskowitz documents the occurrence of leukemia in two cases which he specifically relates back to immunizations. He also indicates that the rise in auto-immune diseases is an automatic result of injecting live virus and foreign antigens into children. He believes the virus from immunizations may be permanently incorporated into the genetic material or DNA of a child's cells. The antibody reaction then turns the immune system against the child's cells, which have been invaded from the viruses from the immunization.

Moskowitz also believes that the timing of the administration of many immunizations is not rational. Two-month-old infants, who possess strong immunity from being breast-fed, have a nervous system far too delicate to be exposed to the pertussis vaccine. In actuality, pertussis is rarely found in infants below five months of age, yet inoculations begin at two months. A high rate of neurological problems from damage to the central nervous system and other problems have been traced directly to the pertussis vaccine.[6]

The current medical fad consists of mixing three or four vaccines together, with plans to inject up to six separate viruses in one immunization. Such repeated vaccinations exhaust the immune system.

Additionally, many side effects from vaccinations result in both immediate and delayed reactions, including permanent disability. These side effects include mental retardation, cerebral palsy, epilepsy, paralysis, learning disability, recurrent respiratory infections, as well as susceptibility to all types of infectious disorders.

In his book, *The Assault on The American Child: Vaccination, Sociopathy, and Criminality*, Dr. Harris Coulter indicates brain injury (including autism), dyslexia, anti-social behavior, and personality disorders as conditions attributable to vaccinations.[7]

Dr. Coulter also warns that more than half of all children who become fussy and feverish following diphtheria/pertussis shots have more than likely suffered some encephalitis (inflammation of the brain) or probable brain damage, even if minimal. (Unfortunately, for children to be fussy and feverish after DPT shots remains the rule rather than the exception.)

In addition, the effectiveness of today's vaccines must be highly questioned. Documentation shows that fifty to sixty percent of children who contracted measles were previously vaccinated for measles. Other statistics show that between sixty and ninety percent of measles occur in adult individuals who were already vaccinated for measles. Nervous system disorders as severe as encephalitis, retinopathy, blindness and seizures have also been traced to measles vaccine.[8]

THE IMMUNIZATION INDUSTRY

Immunization programs are an expensive "industry" costing upwards of one billion dollars a year. The money is made by a few people— the government and pharmaceutical industries.

Every year, drug companies campaign across America. "Don't forget your flu shot!" is the slogan that encourages millions to walk into the clinic, the office, the grocery store, and even to the drive-up window. "Roll up your sleeves!" they say, "but ask no questions."

The thought of people running to the grocery store or street corner somewhere to get a flu shot is crazy. When I hear it, I think of lemmings running into the ocean. Often my patients who come with the worst cases of the flu are the ones who had gotten the flu shot—and they contracted the flu soon after getting the shot.

When people proclaim, "I get my flu shot every year," they have merely succumbed to mass social marketing techniques and worse. They are systematically weakening their immune systems. Do you know the signs to watch out for? The contraindications? Or, the contents of each flu shot? These dangers have been documented by a number of articles published since the 1950s.

In 1974, eighty million people, led by President Ford, rolled up their sleeves and received shots for a flu epidemic that never occurred. Thousands are now paralyzed by Guillain Barre Syndrome. I know because my husband, Dr. Burt Espy, treated a woman who gradually recovered.

Vaccinations, according to Guylaine Lanctot, author of *The Medical Mafia*, "... permit epidemiological studies of populations to collect data on the resistance of different ethnic groups to different illnesses."[9]

What's really in an immunization? In "quality control" hospital research laboratories, researchers may grow cultures to produce immunizations in one room, conduct AIDS research in another, or make polio vaccine in the third laboratory. Cross contamination through unsanitary hospital and research lab coats is often the norm rather than the exception, says Robert S. Mendelsohn in his book, *Male Practice: How Doctors Manipulate Women*. "... Hospitals are prone to handle their laundry so carelessly that those antiseptic-appearing uniforms are often loaded with germs."[10] Some coats are washed only every six or eight weeks and rarely in scalding water. Technicians often walk from room to room, rubbing a sleeve here, or wiping a thigh with something there. As Sherry Rogers, M.D. relates in *Tired or Toxic? A Blueprint for Health*, "Every afternoon at 1:00 we would don our white lab coats (that we rarely washed because we were too tired) and slave over our formaldehyde-soaked cadavers until dinner. Afterwards, still swaddled in the coats, we studied into the wee hours of the morning."[11]

The air in hospital research laboratories provides another fertile avenue of contamination. Yes, many hospitals and labs try to take precautions on some levels, however, *no one truly knows what is in that immunization*. Researchers don't really know either. Cross contamination can be great, and most cultures are at least somewhat suspect.

Another related issue has to do with what a lab culture is grown on. Unfortunately for our little animal friends, most cultures are grown on monkey livers.

Monkeys frequently carry a virus called Simian 40 (SV 40). In fact, when Dr. Albert Schweitzer directed his clinic in Africa, he treated anyone—unless the patient was suffering from a monkey or an ape bite. In those cases, Dr. Schweitzer gently advised, "Go home to your village, be comfortable and die peacefully." Because Simian 40 is so infectious, and he had no way to cure the virus, he didn't want to risk contaminating his other patients.

Could the Simian 40 virus find its way into a lab culture in the U.S.? Yes, it's possible and warrants more close consideration. Lanctot reports: "... in 1960, cultures from the manufacture of anti-polio vaccine were discovered to be infested with Simian 40. As a result, millions of children were contaminated before detection. Today, SV 40 is known to cause immune deficiency, congenital anomalies, leukemia, and malignant illnesses," such as brain tumors.[12]

TO IMMUNIZE OR NOT

You, the public, are not told of the dangers of immunizations. I support you in taking greater responsibility for your health. Individual families should retain the right to choose whether or not to expose themselves or their children to mass immunizations which have a low rate of quality control in production.

Today, it's become much too commonplace to accept immunizations without question. I believe that populations who take immunization programs too lightly face an incredible danger. The possibility of being an unknowing subject in an unwanted experimentation is terrifying. The risk that unforeseen items have been added to the vaccines is too big a risk to take.

In her research, Guylaine Lanctot met with a group of Native American women about the subject of vaccinations. The group's nurse confided that although the federal government had provided her complete freedom in managing the children's healthcare, the government insisted on one strict condition—"*that every vaccination had to be scrupulously applied to all.*"[13]

The federal government's eagerness to require all children to be immunized can be potentially dangerous. The likelihood of these children being injected with substances without their parents' complete knowledge must be addressed. *Parents be forewarned*. Health issues and legal rights' issues are at stake. No one should consent to immunizations without fully exploring the potential dangers.

STRENGTHENING YOUR IMMUNE SYSTEM

Not everyone catches a virus. Lifestyle remains the most important determinant in "who gets sick," followed by genetic predisposition. But the good news is that you can win the fight against genetic predisposition! You can change lifestyle factors and add conditions that the body requires to maintain a healthy immune system!

Once again, the ability of the body to fight disease and avoid illness depends on the health and activity of your immune system "soldiers." Proper nutrient balance remains the major factor which allows the immune system soldiers to remain strong and active.

Immune Nutrients

Anyone who determines that she or he possesses a weak immune system should assume that the body is experiencing nutrient imbalance. Should an immune system demonstrate inadequate functioning, immediate treatment should be instituted even though an individual may not yet prove symptomatic.

Nutrients known to be integral to the functioning of the immune system include vitamins C and E, selenium, vitamin A with beta carotene, zinc, B vitamins, manganese, inositol, iron and copper. Zinc stimulates T-cell production while vitamin A contributes to healthy mucus membranes of the cells. Vitamin E is the oxygenator of the body and also helps in the production of T-cells.

Recently, it's been discovered that bioflavinoids taken with vitamin C assist the body in making more of its own naturally occurring interferon, an essential compound of the immune system. Selenium, found in garlic, provides an important boost to immune system function. It also helps the body hold onto and absorb vitamin E.

Nobel prizewinner Dr. Linus Pauling was a firm believer in the properties of vitamin C. Dr. Pauling reportedly took mega doses of vitamin C every day until his death well into his 90s.

I take a minimum of 6,000 mg. of vitamin C every day and recommend a high dose throughout the day in a sustained release tablet. Along with nutrition, detoxification programs have proved very successful for anyone with a poorly functioning immune system.

To further build health, immune system building nutrients are available. These include Core Level Thymus™ and Core Level Thyroid™ by Nutri-west®, or Immu-Cell™ by Professional Botanicals (see Product Guide). Immu-Cell™ contains milkweed, germanium, CoQ1O, vitamin A, thymus, ginseng and shark cartilage. These products provide wise yet harmless interventions to protect both adults and children, providing immunity without submission to governmental authorities or threat of danger.

Available in a homeopathic form, these immune stimulators may be used in lieu of immunizations or vaccinations to strengthen the immune system, specifically for bacterial and viral immunity. Excellent versions of these, Bacterial Immune™ remedy, and Viral Immune remedy are available from Mountain States Health Products. (See Resource Guide.) In the event that a child has already been exposed to pertussis or other communicable diseases, a new administration of the immune system stimulators can be introduced and may prove helpful.

Consult with a natural healthcare practitioner for any questions you may have regarding the use of natural remedies.

Immune Herbs

Echinacea remains a simple, yet powerful herb for stimulating the immune system. It resembles a daisy, with purple petals and a yellow bulbous center. The petals grow toward the sun and then turn down, making it an extremely pretty herb.

If you decide to grow your own herb garden, the Echinacea root is the most potent part of the plant. Thus I grow plenty of them in my own organic herb garden. Most garden shops sell small Echinacea plants or seeds, which take longer to grow.

With the immune-building herbs Echinacea or astragulas, plus the infection-fighter golden seal, almost any infection can be deterred. In addition, acidophilus (friendly intestinal flora) proves especially helpful if an antibiotic has been taken previously and the body needs rebalancing by replanting the good bacteria that has been lost.

The value of probiotics will be discussed further in Chapter 8, *Leaky Gut and Your Digestion*.

TESTING IMMUNE SYSTEM FUNCTION

The simplest test, designed by Dr. Burt Espy, to determine the status of the immune system is the Copper Test. For this, you'll need to visit a neighborhood hardware store and purchase a small strip of copper, approximately two inches square.

Step 1: Place the copper strip in the energy field (or central abdomen) of the body and perform the Clinical Kinesiology muscle test. A weak muscle response indicates an imbalance in the immune system.

> Copper strip + Muscle test 4+ Strong arm = Functioning immune system
>
> Copper strip + Muscle test + Weak arm = Weak immune system.

Step 2: If the copper weakens the body, obtain a bottle of Echinacea in tincture form. Place the bottle along with the copper onto the abdomen together, and retest to determine if the Echinacea helps to counteract the weakness and make the immune system stronger.

> Copper + Echinacea + Muscle test 4+ Strong arm = Use Echinacea to strengthen immune system.

HEALTHY THOUGHTS, ETC.

Finally, in strengthening the immune system the power of thought remains unmistakable. Many times patients call and say, "I don't think I should come today. I have a cold and don't want to give it to you."

I always tell them, "We have strong immune systems. We work on having strong immune systems. So come!"

Take control of your environment and eliminate toxins such as cigarette smoke, pesticides, vapors, and chemical odors, keeping a harmonious environment in your home.

Also, learn to steer clear of the dangers of chemically altering the immune system. Through educating yourself about natural dietary changes, detoxification, alternative therapies, herbal and other nutrients, you will reap wide-ranging benefits in securing a healthful and normal immune system for yourself and your family for generations to come.

By learning about factors which may have undermined our immune system function in the past, we can better prepare to care for our immune system in the future. The foundation of that knowledge may now be used by the millions of people who unknowingly suffer from the systemic infection, Candida albicans. Chapter 7, *Candida: Causes and Treatment*, provides guidance in identifying Candidiasis along with measures for rebuilding and maintaining the body's immune system following such an overgrowth of unhealthy bacteria.

CHAPTER 6 SUGGESTED READING

Berger, Stuart M.D. *Dr. Berger's Immune Power Diet.* New York: E.P. Dutton & Co., 1986.

Buttram, Harold M.D. and John Chris Hoffman. *Vaccinations and Immune Malfunction.* The Humanitarian Publishing Company, 1985.

Chaitow, Leon. *Natural Alternatives to Antibiotics: How You Can Supercharge Your Immune System and Fight Infection.* Hamersmith, London: Thorsons, 2002.

Coulter, Harris and B.L. Fisher, DPT. *A Shot In The Dark.* San Diego, Calif: Harcourt, Brace, Jovanovich, 1985.

Coulter, Harris. *Vaccination, Social Violence, and Criminality: The Medical Assault on the American Brain.* Berkeley, Calif: North Atlantic Books, 1990.

Fuhrman, Joel. *Eat to Live Cookbook: 200 Delicious Nutrient-Rich Recipes for Fast and Sustained Weight Loss, Reversing Disease, and Lifelong Health.* New York, NY: HarperOne, 2013.

Fuhrman, Joel, M.D. *Super Immunity: The Essential Nutrition Guide for Boosting Your Body's Defenses to Live Longer, Stronger, and Disease Free.* New York, NY: HarperOne; Reprint edition, 2013.

Galland, L. and D.D. Buchman. *Superimmunity for Kids.* New York: Dutton, 1988.

Geison, Gerald L. *The Private Science of Louis Pasteur.* Princeton, N.J.: Princeton University Press, 1995.

Gregory, Scott O.M.D. *A Holistic Protocol for the Immune System: HIV/ARC/AIDS/Candidiasis/Epstein-Barr/Herpes and Other Opportunistic Infections, 6th Ed. Revised.* Calif: Tree of Life Publications, 1995.

Jones, Cindy L.A. Ph.D. *The Antibiotic Alternative: The Natural Guide to Fighting Infection and Maintaining a Healthy Immune System.* Rochester, Vermont: Healing Arts Press, 2000.

Justice, Blair Ph.D. *Who Gets Sick.* Los Angeles, Calif: Jeremy Tarcher, Inc., 1988.

Lanctot, Guylaine, M.D. *The Medical Mafia: How to Get Out of it Alive and Take Back our Health and Wealth.* Miami: Here's The Key, Inc., 1995.

Mendelsohn, Robert M.D. *How to Raise a Healthy Child in Spite of Your Doctor.* New York: Ballantine, 1987.

———. *Male Practice: How Doctors Manipulate Women.* Chicago: Contemporary Books, Inc., 1981.

Neustaedter, Randall. *The Immunization Decision: A Guide for Parents.* Berkeley, Calif: North Atlantic Books, 1990.

Rogers, Sherry A., M.D. *Tired or Toxic? A Blueprint for Health.* Syracuse, New York: Prestige Publishing, 1990.

Simonton, O. Carl, Stephanie Matthews-Simonton and James L. Creighton, Ph.D. *Getting Well Again: The Bestselling Classic About the Simontons' Revolutionary Lifesaving Self-Awareness Techniques, Revised Ed.* Los Angeles: Bantam Doubleday Dell Publishing Group, Inc., 1992.

Wade, Carlson. *How to Beat Arthritis with Immune Power Boosters.* Englewood Cliffs, N.J.: Prentice Hall, 1990.

CHAPTER 7

Candida: Causes and Treatment

Imagine the body as a dynamic "living garden" designed especially for growing its own bacteria, a little yeast or fungus, along with all the good nutrients produced on a daily basis.

The earth itself functions on the same premise. The earth is an organism, harboring billions upon billions of tiny parasites (including you and I)—each parasite doing what it does best. In many instances, this co-existence proves quite functional.

Since the twentieth century, however, we and our earth have become more dysfunctional in relation to the ecological destruction taking place every day. Until recently, this large globe and our human bodies had peacefully co-existed with all the wonderful little parasites and organisms. Dwelling in the twenty-first century, however, means sharing our bodies with as many as twenty separate, unnatural viruses, which, for the most part, lie dormant throughout the course of a lifetime. Now both our bodies and the earth may be threatened unless we begin taking steps to keep them healthy.

More than ever, your "living garden" needs a caring gardener. Who could be better for the job than you! With a few helpful suggestions you can begin to rebalance the earth starting with your own body's ecology.

A healthy immune system depends on maintaining the right numbers of the right organisms in the right places in the body. This chapter is about an unfriendly organism, the yeast Candida albicans, what causes it to overpopulate your intestines and how to deal with it. You will learn:

- how to self-diagnose Candida through simple and effective Clinical Kinesiology energetic testing, in addition to the Candida questionnaire
- what symptoms to expect in Candida
- when to treat this condition
- how to modify your diet
- which alternative therapies to use
- how long to maintain the treatment program
- and how to cope with a Candida "die-off," once you are on the road to balanced health

Healthful diet, nutrients, detoxification and replenishment of healthy intestinal flora are the keys for successfully controlling Candida for life and for rebuilding the integrity of the immune system.

BACTERIA: HEALTHY AND UNHEALTHY

Normally, the human body houses different types of bacteria on the skin, in the mouth, and in the small and large intestine. Some of the body's own B vitamins are produced in the intestines by helpful bacteria.

Orthomolecular biologist Dr. Jeffrey Bland states that over four hundred species of bacteria live in the intestines. More recent research has identified many more species. Estimates now vary from seven hundred to one thousand distinct species that thrive and reside in our intestines, augmenting our immune function. There are more details about this in the next chapter, *Leaky Gut and Your Digestive System*. The weight of these bacteria is 2 ½ to 3 pounds, or equal to the weight of an organ the size of the liver. This bacteria forms the basis of your dynamic "living garden."

Macrobiotic researcher and author, Michio Kushi, calls the intestines the body's "roots." Think of your intestinal roots like soil: a great deal of bacteria and some fungus all help to break down the decomposing matter, making the nutrients from food more available to the body.

The intestines complete this process every day. Additionally, quite a few research studies done on breast-fed infants support Kushi's theory. One study consisted of analyzing stool cultures to detect what organisms and life forms thrive in a healthy newborn baby. In its most natural state, researchers found eighty to ninety percent of the bacteria in a breast-fed baby to be friendly bifidus bacteria.[1]

Microbiology studies also show that the adult human intestinal tract contains a concentration of bifido and acidophilus bacteria, or friendly flora. However, it also contains Escherichia coli, a pathogen or unhealthy bacteria that can make humans quite ill.[2]

In adults with diminished digestive ability, E. coli and other pathogens comprise the most prevalent type of bacteria in the large intestine. Somewhere, in the journey from infancy to adulthood, much of our friendly flora has died out.

E. coli 0157: H-7, the same bacteria that made California children critically ill after eating undercooked hamburger at a fast-food restaurant chain in 1992, should not be prevalent in the healthy intestinal tract. Rather, it should exist as a very small minority.

Dr. Jeffrey Bland proposes an interesting theory regarding the E. coli episode in California. His theory suggests that the true contamination may have stemmed from a strain of super mutant bacteria that developed due to excessive amounts of antibiotics fed to the cattle that provided the hamburger.

Diet explains one of the main reasons unfriendly flora has flourished. It hasn't been proven, per se, but one conjecture offers that bifidus and acidophilus bacteria are extremely vulnerable to antibiotics, while the E. coli 0157: H-7 bacteria remains strong enough not only to survive ... but, as Dr. Bland theorizes, to super mutate and multiply.

Tipping the scale through unhealthy diet, overuse of antibiotics, and other factors throws off the balance of good, protective bacteria—which by sheer numbers alone, normally crowd out offending organisms. However, once you risk leaving the garden gate of your beautiful living garden open, the yeast, Candida albicans may begin to grow.

ANTIBIOTIC EQUALS ANTI-LIFE?

Before we can discuss how antibiotics upset the body's natural immunity and set the stage for the development of Candida albicans, a little background data is important.

One particular category of strong poisons, called antibiotics, kills not only the "bad" but the good bacteria in the body. The word biotic means life form. Antibiotics, therefore, means "against life forms." The whole idea of an antibiotic is to kill off certain life forms. In that context, taking antibiotics is unnatural, especially in the potent form in which pharmaceutical companies produce them.

We've all been sold the message that antibiotics are good medicine. Until lately, science has touted antibiotics as wonder drugs that kill infection and stave off unfriendly bacteria! However, few naturally occurring antibiotics exist, which automatically makes one question. Are antibiotics really the medicine that nature intended to keep us healthy? More and more studies say no.[3] This will be expanded upon in my forthcoming book on drugs, in a chapter devoted to antibiotics and their alternatives.

Origins of Antibiotics

The manufacture of antibiotics began following the discovery of penicillin. Quite accidentally, a small petri dish in a lab was contaminated with a small amount of penicillin mold. In the surrounding area, bacteria that had also been cultured in the petri dish refused to grow. The reason? Both bacteria and mold produce toxins that kill off their competitors.

The same phenomena occurs in the body, on pets, in the ocean, and all over the earth to some degree. As long as an organism maintains a sufficient number of helpful bacteria to counterbalance the effects of potentially harmful bacteria it remains healthy.

Instead of allowing the original, natural concentration used by the penicillin mold to protect itself, new synthetic versions have been designed. Much stronger, and more potent, their whole chemical composition has been altered.

Synthetic penicillin was the first antibiotic on the market. Later, pharmaceutical companies began manufacturing more and more variations— all different chemical renditions of extremely potent poisons.

How Antibiotics "Work"

When people are prescribed antibiotics for a strep throat, the drug also kills off a great deal of the body's good bacteria. It kills the weakest strep first, and the next weakest after more exposure and many days of taking the antibiotic. Most of the time, though, a little bit of strep survives.

The old adage, "Survival of the fittest," applies. The strongest bacteria represent the ones that survive and re-multiply. A little bit of strep on the skin or in the nose is normal in small amounts. The presence of not-so-friendly bacteria in the body is also normal; however, the chemicals prescribed to kill them aren't health-promoting or normal.

Consequently, scientists during the last century and up until the present have unwittingly aided and abetted the creation of mutant bacteria—bacteria that mutates or changes to meet different conditions in the body and environment simply to survive the assault from antibiotics. The strongest bacteria live, reproduce and eventually genetically alter the bacterial gene-pool.

In retaliation, modern medicine pulls out more munitions and produces stronger "guns" with larger "bullets," or, more powerful antibiotics to kill off the now mutated bacteria. The battle being waged in *your* body begins all over again.

Antibiotics do save people's lives in certain critical situations. However, for every sneeze or itchy, runny nose they are unnecessary. Routinely given, antibiotics merely assist in the breakdown of body ecology. When your body is in such an unbalanced state, it opens the door for the yeast Candida albicans to grow, unchecked by your body's natural defense system, your friendly bacteria.

WHAT IS CANDIDA ALBICANS?

Candida describes a physical state in which the immune system becomes compromised by a certain type of yeast overgrowth in the body. Candida shouldn't be confused with the kind of yeast found in bread or baked items, although that yeast is a cousin of Candida albicans. Candida begins when a small percentage of yeast (under less than optimal health conditions) is allowed to grow and become populous, eventually predominating in the system.

Observe moldy bread and you immediately see that in order to feed the mold, nutrients must be extracted—destroying the bread in the process. Obviously bread mold is not the same organism as Candida; however, once Candida becomes ingrained in the system it's just as difficult to extract.

Like mold, Candida represents a type of yeast overgrowth syndrome that entrenches itself in the body. Unfortunately, antibiotics, along with sugar consumption, and other dietary indiscretions provide the perfect conditions for the yeast to grow.

Friendly bacteria are an integral part of the immune system. Once it becomes out of balance from poor diet or antibiotics, Candida may grow out of control and become quite severe. Some of the sickest people on earth suffer from yeast overgrowth syndrome, or Candida. When mild cases are caught and treated early, the changes ultimately save the individual from many future problems. Because this disorder is often quite difficult to diagnose, many cases progress to severe levels before being discovered.

Candida attaches itself to the lining of the intestines by implanting its claw-like "fingers" into the tissue of the intestinal wall. Once ingrained, Candida produces tissue damage in the small and large intestine, which contributes to another serious problem, "leaky gut syndrome." Normally, tiny pores in the membranes of the intestines allow nutrients to flow from the bowel into the blood for absorption into the body. Damage from Candida's grip on the intestinal wall causes normal pores to expand, becoming so large that partially digested food that wasn't quite ready to move, permeates the intestinal wall. Food toxins then flow into the bloodstream, and begin to cause food allergy or sensitivity problems. So, many people with Candida experience food and chemical sensitivities. Some feel as though they're allergic to the twenty-first century. In a sense, this is true.

Doctors prescribing antibiotics have not been taught to look for Candida. Dr. C. Orian Truss, author of *The Missing Diagnosis*, was a pioneering Candida physician. People came to him exhibiting various symptoms, and at first he struggled to make a diagnosis. Nothing fit until he made the connection to Candida.

Dr. Truss discovered several major symptoms of this yeast problem, including: depression, anxiety, irrational behavior, irritability, diarrhea, abdominal bloating, constipation, heartburn, indigestion, loss of self-confidence, lethargy, migraine headaches and even acne.

Women often experience their own set of uncomfortable symptoms including irritation of the urethra, bladder, repeated vaginal yeast infections, PMS, and other menstrual difficulties. Since Dr. Truss's original work, indicators show prostatitis or inflammation of the prostate in men also stems from Candida.

In children, Candida symptoms range from hyperactivity, learning disorders, repeated ear infections, diaper rashes and abdominal discomfort to diarrhea or constipation, poor appetite and erratic sleep patterns.

Originally, Dr. William Crook, author of both *The Yeast Connection* and *The Yeast Connection and the Woman*, and Dr. Orian Truss were demeaned by the medical establishment for their pioneering work with Candida.

Today, their work and research have been overwhelmingly accepted by the general public—and by people who experience Candida.

Causes of Candida

Candida represents an iatrogenic or almost totally doctor-induced disease. It stems primarily from overuse of antibiotics and has also been contracted from consumption of beef, chicken, or milk *containing* antibiotics. If a case of Candida was not drug induced, it likely resulted from unwise lifestyle choices.

Antibiotics fed to dairy cattle contaminate cow's milk, and the antibiotics fed to chickens contaminate the eggs hatched from these chickens. Be wary! You may be in danger of ingesting antibiotics from the food you eat, even though you're determined to avoid antibiotics as a prescription drug.

When the body becomes out of balance with Candida, many other illnesses have license to overtake it.

In a healthy body, the bifidus and acidophilus bacteria grow side by side. If something interferes with the balance, serious problems might arise. You may liken the use of antibiotics to a forest fire which rages out of control burning down the good flora. After such a fire, it is essential to bring renewal to a charred and blackened forest by replanting little seedlings to begin the reforestation. Treatment for Candida also requires replenishment of decimated populations of bifidus, acidophilus, and other vitally important bacteria.

In addition to antibiotics, other drugs prone to stimulate or augment Candida include certain immune-suppressant drugs—a term most people don't often hear. Most have grown accustomed to names such as *steroids*, or *cortisone* instead. Whatever their names, these powerful chemical drugs do suppress the immune system, and do promote the possibility of Candida and more involved problems.

Although indirectly, asthma is also related to Candida. Often, cases misdiagnosed as asthma are really a reaction to severe food sensitivities. In addition, many asthma sufferers are prescribed steroids. This chain reaction of drugs may also contribute to the imbalanced body chemistry which allows Candida to thrive.

Even hormone replacement therapy may be dangerous for a system prone to Candida, since any synthetic hormone throws off the balance of the body's natural hormones.

Hormone composition may be compared with a banana split, with different versions of the banana split representing different hormones. Building an estrogen-hormone banana split, for example, might begin with the "banana," (the basic cholesterol molecule), "several raisins" (natural steroids), a few "cherries" and some "nuts" in a certain pattern. Rearrange the toppings, add other ingredients in other patterns, and the result will be a different hormone.

When healthy and balanced, the body makes all of its own hormones. However, when hormones are created from a synthetic base, the components are qualitatively different from the natural ones, and therefore confuse the body about exactly how to function.

Synthetic hormones are not compatible or in natural balance with the body. Therefore, prescribing estrogen, progesterone, or birth control pills makes Candida worse. This requires the immune system to work even harder.

Another causative factor in Candida stems from the use of cytotoxic drugs. While antibiotics work "against life," cytotoxic drugs refer to "toxic to cell" drugs. What types of drugs are these? Various chemotherapy drugs.

Cancer is the most common disease treated by chemotherapy drugs; however, cytotoxic drugs may also be used for other disorders. Often times, people develop Candida after finishing a program of chemotherapy. In addition, people suffering from debilitating disease and its prolonged stress on the body, are often more prone to Candida.

Immune-System Dysfunction

Candida wears down the immune system and makes it more difficult for the immune system to fight. Of course, many more years of research and study are needed to completely understand Candida and its relationships to other illnesses. However, Candida remains a complex and potentially serious illness.

Dr. Jeffrey Bland, Ph.D., reports that "... one of the first signs seen in HIV-positive individuals who are progressing to AIDS-related complex are nosocomial gastrointestinal infections." These occur as a consequence of compromised function of the intestinal tract as seen in Candida albicans.[4] Other researchers implicate Candida with the onset of Lupus, also a disorder of the immune system. Most autoimmune diseases which have recently come to light have simply been caused by an overburdening of the immune system.

Candida is also a prerequisite for colitis, an inflammation of the large intestine. Cases of Crohn's disease, an inflammation of the small intestine, often reveal that Candida was present first. In short, cure the Candida and it's likely you'll cure the colitis, Crohn's disease, and lupus.

Cases of multiple sclerosis and lupus show marked improvement following treatment for Candida. Multiple sclerosis does have some relationship with the immune system and the integrity of the nervous system—while lupus represents a total immune dysfunction disorder.

People with auto-immune disease are often stymied by their disorders. "Why me?" they question. "How did I get this way?" Although health may often deteriorate quickly, Candida and other immune diseases don't happen overnight.

During critical stages of development, it's quite possible that Candida becomes entrenched in the body, as in the case of Doris.

Doris's Story

Born in the mid-1950s, Doris suffered in infancy with milk allergies as a result of being fed cow's milk instead of breast milk. Doris's busy mother left her lying hour after hour in the crib with a bottle in her mouth. Due to the improper feeding position, milk flowed into little Doris's Eustachian tubes into her ears, and caused an ear infection. Doctors then prescribed antibiotics to get rid of Doris's ear infection. Meanwhile, Doris's milk allergy worsened as her immature digestive system was continually bombarded by the cow's milk, which is too rich for human infants, and poorly tolerated by many adults. This is accentuated by pasteurized milk, and by being deficient in beneficial bacteria.

Again, Doris's mother laid her down in her crib and the cycle began again. Another ear infection, more antibiotics. All the while, the "killing off" of Doris's good bacteria by antibiotics allowed Candida to begin growing throughout her intestinal tract.

Why did Doris's medical doctors fail to see this pattern? Unfortunately, their beliefs and dependence on antibiotic drugs give them few options. Unfortunately, most medical doctors know no other way to treat a patient who is sniffling, wheezing, coughing or suffering from an earache.

Baby Doris grew into a pretty little girl. As she progressed through immunizations and more harmful bacteria in early childhood, the Candida yeast continued to grow. And, what does yeast need to grow? Anyone who has ever made wine or bread knows that a key ingredient must be added to give the yeast something to grow on. That ingredient is sugar. So, it's not surprising that six-year-old Doris loved chocolate candy bars. Because the yeast demanded she bring sugar into her system, candy became an addiction. As a result, her health grew worse and worse. Her bifidus and acidophilus began dying off—bit by bit.

The growth of yeast continued and soon young Doris was diagnosed with a bladder infection. Shortly after that came a yeast infection.

As Doris shyly celebrated her thirteenth birthday, she became noticeably self conscious about a newly-developed problem—acne. Her progression to the standard American teenage diet triggered the Candida in her system to begin producing even more poisons, which meant more work for her liver.

By then, Doris's liver was so overwhelmed that it could no longer adequately filter her body's poisons. She consulted her doctor, who gave her another prescription—for tetracycline.

Never taught to question her doctor, Doris allowed him to take the lion's share of responsibility for her health. "I needed to take this medication. My doctor said so!" she related. So, like so many people, she took the medicine for a year, went off of it and the acne came back. She returned to the tetracycline again and the cycle began again.

If Doris had not suffered through this unhealthy chain reaction, the breakdown of good bifidus and acidophilus bacteria wouldn't have occurred. If she had only known to avoid an unhealthy diet and better understood the dangerous repercussions of antibiotics and other drugs, Doris's body wouldn't have enabled the growth of Candida.

Finally, in her early thirties, Doris encountered a serious health crisis. She began experiencing every symptom imaginable including fatigue, depression, irritability, memory loss, severe menstrual problems, digestive disorders, itching, infertility, psoriasis, vague muscle and joint pains, repeated ear and respiratory ailments—asthma being only one.

Doris, like so many others, was unknowingly set up at a young age to develop all of these problems. Eventually, if she doesn't get some real help, she'll likely end up with a diagnosis of lupus, chronic fatigue immune deficiency syndrome, or multiple sclerosis.

DIAGNOSING CANDIDA

Intervening in Candida involves evaluation of the total body through Clinical Kinesiology testing. Along with the Candida questionnaire and a personal history, Clinical Kinesiology is the simplest method of diagnosis and evaluation of symptoms.

Clinical Kinesiology muscle testing employs a simple handmode (researched and developed by Dr. Burt Espy) for detecting Candida. The index and third finger are curled into the palm, the tip of the thumb and fourth finger are touched together, while the pinky finger rests on the crease of the thumb. This proves to be a difficult position to assume. You may need assistance to ensure the correct positioning. (See the self-testing section at the end of this chapter for specific handmode diagrams and testing instructions.) The Clinical Kinesiology muscle test may then be performed to see if the Candida mode results in a strong or weak muscle test.

Another method of diagnosing Candida involves analysis of stool cultures. This test proves fairly inexpensive and does identify the Candida. In many cases, however, the yeast is not readily apparent through such a simple culture, especially if it is lying in dormant forms in the body.

The Live Cell (living sample of blood) evaluation offers still another way to see the yeast. With the help of a darkfield microscope, the yeast may be seen forming in the blood. This is the only method currently known to distinguish the mycelial or "branched-out" form of yeast in the blood.

An expensive serum antibody test may also be available for doctors to address Candida. The test does have drawbacks, however, and I find Clinical Kinesiology testing to be preferable, due to convenience.

Dormant Forms of Candida

Candida is often difficult to pinpoint. When the presence of Candida triggers the body to form antibodies to the yeast, the yeast takes the form of a spore to avoid attack. Spores resemble tiny buds, as in spores of yeast, or spores of mold. Much like an acorn from an oak tree, a spore represents an easily preserved life form. An acorn sits for years and years, one day germinates, and eventually sprouts into a tree. In the same way, yeast spores in the body may sit dormant for years and one day develop into Candida. Spores either grow into a simple mold, or a mycelial form of mold, much like a tree branching out.

The "branching out" form of Candida yeast attaches itself to and begins breaking down the integrity of the intestinal wall. The yeast in spore form resembles a tiny kernel encased in a hard coating.

The spore doesn't trigger the body to produce antibodies as long as most of the yeast remains in the dormant stage. For this reason, the serum antibody test may not identify the Candida, or the test may reveal only a slight case. In reality, though, the Candida may be quite colonized.

The Role of Parasites in Candida

In recent times, some Candida researchers have indicated that people who have Candida may also carry a parasite. A parasite is a life form that lives off another life form.

"Which comes first, the chicken or the egg?" becomes the question in investigating the presence of parasites in Candida patients. Is the body weakened from having Candida, allowing a parasite into the system, or was the parasite present first … allowing the Candida to grow? Or, because of the parasite, was an antibiotic given which didn't affect the parasite, but triggered Candida?

Symbiotic parasitic relationships are often found in the sea. Tiny fish may live on a big fish, eating bacteria or other organisms that may attack the host fish. In this case, the parasites are helping, not hurting. However, most of the time parasites refer to intrusive protozoa, bacteria, fungus, or even viruses, which live off the host and damage it—not adding any beneficial aspect to the relationship.

Candida is truly an unhelpful parasite when it grows out of control in the body, begins overcrowding and "taking over" just as mold does on a piece of bread.

LIFESTYLE FACTORS THAT AFFECT CANDIDA

Incorporating healthy lifestyle changes make a big difference in fighting Candida. First, the yeast must be killed, your internal living garden replanted, the immune system restrengthened, and diet and lifestyle modified. The most important factor involves withholding the type of food on which the yeast thrives. But remember, the energetically correct food for one person may not necessarily be right for another. Some Candida patients can eat miso and a number of fruits, while other patients cannot tolerate those foods during the time they're battling Candida. Each individual must be tested with Clinical Kinesiology to discover what foods his or her particular body can or cannot tolerate at the time. Then, a program may be designed for each individuals needs, rather than offering everyone the same general guidelines.

What Not To Eat…

Until expert testing helps determine individual food sensitivities, it is wise to leave out sugar, high-fructose corn sweeteners, refined carbohydrates such as white bread and pasta, alcohol, and even honey. This strict diet regimen is required only for a period of time—not forever. It's done simply to give the body a chance to recover.

Vinegar, soy sauce and miso, are a few examples of fermented items that should be avoided by some Candida patients, although other people tolerate these items. Self-testing for food compatibility can be helpful in making this decision.

Restrict the diet from all yeast-containing foods for a minimum of three months. While Candida is different from baker's yeast or brewer's yeast, still, you are advised to adhere to the philosophy that if yeast is growing out of control in the body, any yeast may further upset the immune system. The body begins making antibodies against the yeast, and even the Candida "cousins"—bakers and brewer's yeast—can upset the applecart!

Changing your diet for only three or four weeks and then going off the diet—then back on for three or four weeks doesn't allow for much progress. One patient, Judy, dragged out her Candida "die-off" process for years, because she wasn't able to maintain consistency with her diet. Her Achilles heel is pasteurized dairy foods. Dairy constitutes a major problem because so many food sensitivities and allergies are connected with it. Another layer of her problem was that she loved sugary, sweet yogurt with excess sugar, and chocolate milk.

Making diet changes means commitment; but what better motivation could one ask for than receiving optimal health?

Fermented Foods: To Eat or Not to Eat?

The groundbreaking works of Dr. Orian Truss and Dr. William Crook admonished Candida suffers to avoid fermented foods and beverages as if they represented a type of plague. Today, I see that habitual lack of healthy, wild-cultured fermented foods in our societal diet may be laying the groundwork for Candida to take hold. Including wholesome, naturally-fermented foods in our diet from childhood forward provides more intestinal flora biodiversity and an extra measure of immune system preparedness.

Prior to World War II, it was more common to find grandmother's homemade sauerkraut, pickles and yogurt in the home. After the war and the "modernization" of daily life, Wonder bread, Twinkies, boxed macaroni and cheese, and pizza crowded the fermented food choices right out of homes. Soda pop, Kool-Aid and antibiotics became common place. As a society, we largely gave up the beneficial fermented foods while we began consuming large amounts of devitalized, processed, useless carbohydrates. We exchanged grandmother's stoneware crock of sauerkraut for Betty Crocker's boxed cake mix. More discussion about fermented foods will be found in the next chapter, *Leaky Gut and Your Digestive System*.

So, here you are today trying to determine if fermented foods should be on your menu. I suggest that if your system is not accustomed to healthy fermented foods, keep them to a minimum (or avoid them) until you have taken enough steps to greatly improve your Candida. If your system has had frequent exposure to well tolerated fermented foods, you will likely tolerate them now. Using your self-testing skills for food compatibility will give you the best answer.

I will include dairy foods in this section. That is because the best tolerated and most digestible dairy foods are fermented. These include yogurt, kefir and cheese. A common statement in nutrition circles is "cow's milk is for calves." That is a very true statement. We all have varying abilities to tolerate dairy products. Our food technology weighs in heavily on this issue. When milk (from any source) is pasteurized, it is heated between 145 and 280 degrees Fahrenheit.[5] This kills the normal probiotic bacteria, destroys the inherent enzymes that would help digest the protein components, as well as the fat and milk sugar (lactose). When milk is homogenized, the fat molecules are disrupted and divided into components that no longer fit the molecular structure of your enzymes, and are not efficiently digested. If you include dairy products, they should be organic, raw, and un-homogenized. I will expand upon this in the next chapter.

What To Eat

The majority of your diet should consist of vegetables, whole grains and proteins. I prefer to use primarily plant-based proteins. If you use fish, fowl or red meat (I personally avoid all of these choices) choose organic or comparable quality. Free-range eggs can be a good protein source. Raw tree nuts (if tolerated) are another good protein source, as well as seeds.

In general, grains prove much more favorable as the basis for a healthy diet even though some schools of thought indicate that as the carbohydrates from rice, wheat, barley, oats, and other grains are broken down, the level of blood sugar in the body rises. But I disagree, as long as one has been consistently eating grains and vegetables, and adding enzymes and probiotics. Well digested whole grains (which were never milled into flour) provide a **prebiotic** nutrient source for your friendly bacteria. Sprouting your grains makes them even more digestible. Refer to Chapter 8, *Leaky Gut and Your Digestive System*, page 155.

You can fancy up your grains and vegetables with a wide variety of healthy herbs and spices such as garlic, basil, cilantro, tarragon and oregano.

A diet rich in whole grains (not milled grains or flour products), helps to quell sweet cravings once sugar is eliminated. Incorporating sprouted grains essentially predigests them for you.

Although fruit contains a naturally occurring sugar, fructose, moderate use of energetically compatible fruits satisfy sweet cravings without feeding the yeast.

Sometimes cravings signal what the body truly needs and other times they're a form of disguised message. With no TV commercials to distract or tempt, we could all put more trust in our cravings. Many times, the body signals the need for a particular food; however, the true signals may be misinterpreted by the brain, often because of the artificial foods, preservatives and flavorings. A craving for sweets often indicates a chromium deficiency. A craving for chocolate, specifically, often is symptomatic of a magnesium deficiency.

Engage Your Candida Battle Plan

This segment briefly describes ways to kill off the excess Candida. I always muscle test every new patient for the presence of a Candida overgrowth, and then find which remedies will be the most helpful by using Clinical Kinesiology. Candida is a complex problem and requires a multi-faceted treatment program. Generally, a simple one-remedy approach is not enough. Many of the most effective supplements are synergistic compilations of several herbs, nutrients and enzymes. Active anti-Candida treatment may encompass three to eighteen months. I may change or add items, based on the patient's progress and needs. In many cases, I find that either Expore™ or Total Yeast Redux™ by Nutri-West® are quite effective. Both are powerful synergistic formulations. I also check for parasites using Clinical Kinesiology. If the parasite test is positive, I add a natural parasite remedy.

If you will be searching for your primary Candida killers in a health food store, I am quite impressed with the Renew Life® brand, formulated by Brenda Watson. CandiGone™ is her Candida cleanse. Renew Life® offers potent probiotics (Ultimate Flora™), enzymes, and fiber products to be found in your health food stores.

Typically, digestive enzymes are required at meals because the digestion is compromised. In some cases, I add a protease enzyme away from mealtime to break down the Candida walls. Often the immune system will need boosting. Additional Candida treatments will be discussed next.

Replenish

While it's important to cleanse and detoxify, it's also necessary to replenish the body's friendly bacteria during and following a detoxification plan. Replenishment of natural intestinal flora may be accomplished with several products. Since Candida is essentially due to a lack of protective intestinal (or gut) beneficial bacteria (or flora), one or more probiotic formulations must be included in the program. I often use Total Probiotics™ by Nutri-West®, a comprehensive formula that is enterically coated. In some cases, I use a specific strain of bacteria, Lactobacillus reuteri. This child-appropriate strain is packaged as a coating inside a straw. I often use this for children since it is so easy to administer. In some instances, I use Lactic Acid Yeast™ by Standard Process®, to acidify the intestines and encourage the growth of existing lactic acid bacteria. Your holistic health practitioner can help you with a program of this kind.

Typically, supplemental probiotic formulations provide a food substrate for the living microbes. Most often, their food is powdered cow milk, on which they thrive. Refrigeration of your probiotic source helps to ensure that more of the microbes live longer, since they are in a state similar to hibernation due to the cooler temperature. By refrigerating your probiotic formula, you prolong the life of the microbes and their food source. Keeping them at room temperature stimulates them to be active, and to reproduce, all of which can exhaust the food source over a period of time. If you accidentally leave your probiotic bottle on the kitchen table over a three-day period, little harm is done, but a period of several months is another story. If you buy a probiotic that states "needs no refrigeration," realize that it has lost potency by small increments daily since the date of manufacture.

Liberal use of probiotics is needed. Remember, you are replanting after a devastating "forest fire" has cleared out your native flora. This is one case when more is probably better. That's the kind of replenishment or reforestation needed!

OTHER TREATMENTS FOR CANDIDA

I. Tea Tree Oil:

Women with Candida are prone to vaginal infections. A good item to combat this problem is Australian oil of Melaleuca® alternifolia, or Tea Tree oil. The oil, extracted from a special tree called the Tea Tree, has proven quite beneficial. However, always check to make sure that the oil you purchase meets The Australian Standards Association guidelines which has specified that even the *lowest* quality oil have at least thirty percent of the active ingredient, Terpinen 4-ol. Simply add several drops (6-10) to one quart of warm water in a douche bag and douche daily. Avoid douching during menstruation.

Oil of Melaleuca® alternifolia may be used topically for vaginal infections, or rubbed on skin lesions. For a nail fungal infection, Tea Tree oil combines well with another product, Gentian Violet. Most likely, if growing conditions exist for fungus in the nails, it's probably present elsewhere in the body.

II. Gentian Violet

Older patients may be more familiar with Gentian Violet because it is a treatment that was used years ago. Like its name, the tincture is a very purple liquid. It may be bought in a drugstore without a prescription. For infection on the fingernails or toenails, simply apply the Gentian Violet around the fungal area and allow it to dry.

Gentian Violet kills yeast without harming cells. The tincture does stain anything it touches, however, so be extra careful. One reason it may be unpopular with some people is because of its staining power. However, it has been used effectively as a treatment for nail fungus and even vaginal Candida. If applied vaginally, use gloves to prepare a tampon. After insertion, wear a pad and change both every four hours.

III. Immune System Supplements
Many supplements may be used to build and strengthen the immune system. Some of the more powerful ones include yeast-free multivitamins. (Many B-vitamins are made with yeast so always read the labels.)

The mineral, germanium, represents a good immune system builder. Several antioxidant supplements contain germanium and beta carotene in the same formula. Anyone with Candida requires extra biotin, another B-vitamin. A strong, yeast-free B-vitamin complex with biotin works well. Remember, always take B-vitamins in a balanced formula. Generally, these formulas contain a full complement of B-vitamins in a B-50 or B-100 capsule or tablet. This means that the majority of the components have 50 or 100 milligrams. B_1, B_2, B_6, B_{12}, niacinimide, pantothenic acid, choline, inositol, biotin and paba are the vitamins which prove most important.

Because of problems involving digestion or previous damage to the intestinal tract from Candida, some people cannot absorb nutrients as well as they should. Therefore, a variety of trace minerals such as manganese, zinc, potassium, selenium, silica, boron, molybdenum, and copper should also be included into the dietary and nutrient regimen.

Three excellent professional products for killing off Candida are Total Yeast Redux™, Exspore™ (both by Nutri-West®), and Yeast Fungal Detox. Each of these are comprehensive formulations containing caprylic acid.

Caprylic acid kills Candida. It's also found in olive oil, which more and more people use quite liberally. Caprylic acid may also be found in goat's milk. It's the acid that gives goat milk its pungent smell. Caprylic acid is in coconut oil as well.

IV. Herbs
Echinacea is a strong yet simple herb for building the immune system; it is recommended to help people avoid and recover from different types of illnesses. Fungal, bacterial, viral or parasitic patients benefit from adding Echinacea herb to the diet.

Another powerful herb for combating Candida is Pau d'arco (also called Taheebo and Lapacho) from South America. Pau d'arco, an herb gleaned from the shavings of the bark of the tree, kills Candida specifically while also strengthening the immune system.

Pau d'arco can be used as a tea; however, the strongest form remains the tincture. In all cases, be careful to get certified organic, all natural herbs. That certification guarantees that the trees aren't sprayed or chemically fertilized and the herbs are grown and harvested under specific organic conditions. I have great confidence in Herb Pharm herbs.

V. Flaxseed Oil
Flaxseed oil tops the list of healthful oils in my book. Everyone should take it! Flaxseed oil provides the essential fatty acids needed for hormone production. It also aids in maintaining the integrity of cell membranes.

Every cell membrane in the body stores essential fatty acids. Nowadays, people have become so conscious about not eating fat, that some aren't getting enough fat in their diets. Flaxseed oil is necessary for a healthy body, as opposed to most other types of fats. This natural oil provides the best balance of the high polyunsaturated and

Omega 3, 6, and 9 oils. Fish oil supplements have been touted for helping many body imbalances. Be sure to search for a purified fish oil with mercury and heavy metals removed. Nutri-West® offers Complete Omega 3 Essentials™ and an excellent Flax oil. These are available through the offices of many holistic practitioners. Udo's Choice® is Flax and other vegetarian oils in combination and can be found in many health food stores.

VI. Citricidal®

Citricidal®, manufactured from grapefruit seed extract, produces a potent liquid for killing Candida, fungus, parasites and other organisms. It is also available from holistic practitioners in capsule and tablet form. It kills any "bad guy" in the body. Citricidal® is an effective product that's been on the market quite a few years. It has generated a great deal of interest as a result of its healing properties.

All these powerful remedies work; however, the best case scenario continues to require specific Clinical Kinesiology testing on each individual. While one treatment shows up strongest for one person, a different product or treatment may test more helpful for another.

I encourage you to keep the commitment to use only natural therapies to kill off Candida. As more and more people move in a more holistic direction, I hope usage of all of these types of natural therapies will grow.

Antifungal medications are often prescribed for Candida with the same problem we incur from antibiotics, promoting the strongest organisms to flourish. One of my patients, Marley, was on nystatin, an antifungal, for about one year before she came to see me. She was the most seriously ill Candida patient I'd seen in my office. She had a dull, sallow skin color, dark circles under her eyes, and dry lifeless hair. Marley was seriously emaciated and was not absorbing many nutrients. She was the epitome of "skin and bones" or "looked half dead" descriptions. She looked as if she were fifteen or twenty years older than her chronological age. Marley was fatigued and very depressed. Her natural and holistic treatment extended over eighteen months and she greatly improved after stopping her medication.

CANDIDA DIE-OFF

Before you wholeheartedly begin killing off the Candida, you should be aware of a natural consequence of helping yourself get better—a die-off reaction. This is technically called a "Herxheimer reaction." Natural treatment logically focuses on encouraging or rebalancing conditions in the body which eventually cause the yeast to die. At the same time it's wise to replenish with healthy bacteria at once, and provide them proper conditions to flourish.

Anyone with a great deal of yeast in the system may experience numerous "die-off" symptoms during the progression of the Candida infestation or course of treatment. The yeast organisms carry poison within them. As they die, their membranes eventually rupture as decomposition occurs, releasing the poison or toxins into your system.

The actual "die-off" causes some extreme "I-just-don't-feel-good" types of symptoms. As the yeast continues to die off the toxins may further weaken the immune system leading to infections, allergies, chronic illness and that "sick all over" feeling. This signifies a healing crisis. Although patients sometimes get worse before getting better, once the poisons are flushed through, they continue to get well.

Patients with Candida of the severity of Doris or Marley could experience a difficult "die-off" period. In those cases, a much gentler approach is used. For a Candida patient experiencing a difficult "die-off" it may be necessary to diminish the amount per dose of the nutrients, herbs or supplements being utilized to attack the Candida.

A few patients have become temporarily disabled from working Candida out of their bodies. Their yeast "die-off" proves more intense comparatively to the normal "die-off" episodes that most people experience. Still, even the most severe episodes are usually short-lived.

Detox Following Candida Die-Off

Along with additional nutrients added to the diet, simple herbal detoxification programs prove helpful in the treatment for Candida. Some recommendations include DeTox Tea™ by the Yogi Tea Company® or Renew Life's® First Cleanse™. One of my favorites is Core-Level D-Tox™ by Nutri-West®. I also recommend Total Liver D-Tox™ in combination with Core-Level D-Tox™, both by Nutri-West®. Other companies make similar high quality formulas readily available from reputable health food stores or natural health practitioners.

I recommend a program which contains herbs and various combinations of vitamins and minerals which help cleanse the liver, kidneys and intestines. A good detox program also supplied a digestive aid and suggests a simple method of getting started if a detoxification program has never been undertaken before.

Another cleansing program on the market, Ultra Clear®, has been developed by orthomolecular biologist, Jeffrey Bland Ph.D. His line of probiotic foods consists of powdered predigested protein made of rice proteins and other nutrients which help cleanse the body and rebuild the immune system. Ultra Clear® also makes it much easier for people to continue with their normal responsibilities at home and at work, and do the cleansing program at the same time.

An enema is one of the best natural home detox methods. Enemas help empty the intestines of toxins and large colonies of Candida. The process actually washes them away.

Colon therapy by a trained colonic therapist can also be very helpful. Some colon therapists will instill probiotics into your colon at the end of the treatment. Other natural colon cleansers include various psyllium colon cleaners or Renew Life's® Triple Cleanser™ without psyllium.

Standard Process has a wonderful cleansing program, SP Cleanse. It is quite successful. I also use Total Green™ by Nutri-West in combination with Core Level D-tox™. Your natural healthcare practitioner can guide you with this phase of your program.

TESTS AND QUESTIONNAIRES

A valuable test for discovering the presence of Candida has been developed by William Crook, M.D. Filling out and scoring the Candida questionnaire should enable you and your natural health practitioner to evaluate the possible role of Candida in contributing to your health problems.

Immune and auto-immune system problems are different. Autoimmune disorders are those in which the body's immune system turns against itself. Most of the time, Candida albicans is classified as an immune system disorder, not necessarily auto-immune. If Candida albicans advances untreated, and the same unhealthy dietary patterns continue, the Candida may lead to various auto-immune disorders such as rheumatoid arthritis, multiple sclerosis, lupus, Leaky Gut syndrome, or cancer.

Candida Questionnaire and Score Sheet

This questionnaire is designed for adults and the scoring system isn't appropriate for children. It lists factors in your medical history which promote the growth of Candida albicans (Section A), and symptoms commonly found in individuals with yeast connected illness (Section B and C).

For each "Yes" answer in Section A, circle the Point Score in that section. Total your score and record it in the box at the end of the section. Then move onto Sections B and C and score as directed.

Filling out and scoring this questionnaire should help you and your physician evaluate the possible role of Candida in contributing to your health problems. Yet it will not provide an automatic "Yes" or "No" answer.

Section A: History

1. Have you taken tetracyclines (Sumycin®, Panmycin®, Vibramycin®, Minocin®, etc.) or other antibiotics for acne for 1 month (or longer)?	25
2. Have you, at any time in your life, taken other "broad spectrum" antibiotics* for respiratory, urinary or other infections (for 2 months or longer, or in shorter courses 4 or more times in a 1-year period?)	20
3. Have you taken a broad spectrum antibiotic* drug—even a single course?	6
4. Have you, at any time in your life, been bothered by persistent prostatitis, vaginitis, or other problems affecting your reproductive organs?	25
5. Have you been pregnant...	
2 or more times	5
1 time?	3
6. Have you taken birth control pills ...	
For more than two years?	15
For six months to 2 years?	8
7. Have you taken prednisone, Decadron® or other cortisone-type drugs...	
For more than 2 weeks?	15
For 2 weeks or less?	6
8. Does exposure to perfumes, insecticides, fabric shop odors and other chemicals provoke ...	
Moderate to severe symptoms?	20
Mild symptoms?	5
9. Are your symptoms worse on damp, muggy days or in moldy places?	20
10. Have you had athlete's foot, ring worm, "jock itch" or other chronic fungus infections of the skin or nails? Have such infections been...	
Severe or persistent?	20
Mild to moderate?	10
11. Do you crave sugar?	10
12. Do you crave breads?	10
13. Do you crave alcoholic beverages?	10
14. Does tobacco smoke really bother you?	10

Total Score, Section A _____

* Including Keflex,® amoxicillin, Cector®, Bactrim® and Septra ®. Such antibiotics kill off "good germs" while they're killing off those which cause infection.

Section B: Major Symptoms:

For each of your symptoms, enter the appropriate figure in the Point Score column:
If a symptom is occasional or mild
                                                      score 3 points
If a symptom is frequent and/or moderately severe
                                                      score 6 points
If a symptom is severe and/or disabling
                                                      score 9 points
Add total score and record it in the box at the end of this section.

                                                       Point Score

1. Fatigue or lethargy
2. Feeling of being "drained"
3. Poor memory
4. Feeling "spacey" or "unreal"
5. Depression
6. Numbness, burning or tingling
7. Muscle aches
8. Muscle weakness or paralysis
9. Pain and/or swelling in joints
10. Abdominal pain.
11. Constipation
12. Diarrhea
13. Bloating

14. Troublesome vaginal discharge
15. Persistent vaginal burning or itching
16. Prostatitis
17. Impotence
18. Loss of sexual desire
19. Endometriosis
20. Cramps and/or other menstrual irregularities
21. Premenstrual tension
22. Spots in front of eyes
23. Erratic vision

Total Score, Section B _____

Section C: Other Symptoms**

For each of your symptoms, enter the appropriate figure in the Point Score column:
If a symptom is occasional or mild
　　　　　　　　　　　　　score 1 point
If a symptom is frequent and/or moderately severe　　　　　　　　score 2 points
If a symptom is severe and/or disabling
　　　　　　　　　　　　　score 3 points
Add total score and record it in the box at the end of this section.

Point Score

1. Drowsiness
2. Irritability or jitteriness
3. Incoordination
4. Inability to concentrate
5. Frequent mood swings
6. Headache
7. Dizziness/loss of balance
8. Pressure above ears ... feeling of head swelling or tingling
9. Itching
10. Other rashes
11. Heartburn
12. Indigestion
13. Belching and intestinal gas
14. Mucus in stools
15. Hemorrhoids
16. Dry mouth
17. Rash or blisters in mouth
18. Bad breath
19. Joint swelling or arthritis
20. Nasal congestion or discharge
21. Postnasal drip
22. Nasal itching
23. Sore or dry throat
24. Cough
25. Pain or tightness in chest
26. Wheezing or shortness of breath
27. Urgency or urinary frequency
28. Burning on urination
29. Failing vision.
30. Burning or tearing of eyes
31. Recurrent infection or fluid in ears
32. Ear pain or deafness

Total Score, Section C _____

Total Score, Section A _____

Total Score, Section B _____

Total Score, Section C _____

Grand Total Score _____

The Grand Total Score will help you and your physician decide if your health problems are yeast-connected. Scores in women will run higher, as 7 items in the questionnaire apply exclusively to women, while only 2 apply exclusively to men.

　Yeast-connected health problems are almost certainly present in women with scores over 180, and in men with scores over 140.

　Yeast-connected health problems are probably present in women with scores over 120 and in men with scores over 40.

　With scores of less than 60 in women and 40 in men, yeasts are less apt to cause health problems.

From: Crook, W.G., *The Yeast Connection and the Woman*, Professional Books, Jackson, TIM., 1995. Used with permission.

** While symptoms in this section commonly occur in people with yeast-connected illness, they are also found in other individuals.

Candida Handmode Test

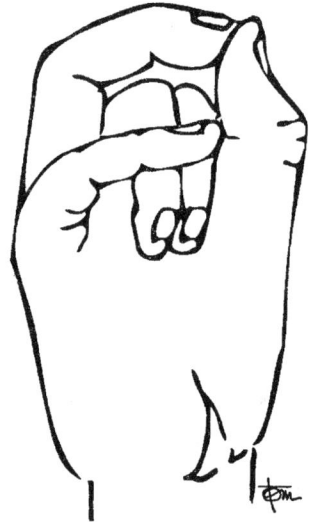

The Candida Handmode test is performed by folding the 2nd (pointer) finger and the 3rd (middle) finger down on the palm. These fingerprints touch the fleshy thumb pad. Then touch the fingerprints of the thumb and 4th (ring) finger together. The tip of the 5th (pinky) finger touches the thumb's crease which is closest to the end of the thumb. You or a friend may have to hold the last finger in place during the test.

The Candida Handmode Test was researched and developed by Dr. Burt Espy.

The following Clinical Kinesiology self-test allows you and a partner/tester to determine whether or not Candida is present in your system. Before proceeding with any testing, first perform the Indicator Muscle Test as instructed in Chapter 1. Once a strong Indicator muscle is determined you may proceed as follows:

Step 1: Assume the Candida handmode as illustrated.
Step 2: Have a partner/tester perform the Clinical Kinesiology muscle test on the test-subjects opposite

Indicator arm muscle.

> Candida Handmode + Muscle test + Strong arm = no presence of Candida.
>
> Candida Handmode + Muscle test + Weak arm = Candida present. Seek further testing and treatment from a trained natural healthcare practitioner.

If Candida is present, you will need to be tested for food sensitivities, so that you can streamline your diet to a compatible menu. Select one or more "Candida Killer" remedies and a potent probiotic.

Lupus Test

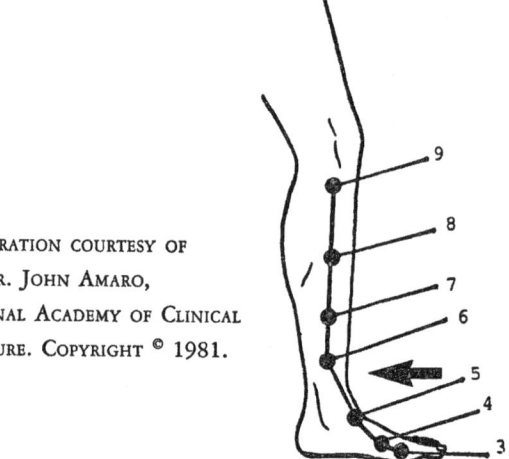

ILLUSTRATION COURTESY OF
DR. JOHN AMARO,
INTERNATIONAL ACADEMY OF CLINICAL
ACUPUNCTURE. COPYRIGHT © 1981.

An acupuncture point to test for lupus can be found three-fourths of an inch above the internal ankle, on the Spleen Meridian, halfway between Spleen 5 and 6.

Step 1: Locate the lupus acu-point and place your finger on the point.
Step 2: Have a partner/tester perform the Clinical Kinesiology muscle test on the opposite arm as follows:

> Touch Lupus Point + Muscle Test + Strong arm = no Lupus present in the body.
>
> Touch Lupus Point + Muscle Test + Weak arm = Schedule further testing with a natural healthcare professional.

Again, should the Candida questionnaire provide a "yes" score and/or the Candida handmode or lupus acupoint result in a weak muscle test, consult a natural health practitioner who can further evaluate your situation. Together you can work with your practitioner to design a program to combat your individual Candida problem. Establishing this relationship will allow your natural health practitioner to monitor or oversee your "home" work while you benefit from his or her professional expertise and recommendations.

Chronic Fatigue Syndrome

Currently, no specific energetic test for chronic fatigue immune deficiency syndrome is available. The cases that I've treated all stemmed from a heart imbalance. The patients may be weak and may have some viral exposure connected to the deficiency; however, in my clinical research, the illness stems from Heart Meridian imbalances. Toxicity often due to Candida or leaky gut is another major contributor to chronic fatigue syndrome.

CONTROL CANDIDA

Understanding lifestyle patterns that help create Candida is the first step to solving this condition. Revamping a deficient lifestyle establishes your path to regaining health. Making a commitment to avoid and strive to eliminate refined sugar, high fructose corn sweeteners, processed foods, antibiotics, anti-inflammatory drugs, etc., will be critical health-building measures to include in your plan. A healthful diet, supplemental nutrients, detoxification and replenishment of healthy intestinal flora are your keys to recovery.

Making the commitment to renewed health and taking control of the treatment enables you to create the energy and build the stamina needed to stop the growth of Candida albicans, ultimately strengthening the integrity of your immune system.

With everything functioning well in the body, plus access to a good diet, clean water, air, exercise and sunshine, many Candida patients may look forward to becoming much healthier people.

Prevent the Progression of Candida

In some cases, the Candida has been so entrenched that actual damage to the intestinal lining has occurred and a condition termed "leaky gut syndrome" has developed. In Chapter 8, *Leaky Gut and Your Digestion*, you will begin to understand this curiously named condition, which causes a myriad of symptoms from headaches to allergic reactions to fatigue, and many others in between. You will also learn about how to promote healing of your innermost organs.

CHAPTER 7 SUGGESTED READING

Boroch, Ann, CNC; foreword by David Perlmutter, M.D., F.A.C.N., A.B.I.H.M. *The Candida Cure: Yeast, Fungus & Your Health—The 90-Day Program to Beat Candida & Restore Vibrant Health, Revised Ed.* Studio City, Calif.: Quintessential Healing, Inc., 2014.

Chaitow, Leon N.D. *Candida Albicans: Could Yeast Your Problem? Revised and Expanded Ed.* Rochester, Vt.: Inner Traditions International, Ltd., 1998.

Connolly, Pat. *The Candida Albicans Yeast Free Cookbook: How Good Nutrition Can Help Fight the Epidemic of Yeast-Related Diseases, 2nd Ed.* New Canaan, Conn.: TC/Contemporary Publishing Group, Inc, 2000.

Crook, William G., M.D. *Chronic Fatigue Syndrome and the Yeast Connection: A Get-Well Guide for People With This Often Misunderstood Illness—And Those Who Care for Them.* Jackson, Tenn.: Professional Books 1992.

———. *The Yeast Connection Handbook: How Yeasts Can Make You Feel "Sick All Over" and the Steps You Need to Take to Regain Your Health.* Jackson, Tenn.: Professional Books, 2002.

———, Carolyn Dean, M.D., N.D. and Elizabeth B. Crook. *The Yeast Connection and the Womans Health, Reprint Ed.* Jackson, Tenn.: Professional Books, 2007.

Gare, Fran, N.D. and Warren M. Levin, M.D. *Beyond the Yeast Connection: A How-To Guide to Curing Candida and Other Yeast-Related Conditions.* Laguna Beach, Calif.: Basic Health Publications, 2013.

Gates, Donna with Linda Schatz. *The Body Ecology Diet: Recovering Your Health and Rebuilding Your Immunity.* Carlsbad, Calif. and New York: Hay House, revised edition, 2011.

Jackson, Natalie. *The Easy Candida Cure: Effective, All-Natural Solutions to Overcome Candida Infection within 30 Days (Candida Diet, Candida Cleanse, The Body Ecology Diet,* Kindle Edition.) Amazon Digital Services, Inc., 2013.

Lorenzani, Shirley, Ph.D. *Candida, A Twentieth Century Disease.* New Canaan, Conn.: Keats Publishing, Inc., 1986.

Martin, Jeanne Marie and Zoltan P. Rona, M.D. *Complete Candida Yeast Guidebook, revised 2nd Ed.: Everything You Need to Know About Prevention, Treatment & Diet.* New York: Three Rivers Press, 2000.

Mintz, Morton. *The Therapeutic Nightmare.* Boston: Houghton-Mifflin, 1965.

Murray, Michael T., N.D. *Chronic Candidiasis: Your Natural Guide to Healing with Diet, Vitamins, Minerals, Herbs, Exercise, and Other Natural Methods.* New York: Three Rivers Press, 1997.

Schmidt, Michael A., Lendon H. Smith and Keith W. Schnert. *Beyond Antibiotics: Fifty Ways To Boost Immunity, 2nd Ed.* Berkeley, Calif.: North Atlantic Books, 1994.

Semon, Bruce, M.D., Ph.D. and Lori Kornblum, foreword by Bernard Rimland, Ph.D. *Feast Without Yeast: 4 Stages to Better Health.* Glendale, Wisc.: Wisconsin Institute of Nutrition, 2002.

The Candida Free Cookbook: 125 Recipes to Beat Candida and Live Yeast Free. Berkeley, Calif.: Shasta Press, 2013.

Trowbridge, John P. and Morton Walker. *The Yeast Syndrome: How to Help Your Doctor Identify and Treat the Real Cause of Your Yeast-Related Illness.* New York: Bantam Books, 1986.

Truss, C. Orian, M.D. *The Missing Diagnosis.* Birmingham, Ala.: Missing Diagnosis, Inc., 1983.

———. *The Missing Diagnosis II.* Birmingham, Ala: Missing Diagnosis, Inc., 2009.

CHAPTER 8

Leaky Gut Syndrome

One crisp fall day, Inga came to my office lugging a box full of supplements and a small bag full of prescriptions drugs. Her story was long and detailed. Here is the essence in her words:

> During my young life and when I was of school age, I was underweight and constantly sick with stomach/intestinal disorders, sinusitis, tonsillitis, twitches, cystic acne, headaches and various aches and pains that would just show up from time to time. Years later, after extensive emotional stress, constant itching on my neck and both of my arms showed up even though my skin looked normal. My health quickly seemed to worsen, and it seemed as if new symptoms appeared every week or so. I was seeing multiple different doctors for uncontrollable proctitis and colitis, frequent flu infections, colds, constant sinusitis, migraines, aches and stiffness, continued acne, hair loss, severe depression, anxiety, debilitating memory loss, frequent fainting spells, menopausal problems and a multitude of other ailments. Despite being on 3-7 prescriptions, I still felt horrible all the time. I didn't know what feeling good even meant. I often wondered if life was really worth living.

During Inga's exam I noted that she had very red, puffy cheeks, and extremely swollen fingers and knees. All these areas on Inga's body were warm to the touch and quite tender, obvious signs of systemic inflammation. Her abdomen was bloated and uncomfortable. Even though she often had diarrhea, she never felt like she had fully eliminated. Inga also revealed that her job, painting houses, exposed her to toxic fumes all day long and she rarely wore a protective mask. Inga was extremely fatigued all the time and did not prepare actual meals very often. Instead, she subsisted on premade processed foods, soda pop and candy bars.

Her exam revealed several important and related findings. These were: impaired immune function (weak copper test—see Chapter 6), weak digestion, the presence of Candida (see Chapter 7, Candida finger mode test), and the presence of leaky gut syndrome.

These findings correlated with her history of multiple antibiotic prescriptions from childhood forward, several courses of steroids, daily chemical and toxin exposures from paint fumes, and poor diet choices. Each of these causative factors could nudge a person to the brink of leaky gut syndrome. The combination of these factors pushed Inga over the brink to the depths of advanced leaky gut syndrome.

Although Inga had a multitude of seemingly unrelated symptoms appear simultaneously, or near simultaneously, none of her many allopathic doctors suspected that any of these ailments was related. Instead, she was being treated for a multitude of symptoms rather than one primary causative factor. There was no doubt in my mind that Inga was in the throes of a progressively worsening case of leaky gut syndrome. This syndrome may disguise itself with various "masks" and mislead both the patient and the doctor.

Inga's treatment plan included a total renovation of her diet. Sugar, pop and processed foods were abandoned. Inga used her protein drinks for two, sometimes three, meals a day to detoxify and rebuild her system. She also included salads, fruits, and raw or steamed vegetables in her new cleansing diet. Inga's program utilized probiotics, digestive enzymes, and various herbs, vitamins and minerals. She also used one especially powerful healing and rebuilding substance, Xango® juice, which contains xanthones. Xanthones potentiate healing and cellular repair at a rapid rate, calm the nervous system and can quell depression.

Inga put her heart into her healing process and progressed beautifully. Many therapeutic modalities were incorporated into her whole-person treatment program. Near the end of Inga's intensive therapy she joyfully stated:

> I am now a purified, well, whole human being—physically, mentally, and emotionally. I cannot begin to express my elation at how well I feel. I am free of toxins, parasites, and prescription medicines, full of energy, and four sizes smaller. ALL OF THIS ONLY TOOK FOUR MONTHS!

Inga's story should give you hope that recovery from such a dire situation is achievable.

WHAT IS LEAKY GUT?

For clarity it is best to define each word of "leaky gut syndrome" individually. Syndromes, with the exception of genetically determined syndromes such as Down's syndrome, are less rigidly defined than diseases. Non-genetically determined syndromes generally exhibit a constellation of symptoms that often seem unrelated, but commonly occur together. Often syndromes do not have conclusive laboratory, imaging or pathology findings that clearly define them. As they may seem ambiguous or controversial to the allopathic medical community, syndromes are often difficult to diagnose.

The term "gut" may strike you as a slang or improper expression, but in actuality, it is the appropriate medical term. "Gut" traditionally refers to either the digestive tract in its entirety, or it indicates the intestines specifically. In fact, *Gut* is the name of a famous gastrointestinal (digestive system) medical journal. For the purposes of this chapter, gut will refer to the small intestine.

The adjective "leaky" is not ambiguous. By thinking of a leaky roof or a leaky garden hose, you are on the right track.

Leaky gut syndrome infers dysfunction of the lining or mucosal membrane of the small intestine. This leakage allows problematic substances to seep from the processing areas of the small intestine prematurely into the bloodstream. In order to better understand this, envision the screen door in your home. Properly working screen doors allow fresh air, sunlight and the pleasant fragrances of nature into your home while screening out unwanted insects and debris. "Increased intestinal permeability" is synonymous with leaky gut syndrome and is often the term used in professional medical journals. In your body, the gut lining (like a functioning screen door) should be a semi-permeable membrane, filtering out many particles and substances. When it becomes damaged, its permeability increases, and the gut lining's filtration effectiveness decreases.

When your intestinal mucosal lining is healthy, it screens unwanted or harmful items such as pathogenic (disease causing) bacteria that may be unknowingly ingested, toxins exuded from those bacteria, viruses, parasites, foreign materials, environmental toxins and incompletely digested food particles. A healthy small intestine does not leak. The food substances remain in the processing area long enough to be properly digested, and your body is able to fully utilize the digested nutrients.

Let's now imagine that the screen door is damaged and has several gaping holes. Mosquitoes, flies, grasshoppers and anything blowing in the wind will blow into your home. By the same token, if your intestinal lining is damaged enough to be "leaky," all sorts of unwanted debris and "bugs" can travel right into your bloodstream.

If you have leaky gut syndrome, your nutrient absorption will decrease since the digestive process is shortened. The particles of fats, protein, and carbohydrates that had not broken down enough to become fuel for your body are seen as antigens (a foreign or toxic substance) by your immune system. This will cause excess immune activity, which will ultimately wear down your immune system. It may also cause you to be sensitive or allergic to more and more foods. And of course, allowing bacteria, viruses and parasites into your blood could have a variety of serious, negative consequences.

Leaky gut syndrome is neither a simple nor a consistently defined malady. It manifests with a jumbled variety of symptoms and conditions that vary greatly from one affected person to the next.

The presence of digestive malfunction, inflammation and decreased immunity are the most characteristic symptoms.

The chart (on page 146) diagrams the multitude of symptoms and issues commonly associated with leaky gut syndrome. Some individuals may suffer from only three symptoms, while others may endure thirty. For clarity, some symptoms are listed in more than one category.

SNAPSHOT OF YOUR DIGESTIVE SYSTEM

Understanding your digestive tract and its normal functions is an invaluable step to approaching the subject of leaky gut syndrome. Let me introduce you to your own digestive system.

Your mouth is the entrance portal to your digestive tract. **Amylase,** a starch based digestive enzyme, is released into the saliva. This begins softening the food, which must be broken down to molecular size to be utilized. A certain volume of food or substrate—known as **chyme**: an acidic fluid consisting of partially digested food and gastric juices that travels from the stomach to the small intestine—must collect in the stomach before the next set of chemical processes is thoroughly activated.

At precisely the correct time interval for that load of chyme, your stomach will secrete hormones to activate the next digestive step. The gallbladder and pancreas are alerted to gear up. The **duodenum** (the first segment of your small intestine) is signaled to expect the arrival of the acidic chyme.

Once the chyme leaves the stomach and enters the first segment of the small intestine, the duodenum, the chemical processing begins in earnest. Your duodenum's mucosa is quite vulnerable because it receives the acidic chyme from the stomach and receives alkaline bile from the

Symptoms and Conditions Related to Leaky Gut Syndrome

Gastro-Intestinal
- Bloating
- Flatulence
- Constipation
- Diarrhea
- Liver dysfunction
- Gluten intolerance
- Food sensitivities
- Malabsorption of nutrients
- Irritable bowel syndrome
- Inflammatory bowel disease
- Crohn's disease
- Ulcerative colitis
- Abdominal discomfort

Inflammation
- Swelling—muscles, face, hands, feet, joints, soft tissues, etc.
- Intestinal tract inflammation
- Fibromyalgia
- Organ dysfunction—liver, thyroid, heart, pancreas, etc.

Respiratory System
- Asthma
- Cystic fibrosis
- Nasal congestion
- Sinus issues
- Chronic sinus infection
- Shortness of breath

Nervous System, Brain and Mind
- Autism
- (Apparent) Hyperactivity
- Multiple sclerosis
- Confusion
- Mental fogginess
- Poor memory
- Mood swings
- Depression
- Headaches
- Migraines
- Anxiety
- Insomnia
- Schizophrenia

Total Body or General Symptoms
- Chronic fatigue
- Constant hunger
- Weight gain
- Difficult weight loss
- Insomnia
- Accelerated aging
- Body or joint aches and pains
- Fibromyalgia
- Multiple chemical sensitivities
- Sensitive to weather changes
- Arthritis
- Malnutrition
- Hormonal disruption (i.e. worsening of PMS, menopause, andropause etc.)

Skin Issues
- Flushing—especially of face
- Acne
- Dermatitis
- Eczema
- Psoriasis
- Rashes
- Itching
- Hives
- Rosacea
- Hair loss

Decreased Immune Function
- Repeated bouts of colds, flu, sore throats, abscessing teeth, candida
- Fevers of unknown origin
- Food sensitivities and allergies
- Environmental sensitivities and allergies

Autoimmune Disorders***
- Systemic lupus erythematosus
- Chronic fatigue syndrome
- Hypothyroidism
- Hashimoto's thyroiditis
- Multiple sclerosis
- Inflammatory bowel syndrome
- Ulcerative colitis
- Crohn's disease
- Asthma
- Diabetes type II
- Rheumatoid arthritis
- Fibromyalgia
- Reiter's syndrome

*** A chronic state of inflammation and immune dysfunction may evolve into an autoimmune disorder.

liver and gallbladder, as well as potent enzymes from the pancreas. The largest percentage of chemical digestive function occurs here, in the duodenum, the shortest segment of the small intestine.

The next stop along your digestive tract is the **jejunum**. Here, the villi—microscopic finger-like projections of the intestinal surface—facilitate nutrient absorption. The intestinal lining of the jejunum has more villi than the other segments of the small intestine. The various nutrients (and toxins if you allow them passage through the mouth portal) seem to easily glide through the epithelial lining of their chosen villi to the safety of the nearest capillary. From here, the nutrients are routed all over the body. They all go through a checkpoint at the liver and may receive further processing. The **ileum** is the third and last segment of the small intestine. The ileum is ready for action and essentially reprocesses the chyme, attempting to glean the last nutrients for your body.

After moving directly through the **ileo-cecal valve** and brushing alongside the appendix, the chyme lands in the **cecum**, the first segment of the large intestine. All useable remaining nutrients are extracted, leaving only waste material.

The stool is propelled around a turn to the transverse colon. The action known as "peristalsis" moves the ever firming mass of waste and dead or dying bacteria that have reached the limits of their longevity toward the exit. Peristalsis takes the waste around another bend to the descending colon. This whole digestive excursion is now drawing to a close.

Ultimately, the processed stool is collected in the rectum for brief storage before elimination.

Your digestive system functions to process fuel in the form of ingested food and liquids. The various nutrient components of the diet are broken down into useable sizes and shapes at a molecular level. These components are selected and moved from the processing area of your body to the appropriate "end users," which are specific cells, tissues or organs.

Both mechanical (chewing and churning), and chemical (enzymes and acids) methods accomplish the fuel "combustion." Breaking down the fuel adequately yields energy, nutrients and wastes. Your digestive system inherently knows how to process, direct and utilize the valuable nutrients, and how to rid itself of the "leftovers." The intricate balance of functions and mechanisms incorporated in making fuel useful to your body is remarkable.

Numerous organs, some with multiple segments, interact like the instruments in a symphony with deft precision to accomplish the task of digestion.

Surprisingly, the digestive system is considered to be external to your body. Most of your digestive tract is a long hollow tube with openings to the outer world at each end. Your mouth is the entrance portal to your digestive tract, while your anus is the exit. These openings to the outer world can also allow bacteria and other microbes inside the hollow space.

You could consider your intestinal tract to be akin to a subway transportation system. Air from the great outdoors freely moves in and out of the subway tunnels just as your microbial friends (and a few bad guys) travel in and around your body. Of course, promoting greater numbers of friendly

---

Name That Microbe

Many terms have been used to describe these friendly microbes: normal bacterial flora, natural flora, intestinal flora, intestinal beneficial flora, intestinal microbiome, biofilm, friendly microbes, *probiotics* and others. Essentially, these terms are all equivalent for general purposes.

bacteria, while limiting harmful bacteria, builds your health.

To further understand leaky gut syndrome, we will focus specifically on the small intestine and its vitally important, yet delicate, lining.

The Delicate Lining

The mucosal lining of your small intestine is exceptionally soft (think velvet) and was designed to have maximum absorptive surface area. The mucous membrane lining is designed with a ripple effect. The rippled tissue is covered with millions of microscopic **villi** that project from the mucosal tissue into the **lumen** (or hollow space) of the "hollow tube," your small intestine. The primary job of the villi is to help absorb nutrients from food.

The vast number of villi, and the larger folds of tissue on which they perch, allow your body the greatest possible opportunity to extract the maximum amount of nutrition from the healthful foods you eat. The calculated dimensions of the absorptive surface of the intestinal tract mucous membrane are thought to be 5,400 square yards (4,500 square meters).[1] That is almost as big as the surface area of football field, and provides an amazing surface area for your nutrient absorption. Your body was designed for optimal performance! This normal process is progressively diminished by any degree of damage to the intestinal lining. If your diet includes, toxins, chemicals and preservatives, your villi will innocently labor just as diligently to bring those into your system as well. The villi are truly microscopic; even so, your body has **micro villi** that are even smaller. They are positioned on the villi in key areas for extra absorbent power.

This is a schematic of a small sampling of your villi.

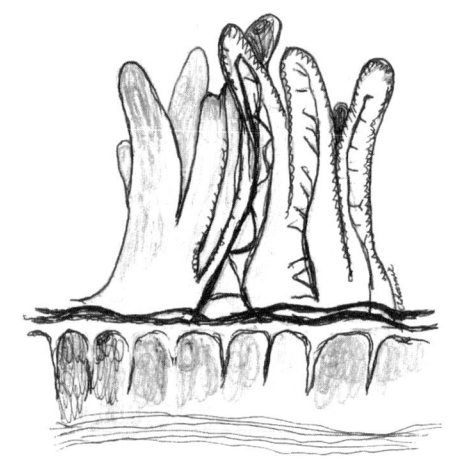

These minute villi seem like tiny fingers. In fact, they function like fingers. Your villi "massage" and "knead" your digesting food substrates in order to aid in nutrient absorption as it is being moved along the digestive pathway.

Between each two villi, at the troughs, is an area of epithelial cells called **desmosomes**. Think of these as little doorways that are closed most of the time. Imagine the potential space between the door and the doorjamb to be the cellular junction—termed **"tight junctions."** When all is well with your intestinal lining, the tight junctions are truly tight-fitting. When all is *not well* with your intestinal lining, the junctions are loose, allowing items from the external environment to enter and disturb your digestive function. The result—misery and leaky gut syndrome.

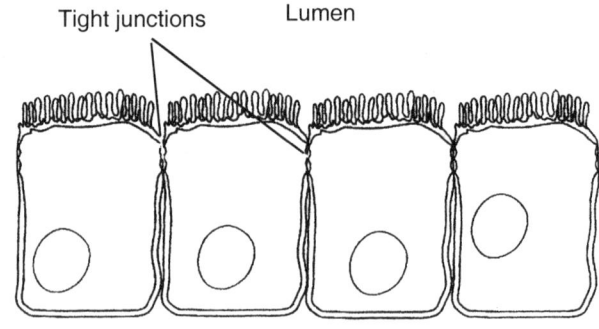

Typically, necessary nutrients and normal biochemical agents move through the intestinal lumen (hollow space) to the mucous membrane shield that protects the villi. The mucous membrane and villi are termed the **brush border**, since the villi look like the bristles of a hairbrush. The protective covering could be imagined as hair gel covering the bristles. We can imagine the gel to be a protective covering consisting of a series of miniature screens or sieves. When the brush border (mucous membrane, villi, and gel) is intact and functional, molecules or particles that are too large for your cellular "factories" to deal with are kept out of the work areas. The screening mechanisms filter out undesirable chemical substances as well. The screening material is composed of many biochemicals such as enzymes, bile, acids, antigens, and ionic (mineralized) fluids.

> ## The Brush Border
>
> Cellular components are also part of your brush border screening network—notably various immune cells, such as white blood cells, immune IGA cells and mast cells. Hoards of colonies of your friendly bacteria or probiotics are also required for a healthy brush border.

Glycoproteins and mucopolysaccharides are components of both your screen and active transport systems as well. These are biochemicals produced in your body from pieces of proteins and carbohydrates, and are easily replenished as needed. Mucous secreted by your own intestinal cells is the medium and carrier for these components.

This rich mucosal layer also functions as the active transport mechanism to move desired nutrients inside the villi, and on to the bloodstream. The screening process, when well functioning, removes large molecules, offensive particles (as determined by your antibody screeners), as well as harmful bacteria and parasites. When damage to your intestinal lining, or a leaky gut scenario exists, then any or all of these renegades may gain access to the interior of your body.

The Onslaught

When leaky gut syndrome has developed, it is as if a malevolent force flings open the desmosome doors, pulling the tight junctions asunder and giving full access to all renegades in the area. Large molecules of partially digested proteins, starches and fats are the ring leaders of the renegade marauders. These unwelcome guests storm the doorways (desmosomes and tight junctions), climb into the elevators (capillaries within the villi), and travel all over your body. They begin triggering your immune system, and then antibody production goes wild.

Many varied symptoms then occur as a result of inflammation and antigenic triggering by a multitude of substances your body views as either foreign or incompatible. Food and pollen sensitivities and allergies develop. Leaky gut syndrome is induced in two primary ways, the first, insidiously and incrementally due to various lifestyle factors. The second develops rapidly, due to the use of drugs.

Drug-induced leaky gut syndrome is precipitated by orally administered or injected steroids, non-steroidal anti-inflammatories, chemotherapy, radiation therapy or antibiotics. Hormone replacement therapy and birth control pills kill off intestinal flora and may result in leaky gut syndrome as well. In the case of anti-inflammatory drugs, chemotherapy, radiation therapy and strong antibiotics, we can visualize the results to be similar to using an electric sander on the delicate brush border of your intestines—widespread devastation.

In this instance, the mucosal protection, the mucopolysaccharides and the glycoproteins have been decimated. The microvilli are damaged, the villi are injured. With the mucous membrane screens, the protective gel and the "security personnel" gone, the tight junctions are vulnerable. Your friendly bacterial colonies have lost their lodging quarters and their mucoid food source, so they die and their corpses move downstream in the intestinal tract toward the exit in excessive numbers.

During such an onslaught, you've reached the point at which you truly need more protective, friendly bacteria, yet their populations are **diminishing** due to the leaky gut process. Your friendly probiotic bacteria actually help to fight off foreign invaders with two distinct strategies. The first is to heavily compete with the newcomers for space, food and nutrients. This "war strategy" makes the inclusion of supplemental probiotics in your treatment plan doubly important. The second way that both your inherent good bacteria and your supplemental probiotics help fight off the bad bacteria is by oozing out toxins (exotoxins) that damage or kill pathogenic bacteria, and do not harm beneficial bacteria.

> Probiotics are life-promoting beneficial bacteria that inhabit your healthy intestinal tract.

The greater your exposure to the previously mentioned medications, the more extensive the devastation to your mucosal membranes and villi. Your tight junctions become more and more like gaping openings. Pathogenic bacteria, their secreted toxins, parasites, and more antigenic factors walk in the open and unguarded doors. These invaders flood your bloodstream and gain access to the formerly forbidden inner recesses of your body.

In less dramatic cases, and insidious process may be precipitated by milder provocateurs.

The Importance of Healthy Flora

Flora play an important role in our ability to fight infectious diseases, providing a front line in our immune defense … Some flora have anticancer and antitumor properties. Friendly flora also manufacture many vitamins, including B-complex vitamins…plus vitamin A and vitamin K. Lactic acid-secreting acidophilus and bifidus increase the bioavailability of minerals which require acid for absorption: calcium, copper, iron, magnesium, manganese.
—Lipski, Elizabeth, MS, CCN. *Leaky Gut Syndrome.* Los Angeles, Calif: Keats Publishing, 1998, 36-37.

These may include insufficient digestive enzymes; frequent ingestion of allergenic foods and/or alcoholic beverages; consistent exposure to environmental toxins; dermal (skin) absorption of toxins from lotions, sunscreen, cosmetics; immune system deficiencies; an overload of numerous food additives, or GMO-tainted foods. Chronic infections such as Candida, intestinal parasites and AIDS may also damage the mucosal lining as well as most allopathic (orthodox medical) treatments for these conditions.

DO I HAVE LEAKY GUT?
Probably. Most of us have this dysfunction to a mild and bearable degree at least. With illness, medications, food poisoning, heavy metal and/or chemical exposure, the leaky gut process can escalate to debilitating proportions. If you have digestive difficulties, chronic inflammation, food sensitivities, food allergies, seasonal allergies, and/or candida, you likely have a leaky gut scenario that merits attention.

The Leaky Gut Questionnaire

You can simply and painlessly begin to assess your potential issue with leaky gut by utilizing this simple Leaky Gut Questionnaire and score sheet.

Instructions
This questionnaire is designed for adults and the scoring system isn't appropriate for children. It lists factors in your medical history that may allude to a diagnosis of leaky gut (Section A), symptoms commonly found in individuals with leaky gut (Section B), and drug use which may cause leaky gut (Section C).

For each "Yes" answer in Section A, circle the point score and then total and record it at the end of the section. Then move onto Sections B and C and score and record as directed.

Filling out and scoring this questionnaire should help you and your physician evaluate the possible diagnosis of leaky gut, yet it will not provide an automatic "Yes" or "No" answer.

Section A History

1. I have Celiac Disease (inability to digest gluten).	100
2. I have been diagnosed with Alcoholism	30
3. I have been diagnosed with Arthritis	30
4. I have been diagnosed with Asthma	30
5. I have been diagnosed with Autoimmune Disease (such as Lupus, Ankylosing Spondylitis, Hashimoto's Disease, etc.)	30
6. I have been diagnosed with Crohn's Disease	30
7. I have been diagnosed with Diabetes	30
8. I have been diagnosed with Migraines	30
9. I have been diagnosed with Multiple Sclerosis	30
10. I have been diagnosed with Ulcers	30
11. I have been diagnosed with Ulcerative Colitis	30
12. I have Candida, or I have had Candida.	30
13. I have Parasites, or I have had Parasites.	30

Total Score, Section A _____

Section B Major Symptoms*

1. I know that I have difficulty with my digestion.	40
2. I have food sensitivities and/or food allergies.	40
3. I am sensitive to weather changes.	30
4. I am often fatigued / just don't have enough energy.	30
5. I often have muscle aches and pains for no obvious reason.	30
6. I often have joint pains.	30
7. I am bothered by skin rashes, breakouts, etc.	30
8. I frequently have diarrhea, and/or abdominal pain.	30
9. My memory is poor.	20
10. I often feel "yucky" or even toxic.	30
11. I sometimes have fevers for no known reason.	20

Total Score, Section B _____

*While symptoms in this section commonly occur in people with Leaky Gut, they are also found in other individuals.

Section C Drug Use

1. I now smoke tobacco, or I have smoked tobacco for 5 years at some point.	30
2. I drink 4 or more alcoholic beverages per week.	30
3. I often take steroidal anti-inflammatory drugs (prednisolone, prednisone and medrol, beclomethsone, budesonide, flunisolide, fluticasone and triamcinolone) and/or non-steroidal anti-inflammatory drugs (NSAIDs) (aspirin, Advil, Tylenol, etc.)	80
4. I have taken antibiotics several times.	50

Total Score, Section C _____

Total Score, Section A _____

Total Score, Section B _____

Total Score, Section C _____

Grand Total Score _____

The Grand Total Score will help you and your physician decide if your health problems can be diagnosed collectively as leaky gut.

Leaky gut is almost certainly the diagnosis with a grand total score higher than 270.

Leaky gut is probably the diagnosis with a grand total score higher than 180.

With a grand total score less than 90, leaky gut is less apt to be the diagnosis or might be a mild or recovering case.

Other Tests

If your questionnaire score is high, you wish more investigation, or your "gut level feeling" guides you to seek more evaluation, two other tools are available, typically with your health practitioner's guidance.

1) The Intestinal Permeability Test

The Intestinal Permeability Test is a laboratory test that can be performed to shed light on this problem. All lab tests have shortcomings, but this one is typically reliable. If you want to have this test, first find an "outside the box" doctor and ask if they now have a relationship with a lab that performs this test, and a source for the required test reagents.

This test determines the relative amounts of two non-metabolizing sugar molecules—mannitol and lactulose—passing through the intestinal lining. When undergoing this test, the patient drinks measured amounts of lactulose and mannitol and gives a urine sample after six hours.

Since mannitol is a small molecule that readily passes through the intestinal wall, it is a good marker for how well nutrients are being absorbed. On the other hand, lactulose is a larger molecule, and requires larger holes in the lining to pass through. Elevated levels of both molecules in the urine test suggest increased intestinal permeability, a finding consistent with leaky gut.

2) Clinical Kinesiology Finger Mode

I always complete a thorough health history and exam for each patient. I always tell patients that I function as a detective, gathering clues. All of this gathered data helps a good doctor formulate the next question. Since I knew that leaky gut syndrome was an important dysfunction, I set about to research a reliable finger mode that would communicate to the patient's body. I have been using this finger mode since 2000 and find it quite useful. You may use this on your own or ask your trusted Clinical or Applied Kinesiology practitioner to test you using this tool. If using this finger mode weakens the indicator muscle, suspect leaky gut problems. You or your practitioner can also cross reference (or two point therapy localize—review Chapter 1) various supplements or treatments for applicability to your case.

LEAKY GUT HANDMODE TEST

The leaky gut handmode is performed by folding the 4th and 5th fingers down to the palm, touching the hollow space between the thumb's pad and the pad below your smallest finger. Securely touch the finger prints of the thumb and 3rd (or middle finger). Extend the 2nd (or pointer) finger straight, not touching any part of your hand.

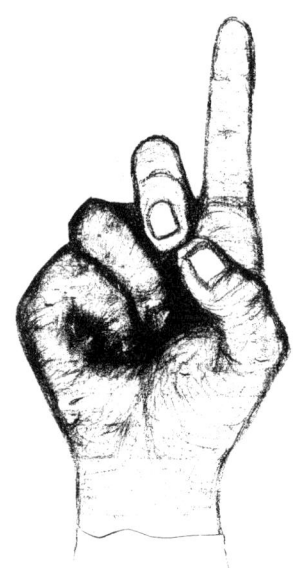

*The leaky gut hand mode was researched and developed by Dr. Susan Levy.

The following Clinical Kinesiology self-test allows you and a partner/tester to determine whether or not leaky gut syndrome is present in your system. Before proceeding with any testing, first perform the Indicator Muscle Test as instructed in Chapter 1. Once a strong indicator muscle is determined, you may proceed as follows:

Step 1: Assume the Leaky Gut handmode as illustrated.

Step 2: Have a partner/tester perform the Clinical Kinesiology muscle test on the test-subject's opposite indicator arm muscle.

> Handmode + Muscle test + Strong arm= No presence of Leaky Gut
>
> Handmode + Muscle test + Weak arm= Leaky Gut is present. Seek further testing and treatment from a trained natural healthcare practitioner. Observe dietary and nutrient recommendations.

If leaky gut is present, you will need to use one to several appropriate healing and soothing remedies. Probiotics will be very helpful. Healthy lifestyle measures are a must.

FOODS TO FIX YOUR MUCOSA

Healing your intestinal lining, or mucosa, may first begin with eliminating irritating "foods." These so called foods include alcohol, soda and caffeine; processed, fried, GMO, and "junk" foods, etc. While many things may need to be eliminated from your diet, there are three main food groups that can help to heal your leaky gut syndrome as well: one group that I am calling "soothing" foods, foods that do not require intense work to digest, another is foods that contain prebiotic components and nurture your healthy intestinal bacteria, and a final group that is naturally fermented foods, which are in a sense, predigested.

YOUR DIGESTIVE SYSTEM SPEAKS

Your digestive system chemistry lab was designed to function perfectly, and it usually will if you follow the owner's manual. The instruction manual (if only it existed) should read:

1. Only eat healthful, unadulterated foods.
2. Don't dilute your digestive juices with a quart of liquid with the meal; moderate amounts are acceptable.
3. Heartily drink pure water between meals.
4. Eat breakfast (genuinely nutritious, wholesome, and non-sugared).
5. Eat your final meal of the day at least 3 hours before bedtime.
6. Chew moderate-sized bites of food well, liquefy each bite if possible.
7. Eat in a calm and relaxed state.
8. Try mildly under-eating to avoid overeating.
9. Listen carefully to your digestive system when it says, "Please don't make me try to process THAT again." Give your gut a break.
10. Obey if you hear, "Don't give me acid blocking pills because then I can't absorb important minerals and vitamins and I'll just make extra acid since I'm programmed to do so. Before this fight is over, you may totally wear me out or cause us an ulcer."

Be nice to your digestive system and she or he will be nice to you.

Fermented Foods

Milk-based Foods

If you are not vegan by choice or belief, and are not terribly lactose intolerant, using homemade raw-milk yogurt or kefir could be quite beneficial in helping heal your leaky gut. If you experience a mild degree of lactose intolerance, adding probiotics in supplement form to your daily regimen may reduce your level of lactose intolerance.

Look for organic, pasture-grazed yogurt in your health-food store or food co-op. *Straus* is a reliable brand; it is organic and Non-GMO verified. The majority of American states prohibit the sale of **RAW** milk. It seems the bureaucrats prefer the overheating of milk to the healthful raw milk and raw milk products that have sustained generations in many countries. Heating milk in the process of pasteurization will kill all the good bacteria, kill all of the enzymes, denature the proteins (making them doubly indigestible), and ultimately promote less clean and sanitary milk handling procedures (since no one will know how contaminated the commercial milk is after it's pasteurized).

With that being said, the raw-milk yogurts or kefirs (a more liquid consistency) are beneficial, yet I don't classify them as being of **THERAPUTIC** strength in serious cases of leaky gut syndrome. Adding a powerful probiotic to your daily supplement regimen for months to a few years is typically requisite. Why not proactively use probiotics to prevent numerous maladies? The addition of beneficial bacteria from food sources is a good practice, yet it is similar to adding a thimble full when, in reality, you need a bucket full of probiotic culture when combating a symptomatic leaky gut syndrome situation. Frequent or periodic use of cultured raw milk products is a purposeful **lifelong lifestyle enhancement** to consider. Using cultured raw milk products and other fermented foods is an excellent measure to **prevent** leaky gut. Incorporating these into your leaky gut recovery diet is quite beneficial.

When you make your own yogurt—or kefir—from raw (**UN**pasteurized, **UN**homogenized) milk, you begin the process of creating a fermented food with a wholesome, unadulterated food substance. Check out the Milk Composition Chart in Chapter 13: *Optimizing Your Children's Health*, on page 247. You should know that milk from water buffalos and donkeys are now used as hypoallergenic alternative milk sources for those who have developed cow or goat milk sensitivities. If lactose intolerant people use probiotics and enzymes as supplements on a daily basis, they improve their tolerance to milk products. If the milk is sourced from a goat, cow, or other mammal that you "know," so much the better.

Non-milk Foods

If you cannot or prefer not to use the raw-milk-based fermented probiotic food sources described, you have numerous alternatives:

- Water kefir (a kefir grain starter fermented for a few days in water)
- Coconut water kefir (as above with purchased coconut water)
- Homemade raw sauerkraut (refrigerated for long-term storage—up to many months, but never heat to serve)
- Raw fermented vegetables (vinegar is never used in **raw** lactic fermentation) such as:

    – Beets
    – Broccoli
    – Cabbage (White, Red, Savoy)
    – Carrots
    – Cauliflower
    – Celery and Celery Root
    – Cucumber
    – Leeks
    – Onions
    – Peppers (Bell, Pimento, etc.)
    – Pumpkin
    – Radish
    – Rutabagas
    – Squash

- Fennel Tops and Root
- Garlic
- Kohlrabi
- Tomato
- Yams

- Miso, tempeh, or nattō (very difficult to process at home—purchase organic, preferably non-soy or soy that is NON-GMO verified)
- Kombucha tea (fairly easy to make, but **VERY** easy to contaminate and grow unidentified and unwanted microbes). I suggest purchasing it at a health-food store. I love the Synergy® brand—it is high quality and organic.
- Amazake (fermented brown rice beverage—get alcohol free). Grainessence® has produced this for years, and uses organic rice.
- Rejuvelac—(fermented water remaining after soaking and sprouting whole wheat berries or other grains such as rye, barley, millet, buckwheat, quinoa, brown rice, or whole oats for a few days). To use, strain and refrigerate the liquid—use a few ounces per serving. Ann Wigmore, the mother of the wheatgrass (1909-1993) and raw foods movement, made Rejuvelac famous. Rejuvelac is essentially gluten free, regardless of which grain is used to produce it. These sprouts can be used raw on salads, to garnish soups, or other entrees. Another option is to mash them together and dehydrate at 110°F or less for several hours and use as a cracker.

If you purchase sauerkraut, never buy canned—it was quickly processed and then boiled so no probiotics remain. My favorite commercial raw sauerkraut is Bubbies®. If you buy live culture sauerkraut, it will be in the refrigerated section of your health-food store, and must be refrigerated at home. Raw sauerkraut will literally last for years unopened and refrigerated, and many months once opened.

> ## On Sauerkraut
>
> Klaus Kaufman, German doctor of science and author of several health books, has this to say about sauerkraut (see Suggested Reading):
>
> It is truly a broom for the stomach and intestines. It takes away the bad juices and gases, strengthens the nerves and stimulates blood formation. You should eat it even if other cabbage is forbidden in your diet. Eat it moderately, well-chewed, and do not drink anything with it.
>
> Hippocrates, the father of medicine, demanded that our nourishment be curative, and that our cures be nourishing. In modern times, his words still have urgency and significance.
>
> Lactic acid-fermented vegetables supremely fulfill Hippocrates' ideal of nutritious and curative nourishment. They are not only tasty, but they also exert stimulating and healing effects.

When you are healing from a leaky gut problem, focus on enriching your diet with raw fermented foods and beverages as mentioned above. Typically these foods contain lactic acid that feeds and sustains many types of probiotic bacteria. Cabbage and sauerkraut are delectably advantageous. Cabbage grows on the soil surface and is rich in soil based organisms—certain strains of beneficial bacteria. It is one of the richest sources of vitamin U (known to heal ulcers and other mucus membrane defects).

Other fermented food sources (such as pickled ginger, daikon radish, plums, cucumbers, beets, etc.) come from Japanese and European traditions using vinegar. The traditional Japanese fermentation vat is wooden and stored under the floorboards of the family home. In rural areas it is common for the same vat and culture liquid to be constantly used for 200-400 years.[2] Likely these fermented food items have little lactic acid bacteria, but have other bacteria cultures that are beneficial. These fermentation methods are reliable for food preservation.

If you muscle test with a "Yes" response to pickles, umeboshi plums and other vinegar pickled items, uses these as condiments rather than staples.

Prebiotics—Foods That Feed You and Your Microbes

Prebiotics are food constituents that nurture and nourish the probiotic bacteria within your intestines. To further expedite your leaky gut syndrome recovery diet, you can include specific foods that contain these prebiotic properties. Providing prebiotic foods to your intestinal bacteria is equivalent to giving them 5-star accommodations.

One very important prebiotic is inulin. Inulin is a polysaccharide based on fructose that is present in the roots of certain plants and is often used to test kidney function. It helps make a better environment for your beneficial bacteria. Foods containing inulin include:

- Artichoke
- Chicory root
- Dandelion root
- Jicama

Fructooligosaccharides (FOS), sometimes referred to as oligofructose or oligofructan, is a potent prebiotic. This compound occurs naturally, is often used as an alternative sweetener, and provides food for your beneficial bacteria. When you see FOS as an ingredient, it may have been derived from a soy source. If you use a food or supplement with a soy based FOS, look for the GMO-free verification symbol on the label.

FOS food sources (all non-soy) include:

- Bananas
- Barley
- Fruit
- Garlic
- Jerusalem artichoke
- Onions
- Whole milk
- Whole milk yogurt and Kefir

Other prebiotic foods to include in your leaky gut syndrome recovery diet:

- **Beans and legumes** of all types (examples: aduki beans, black beans, cantenelli beans, garbanzo beans, kidney beans, lima beans, lentils, navy beans, pinto beans, and red beans).
- **Berries** (examples: blackberries, blueberries, cranberries, gogiberries, loganberries, marionberries, raspberries, and strawberries). These berries also provide anthocyanins, which are protective phytonutrients, and malic acid, a natural fruit acid that works to quell inflammation.
- **Greens** (examples: arugula, bok choy, chard, collards, dandelion greens, kale, lamb's quarters—considered a garden weed—mustard greens, spinach, stinging nettles, tat soi).
- **Miso**
- **Onions**
- **Tomatoes**
- **Whole grains and seeds**: unhulled, unmilled; choose gluten-free or low gluten (examples: amaranth, brown rice, buckwheat, chia seed, flax seed, hemp seed, quinoa, millet, sorghum, sesame seeds, teff and wild rice).

Selecting from these foods adds fiber and rich sources for vitamins, minerals and phytonutrients. Chia, hemp seeds and arugula provide omega-3 essential fatty acids. You gain multiple benefits while making a better home for your beneficial bacteria when regularly incorporating these foods in your diet.

Soothing Foods

Quercetin is a natural anti-inflammatory agent that blocks histamine (i.e., inflammatory) reactions in your body. Including soothing quercetin-rich foods in your leaky gut syndrome recovery diet will be highly beneficial. Food sources of quercetin include:

- Apples
- Broccoli
- Capers
- Garlic
- Grapes
- Green tea
- Kale
- Kiwi
- Leafy greens
- Onions
- Tomatoes

Okra is a food that has mucilaginous healing and soothing qualities. Think of okra (except when it's deep fried) as an intestinal comfort food. Soaked flax and chia seeds soothe your intestines as well. Include these foods in your leaky gut recovery diet.

These herbs are available in bulk and each can be used as a tea. They are also available as tinctures or capsule products. I prefer organic tinctures. Herb Pharm® always provides excellent quality.

There is an abundance of healing herbal and nutrient help available. Consult with your Clinical Kinesiology or Applied Kinesiology practitioner

Suggestions About Supplement-Taking

Taking only a multivitamin or a few supplements on an empty stomach, especially in the morning, may cause nausea. If nausea occurs under these circumstances it is likely that the supplements are not being digested and utilized, and your stomach is confused about what to do next. Certain supplements and nutrients are best taken *away from* meals, and will be labeled as such. I find that the greatest number of vitamins, minerals, phytonutrients, and a multitude of other nutritional supplements will be best absorbed if consumed *during a meal*. Chewing all supplements that are appropriate to chew (no capsules, time released or very hard pills) will yield a higher amount of absorbed nutrients since they go through a digestive cycle with food. I recommend interspersing them throughout the meal.

Herbs to Help Heal Leaky Gut

Demulcent Herbs	Other Herbs
Aloe Vera	Bittersweet
Cumin	Black Pepper
Mallow	Bosweilla (Frankincense)
Marshmallow	Calendula
Meadow Sweet	Chamomile
Mullein	Dandelion
Panex Ginseng	Fennel
Plantain	Ginkgo biloba
Slippery Elm	Goldenseal
Willow Bark	Licorice (Deglycyrrhized)
	Mastic gum
	Oregon Grape
	Turmeric
	Uno de Gato (Cat's Claw)

Nutrients That Help Overcome Leaky Gut

Vitamins	Minerals	Digestive Enzymes	Amino Acids	Miscellaneous
Folic Acid (B9)	Zinc	Plant Based Enzymes	L. Glutamine Powder	Colostrum
Pantothenic Acid (B5)	Magnesium	Lactase	Proline	Gamma Oryzanol
Vitamin A	Sulfur	Hydrochloric Acid (Betaine HCL)*	Glycine	Homeopathics to support Intestinal Tissues Small and Large Intestine Sarcode by Mountain States Health Products, Inc. Mucosa Compositum by Heel
Vitamin C		Pepsin*		Medium Chain Triglycerides (MCT)
Rutin		Okra Pepsin by Standard Process®		Quercetin
Vitamin U				Xanthones found in Xango® or mangosteen juice
Vitamin E				Fiber—one or several: psyllium, flax seed, oat bran, acacia, pectin cellulose, beta glucans
				Essential fatty acids—flax oil, omega 3 oil (purified)
				Total Leaky Gut® by Nutri-West®
				Luvos** (clean dirt)—an old German remedy soil gleaned from ground where truffles grow
				Bacofloro**- Bacillus Coagulents
				Alpha Lipoic Acid
				N-Acetyl Glucosamine (NAG)
				Chlorophyll

**From Marco Pharma International 1-800-999-3001

*Withhold in acute cases

to determine your best protocol. I suggest at least three remedies and one or more probiotic formulae. When selecting herbs, I suggest organic and wild-crafted choices whenever possible.

DO I NEED TO TAKE PROBIOTICS?

As we have noted, probiotics are life-promoting, beneficial bacteria that inhabit your intestines. The variety and number of probiotics dwelling and working in your intestines play a significant role in your health. Large numbers of the correct probiotics boost your immunity, produce certain vitamins, and help to kill or deter pathogenic (disease causing) organisms. If you have leaky gut syndrome, you have a deficiency of health-promoting probiotic bacteria. Increasing the numbers of necessary probiotics will move you away from leaky gut syndrome and toward improved health.

The answer to the question, "Do I need to take probiotics?" is Yes! Yes! and Yes! You can find probiotics in powder, liquid, capsule, and pearl forms, or even coating the inside of a special drinking straw.

Many formulations are available. Choose a high dosage one. Be sure that several strains of beneficial bacteria are present (many experts recommend that at least seven distinct varieties are present). I suggest that many people have two formulations available, one for morning and one for evening. This is one way to plant "seeds" of several varieties. You may also wish to rotate formulations as you obtain refills.

Several strains of beneficial bacteria, listed below, have been identified and labeled as "resident strains." This means that these strains are expected to be permanent residents in your microbiome (your personal intestinal ecosystem of friendly probiotic bacteria). Attempt to supplement with these even if it takes two formulations to include all seven strains.

The resident strains are:

- Lactobacillus acidophilus
- Lactobacillus salivarius
- Bifidobacteria bifidum
- Bifidobacteria infantis
- Bifidobacteria logum
- Streptococcus faecalis
- Streptococcus faecium

There is no need to limit yourself to these few. Some research indicates that we have at least 1,000 beneficial bacterial strains in our healthy microbiome. Some of these are considered "transient" because they come and go. Some transients prepare the environment for "residents."

Probiotics — A Way of Life

"Adding food sources and supplemental probiotics should be considered as much as a lifestyle principle as brushing your teeth. By the way, probiotic toothpaste is available, and is better for your heart and total body health than antiseptic mouthwash which kills your proactive beneficial bacteria." — Vikas Kapil, et al.[3]

If Antibiotics Are Necessary

If at any point you take antibiotics, do so only because they are **truly necessary.** The wisest action you can take is to ask for a preliminary test to help guide your doctor concerning the applicability of antibiotics. Most upper respiratory infections are viral, which means antibiotics are inappropriate and actually harmful to your gut flora. If you are concerned about having a strep infection, a rapid strep test for home use is available at most pharmacies and many online sources.

For suspected urinary or wound infections, it is best to undergo a culture and susceptibility test. This is a common laboratory test used to identify a specific bacterial culprit. Once the type of bacteria is identified, it is then paired with various antibiotics to determine which one is the most effective at eliminating the infection. Two to four days are required for the testing process. During this waiting period you can use herbal, nutrient and homeopathic remedies to help strengthen your own immunity. You will be able to learn about many helpful alternatives in my book about drugs.

Undergoing this laboratory test can ensure that the most appropriate antibiotic can be prescribed. To protect your microbiome when taking an antibiotic, also take a probiotic about three-four hours after each antibiotic dose, to begin replenishing your normal bacterial balance. When you have completed the course of antibiotics, continue to take the probiotics for several months at a greater than normal dosage. After repeated courses of antibiotics, or very strong antibiotics, replenish with high dose probiotics for at least two years.

In this chapter we have covered a great deal about what is required to help your intestinal health. It is now up to you to incorporate healthy lifestyle measures and a therapeutic dietary plan into your daily life. You may need guidance in selecting a nutrient and herbal protocol, but the material contained here provides a basis for understanding leaky gut syndrome and how to heal from this dysfunction, as well as vital information about how "invisible" microbes can impact your health. You now have many tools in your toolbox to stop your "leak."

The next chapter will focus on how invisible electromagnetic influences and electrical energy, buzzing all around your body, comes inside and causes mayhem. Electromagnetic pollution is an invisible, yet powerful, force that alters cells in your body, and disturbs acupuncture meridians and organ systems. Chapter 9, *Unfriendly Energy: Electromagnetic Pollution*, discusses invasion from unhealthy external energy and provides recommendations for maintaining the integrity of the body by minimizing exposure to these unhealthy electromagnetic fields or EMFs.

CHAPTER 8 SUGGESTED READING

Adams, Case, Ph.D. *Increased Intestinal Permeability aka Leaky Gut Syndrome: The Science of Achieving Digestive Health*. Wilmington, Delaware: Logical Books, 2012.

Aranga, Teri, Claire Viadro, M.P.H., Ph.D., and Lauren Underwood, Ph.D. (editors). *Bugs, Bowels, and Behavior: The Groundbreaking Story of the Gut-Brain Connection*. New York: Skyhorse Publishing, 2013.

Chesman, Andrea. *The Pickled Pantry*. North Adams, Mass: Storey Publishing. 2012

Chutkan, Robynne, M.D., FASGE. *Gutbliss: A 10-day Plan to Ban Bloat, Flush Toxins, and Dump Your Digestive Baggage*. New York: Avery, 2013.

Davis, William, M.D. *Wheat Belly: Lose the Wheat, Lose the Weight, and Find Your Path Back to Health*. New York: Rodale, Inc., 2011.

Davis, William, M.D. *Wheat Belly Cookbook: 150 Recipes to Help You Lose the Wheat, Lose the Weight, and Find Your Path Back to Health*. New York: Rodale, Inc., 2013.

GAPSdiet.com. Internal Bliss – *GAPS Cookbook (Recipes designed for those following the Gut and Psychology Syndrome Diet)*. Omaha, Nebr.: International Nutrition, Inc., 2nd edition, 2010.

Ingraham, John L. *March of the Microbes: Sighting the Unseen*. Cambridge, Mass: The Belknap Press of Harvard University Press, 2010.

Kaufmann, Klaus DSc, and Annelies Schöneck. *Making Sauerkraut and Pickled Vegetables at Home: Creative Recipes for Lactic-fermented Food to Improve Your Health*. Summertown, Tennessee: Books Alive, 2002

Lipski, Elizabeth, M.S., C.C.N. *Leaky Gut Syndrome: What to do About a Health Threat that Can Cause Arthritis, Allergies and a Host of Other Illnesses*. Los Angeles, Calif.: Keats Publishing, 1998.

McKenna, Maryn. *Superbug: The Fatal Menace of MRSA*. New York: Free Press. 2010.

Pagano, John O.A., D.C. *One Cause, Many Ailments: Leaky Gut Syndrome: What It Is and How It May Be Affecting Your Health*. Virginia Beach, Virginia: A.R.E. Press (Association for Research and Enlightenment), 2008.

Taylor, John R. N.D., and Mitchell, Deborah. *The Wonder of Probiotics: A 30-Day Plan to Boost Energy, Enhance Weight Loss, Heal GI Problems, Prevent Disease, and Slow Aging*. New York: St. Martin's Press, 2007.

Watson, Brenda, N.D.; Smith, Leonard, M.D.; Holt, Stephen, M.D. (Foreword); Stockton, Susan, M.A. (Collaborator). *Gut Solutions: Natural Solutions to Your Digestive Problems*. Palm Harbor, Florida: Renew Life, 2004.

Yamaguchi, Eri. *The Well Flavored Vegetable: Novel and Traditional Vegetable Recipes from Japan*. New York: Kodansha International, 1988.

CHAPTER 9

Unfriendly Energy: Electromagnetic Pollution

Throughout her twenty-year broadcast writing and producing career, one of my patients, Carol Lehr, worked in television stations and production studios that emit incredible amounts of electromagnetic pollution. This is commonly termed EMF (electromagnetic frequency), which alludes to an excess of or adverse effect from the electromagnetic frequencies moving through and "spilling" over into the area. On a daily basis, errant energy from all manner of television broadcasting equipment, including TV monitors, video switcher panels, satellite dishes, computer editing and production units has whirred in Carol's close proximity. This high concentration of electricity continually focused a great deal of electromagnetic pollution directly to Carol as she worked in the confines of these technical areas.

In 1991, Carol began to experience mid-back and neck muscle spasms and other vague stress-related symptoms. Eventually, these became so severe that she considered giving up her profession. Instead, she chose to be evaluated by Clinical Kinesiology. Carol's muscle tests consistently indicated electromagnetic and geopathic (invisible energies emanating from the Earth affecting the body) imbalances stemming from a heart imbalance.

Treatment with acupuncture and magnets temporarily strengthened Carol's Heart Meridian. However, returning day after day to the same environment at the television station simply unbalanced her meridians once again. The decisive factor that eventually "cured" Carol's heart imbalance and allowed her to continue her career was the addition of a Comfort Clock to her work space. A Comfort Clock is an EMF-clearing device from Mr. Lesser of AdvancedLiving.com.

It's obvious to Carol that, with her body's high degree of sensitivity, she needs protection from the electromagnetic pollution that bathes her and many others every day.

EMFS AND YOU

What is this thing called electricity? More importantly, how have we come to live in a world so dependent upon it without previously questioning its effects on our bodies? Living in an increasingly high-tech society, it's more important than ever to evaluate the risks of electromagnetic pollution, including the link between exposure to electric and magnetic fields (EMF's) and susceptibility to a number of disease states.

On May 31, 2011, in Lyon, France, the World Health Organization's (WHO) International Agency for Research on Cancer (IRAC) classified radio frequency electromagnetic fields as possibly carcinogenic to humans. This is one example showing the international scientific community having copious amounts of research findings about harmful non-thermal effects on the human body from RF (radiofrequency) radiation. Sadly, regulators only consider thermal (tissue heating effects) in formulation of the safety guidelines. In America, the unhealthy, non-thermal effects occur below the FCC (The Federal Communications Commission) lawful limits, and therefore, the public is not legally protected from RF or EMF pollution which may have neurological, carcinogenic, genetic, or other adverse effects.

Despite growing scientific evidence, it's shocking that no public advocates in the form of government health officials or agencies exist in regulating EMF pollution. Instead, those in opposition to the regulation of EMF's include every political power base in America, from computer manufacturers to consumer electronics industries to real estate, insurance, and—principally—utility companies. The lack of protective regulation is reason enough to be concerned.

This chapter will provide you with an understanding of EMF interaction and effects on the electromagnetic body. It will encourage you to guard against electromagnetic imbalances through new awareness of body symptoms stemming from EMF pollution. You will be alerted to warnings about the newest and most dangerous electromagnetic polluters of the body, including the magnetic resonance imaging device (MRI), computers, microwave ovens, and hand-held electronic devices, Wi-Fi sources, "smart" electrical meters, and powerful microwave transmission towers.

Suggestions and recommendations for minimizing exposure to electromagnetic pollution will be offered here, as well as information about unprecedented new methods for diverting or converting unhealthy energy through environmental surveying, EMF monitoring and EMF-clearing devices.

You will discover how easy it is to self-test for EMF exposure through Clinical Kinesiology energetic testing, enabling quick determination of electromagnetic imbalances from overexposure to EMF pollution.

Finally, this chapter will consider invaluable alternative treatments for rebalancing energetic imbalances using acupuncture or therapeutic magnets and simple lifestyle measures to help stop short-circuiting the body's energetic system.

THE ELECTROMAGNETIC BODY

Envisioning the electromagnetic body requires some firsthand knowledge of its atomic structure. In today's fast-paced society, most people have had little opportunity to stop and consider their own "electric" body.

Jog your memory a bit. Try to recollect a high school chemistry class and recall the design of an atom. First of all, the average diameter of an atom is 100 billionth of a millimeter, or 10^{-7}. Infinitely small, an atom is comprised of mostly empty space, energy and a tiny amount of matter.

To put the size and attributes of an atom into clearer perspective, imagine the earth as the size of an orange. In relation, the entire orange/earth's atomic matter would amount to the size of several cherries, the nucleus of each cherry no larger than a grain of salt. Likewise, electrons orbiting the cherries would resemble specks of dust. The rest of the "orange" would be empty space and energy.

The human body is composed of the same atomic structure as the earth/orange: mostly empty space and a small amount of matter or energy. Electrical energy... *and* magnetic energy; the two are inseparable.

Electrons orbiting between atoms and around the atom's nucleus create the energy patterns or energy in motion that sustains most of life. You, I, and everything else are made of oscillating fields of energy. All energy circulates in waves or pulsations. Certain *frequencies* describe how oscillating waves may be organized or patterned.

Robert Becker, M.D. (1923-2008), author of two groundbreaking books, *The Body Electric* and *Cross Currents*, was a prominent researcher who recognized a link between electromagnetic fields and illness. Becker reported that electromagnetic fields flow in living organisms producing magnetic fields which also extend outside the body. These natural body fields can also be influenced by external magnetic fields.[1] Consequently, when two waves of energy meet, if they're not congruent or precisely the same frequency, size and intensity, the stronger energy field may overpower or destroy the weaker. In addition, when two waves of energy at the wrong interface collide, they may "cancel out" one another.

Magda Havas, Ph.D., an Associate Professor of Environmental and Resource Studies at Trent University, is one of the world's leading experts on the biological effects of environmental contaminants.

Epidemiological studies of cancer have focused on two primary populations: children in residential settings and adults in occupational settings. The main cancers associated with EMF exposure are leukemia, nervous system tumors and, to a lesser extent, lymphoma among children; and leukemia, nervous system tumors, and breast cancer among adults.[2]

Throughout Magda Havas's studies, she has demonstrated the correlation between childhood cancer, specifically leukemia, and exposure to EMF. She has also found a "link between EMF exposure leukemia, brain tumors, and breast cancer"[3] in adults.

By understanding the energetic quality of the human body, of all matter and everything surrounding it, you may better understand how a correct balance of energy brings good health, vitality and well-being. Without such balance, the risk for electromagnetic illness becomes much greater.

Throughout the body, the same energy flows continuously. Maintaining energetic balance and health may be best obtained by surrounding oneself with naturally occurring energy forms, such as those within nature—like trees, rocks, peaceful meadows, forests, and rushing streams. On the other hand, introducing the body into disharmonic energy fields such as those created by high-voltage power lines, microwaves, electric appliances, cellular phones, computers, tablets, home security systems, Wi-Fi transmitters, radios, televisions, smart meters, and cellular transmission towers, may prove quite harmful. Various military and warfare radiofrequency applications are terrifyingly powerful.

In *Longevity: Fulfilling Our Biological Potential*, author Kenneth Pelletier says there appears to be "... a vital link between the electrical potentials of the human organism and those of the physical environment. Electromagnetic fields which pervade the environment have pronounced effects on the human body."[4]

Ann Louise Gittleman has researched this topic and presents relevant information in her book *Zapped*. On page 29 she clearly illustrates DNA and cellular damage when thermal effects (the only regulated effects) were absent. In other words, the regulations are not designed to protect anyone from the most serious and problematic aspects of these energy fields.

> Our bodies have an amazing defense system. Just as cell membranes offer some protection from EMFs (though not enough), a healthy cell membrane will also self-heal. But, before it repairs the tear, it may release a digestive enzyme called DNAase, which can destroy or damage DNA, potentially turning your genetic material into a precursor to disease by altering its important directions on how and when to grow, divide, and die. Studies using cell phone signals have found evidence of just that effect. For instance, in one Greek study of fruit flies, whose short life span makes them the perfect subject for basic genetic research, researchers found that exposure to mobile phone signals for only six minutes a day for six days actually fragmented the genetic material in the cells that produced the flies' eggs, and half of the eggs died.[5]

Clinical Kinesiology testing shows, categorically, that most human-made energy forms prove incompatible with the human body—interfering not only with individual cellular processes, but with the delicate energetic system as a whole.

HEALING ENERGY IMBALANCES

Robert Becker defines energetic healing as a type of therapy that taps into an invisible common source, "... the body's internal energetic control systems ..."[6] Energetic healers, like mechanics, must be able to pinpoint short circuits in the body's energy system. According to Becker, energy therapy such as acupuncture allows the healer "... to produce external electromagnetic energy fields that interact with those of the patient. The interaction could be one that 'restores' balance in the internal forces or that reinforces the electrical system so that the body returns toward a normal condition."[7]

Dr. Alan Beardall understood this unique pre-arranged pattern of body energy when he formulated Clinical Kinesiology diagnostic testing from the centuries-old Chinese acupuncture philosophy. Clinical Kinesiology testing utilizes the body's energetic feedback system to interpret the body's reaction to specific electromagnetic pollution. In addition, testing provides the means for rechanneling naturally occurring energy in the body for healing purposes. Because every individual's electromagnetic body reacts differently, it's important to begin to appreciate your own body as the delicate bundle of energy (with a specific vibration) that it is.

Clinical Kinesiology diagnosis incorporates various electromagnetic therapies which may be used to rebalance the body. Acupuncture gently "boosts" the body through needles which administer energy in amounts similar to those released by the body's own energetic system. In the practice of Therapeutic Touch, healers direct and modulate their own internal energy systems to produce external electromagnetic energy fields that interact with and augment those of their patients.

These sources of energy are resonant and compatible with your body's inherent energy system. Your body's chi' (your internal electrical system) is both subtle and delicate.

EMFs: THE SCOPE OF THE PROBLEM

Early Model T and Model A cars were built using engines that required gasoline. At the time, inventors knew little about pollution from fossil fuels.

Their all consuming focus? "How do we make this automobile run and move forward?" Now, one hundred or more years later, we're realizing the dangerous effects that auto emissions, specifically carbon monoxide, have on our health. The same concerns have recently surfaced regarding the correlation between electromagnetic fields and illness.

Over the years, experimenters have manufactured conductive wires and routed electrical energy in definite frequencies for productive purposes. Yet, as they continued to make discoveries further advancing technology, they have failed to address the far-reaching negative effects that this unknown technology exacts on the human body. Electrical engineers did not know that diverting, controlling, and transporting electrical energy for a multiplicity of purposes in the modern world would result in electromagnetic spin-off, pollution and other negative side effects. The door has been left open! Now, potential risks from such unharnessed electromagnetic fields, or EMFs, affect nearly everyone.

Indeed, it's not simply the dramatic increase of EMF-emitting sources that is ominous, but the exponentially increased exposure of virtually all humans and all life forms to them. Those who try to limit their EMF exposure are unknowingly plagued by second-hand EMF exposures emanating from their neighbor's Wi-Fi, and even a passing car's cell phone, GPS, or satellite radio transmission.

> There is no doubt that the level of low frequency radio waves is increasing in our environment and that, as a result, most of us are living in an electronic smog… With the increasing popularity of wireless Internet, the sense of urgency has become stronger…The European Environment Agency (EEA) called for immediate action to reduce exposure to radiation from Wi-Fi, cell phones and their transmission towers.[8]

With the increased popularity of cellular phones, tablets, computers, Wi-Fi and other EMF producing intruders, children living in today's world are exposed to these electromagnetic pollutants more than any preceding generations.

Recognizing the negative effects of electromagnetic pollution, spin-off, or excess is only the first step in helping to avoid this modern threat to health. Dr. Becker concluded his research saying, "… the exposure of living organisms to abnormal electromagnetic fields results in significant abnormalities in physiology and function."[9]

We are only beginning to discover the down sides to our advanced technology. While suspected by radar operators since the mid-1940s, the effects of electromagnetic pollution on the environment and the human body are finally being recognized. Epidemiologists and other scientists in America, Sweden, Canada, Finland and most all industrialized countries contribute new findings on EMF pollution weekly. As a result, the body of evidence is mounting.

The Government's Role

During the 1990s, the U.S. Department of Energy established the EMF Rapid Program and allocated $65 million for EMF research. However, the allotment required that the private sector contribute matching funds. Electric companies, expected to be the principal contributors, became increasingly nervous about the scientific findings. So nervous, in fact, that their continued financial support for new studies plummeted and they turned to lobbying members of Congress against EMF regulatory increases.[10]

The industry protective atmosphere in today's Congress does not bode well for the release of new findings. Not only slow to react, the American government has, in some cases, concealed information on electromagnetic pollution.[11] Federal agencies continue to downplay the connection between electromagnetic pollution and disease and have yet to establish any meaningful safety standards. American regulatory agencies cling to the irrelevant and antiquated premise that thermal (heat) changes produced in a living organism is the only parameter to observe or regulate. This excludes considering changes in physiology, cellular function or DNA damage, which all could predict cancer and other degenerative diseases if examined and documented.

The U.S. Telecommunications Act of 1996 has not been modernized to reflect copious amounts of valid scientific data proving harmful effects of radio frequency (RF) and other electromagnetic frequency (EMF) exposures. The Federal Communications Commission (FCC) does little to enforce them.

The EMR Policy Institute, a non-profit, watchdog corporation, has undertaken the use of calibrated RF survey equipment to analyze industrial and communications sites. With limited resources, they have discovered hundreds of sites emitting harmful frequencies far in excess of the inadequate legal mandates. This endangers the workers at these facilities, as well as all residents and passersby in the neighborhood.

Jerry Phillips, Ph. D., director of the Science Learning Center and professor of chemistry at the University of Colorado, asserted that few scientists understand electrical fields and their biological effects. He attributes the sparsity of valid studies to the fact that the subject matter is elusive, nebulous and convoluted. While addressing the EMR Policy Institute in 2009, Dr. Phillips further stated that valid studies performed by qualified and knowledgeable scientists are dismissed and rejected by their colleagues, who greatly outnumbered them. The "mainstream" scientists state that no known evidence exists of RF or EMF frequencies being harmful to humans. The fact remains that harm and evidence have been presented, but it is not understood by the mainstream majority. This makes changing regulations a slow and tedious uphill battle.

In *The EMF Book*, Mark A. Pinsky cites a widely publicized 1990 EPA (the U.S. Environmental Protection Agency) draft report which recommended classifying electromagnetic fields as a "probable" human carcinogen (cancer-causing agent). Pinsky reports that the first Bush administration "… toned down the EPA's recommendations," sparking media and public outcry following the alteration of the document.[12]

After the advent of the watershed Swedish studies in the 1990s, the head of the EPA, Carol Browner, again looked at EMFs as a carcinogen. This was described by its chief author, Dr. Robert McGaughy, as the strongest official indictment at that time of EMF as a cancer promoter. We can only hope that the 2011 statement of the International Agency for Research on Cancer (IARC) will be heeded.

Also in the 1990s, the U.S. Congress's National Council on Radiation Protection and Measurements (NCRP) committee report on EMFs was completed after nine years of study and consideration. Dr. Joe Elder, EPA's program officer for the NCRP study, called the 800-page draft "… the first comprehensive review of the world's literature on EMF health effects."[13] This report recommended adopting an ALARA (as low as reasonably achievable) EMF standard limiting all new day care centers, schools, playgrounds, new housing, office and industrial development to *two milligauss (mG)*.[14] EMF savvy scientists realize this parameter is too high, since health consequences are documented at one mG.

In America, milligaus are the units of measurement for magnetic fields. While the Federal government still chooses "not to regulate power frequency EMF levels. Some guidelines are established by other entities." For example, the "State of Florida limits EMF levels to 150 mG at edge of right-of-way."[15] This is an absurdly high allowance, which limits liability to the EMF source, and offers **NO** protection to the public.

CANCER IN CHILDREN

Cancer currently ranks as the number one cause of death by disease in children between the ages of one and fourteen. One third of those deaths are attributed to leukemia. In light of EMF research, considerable evidence suggests that children may exhibit the highest sensitivity and/or susceptibility to electromagnetic hazards.

A pioneering study, conducted by epidemiologist Dr. Nancy Werthheimer at the University of Colorado in 1979, explored the effects of electromagnetic pollution on children. By studying children's death certificates, and later plotting their residences, Werthheimer determined that children who lived near high-power electric lines were two to three times more likely to develop leukemia or brain cancer compared to children living in other areas.[16]

A 1988 follow-up study by Dr. David Savitz also confirmed a possible relationship between magnetic fields from high-voltage electrical lines and childhood cancer. Since then, more and more studies evidence that low-frequency magnetic fields have significant behavioral and central nervous system effects, as well as a stimulating effect, on cancer cell growth.[17]

In 1992, Sweden, a pioneering country in the evaluation of electromagnetic pollution, studied 500,000 children in the most exhaustive EMF residential study ever. Drs. Anders Ahlbom and Maria Feychting found that children living near transmission lines, where they received three milligauss of exposure, were nearly four times as likely to get leukemia. Given the quality of the study and Sweden's Cancer registry, this was considered to be a major breakthrough.[18]

Headway is still being made in various countries around the world limiting and removing harmful EMF and RF devices. All across Europe, in England, France, Germany and Russia, various committees as well as certain government institutes are disconnecting Wi-Fi in schools and libraries due to concerns about EMF related health consequences. Various libraries in Paris, as well as a number of universities have removed Wi-Fi networks. The Frankfurt City Government has banned the installation of Wi-Fi and the German Government has recommended against its installation, as well as the removal of cordless phones in schools. The Austrian Medical Association continues to press for the ban of Wi-Fi in schools. The Swiss government has issued public warnings against the toxic radiation emitted by various devices including cellular phones, laptops, computers, tablets and even baby monitors.

Women and EMFs

Along with children, studies suggest that women may also be more susceptible to exposure to EMFs, citing recent links to pregnancy risks, breast cancer and Alzheimer's disease.

In 1986, Wertheimer and Leeper reported that pregnant women who used electric blankets or waterbeds with electric heaters experienced a significantly higher rate of miscarriages and slower fetal development.[19]

Another study released in June of 1994 by University of North Carolina researchers, indicated that women exposed to electrical or magnetic fields on the job had a thirty-eight percent higher incidence of breast cancer than other women.[20]

Also released in 1994, were findings from three studies conducted in Finland and Los Angeles by University of Southern California researchers. USC's Dr. Eugene Sobel and collaborator, Loma Linda University neurologist Zoreh Davanipour, report that EMFs play an important role in Alzheimer's disease.[21]

People with higher occupational exposures to EMFs were three times as likely to develop Alzheimer's as those with low or no occupational exposure. The study suggests that EMFs could affect communication among nerve cells resulting in neurological diseases. Interestingly, the highest EMF exposure common to both the residential and commercial participants came from sewing machines. Much greater exposure levels from multiple sources bombard virtually all of us today.

Magnets and the Electromagnetic Body

In support of these findings, a Caltech geobiologist, Joseph Kirschvink, made the startling discovery that humans have internal magnets in their brains in the form of magnetite. Like pigeons, fish, and even worms, humans contain a built-in guidance system. This finding, coupled with yet another discovery: a new ferrous (iron-like) material found in each cell of the body, may provide new links between electromagnetic fields and the onset of disease.

The scientists believe that when exposed to strong electric fields, the brain's tiny magnets may re-orient themselves in some way, disrupting the normal flow of materials in and out of cells. This, in turn, affects the health and rate of activity of the cells. Because of this interaction, certain types of therapeutic magnets may be used to heal the body. (Note: Differing methods of applying therapeutic magnets do exist, however. Problems can occur when the body exhibits an electromagnetic imbalance needing one type of magnetic influence, such as a south pole magnet, but instead, receives a north pole magnet. For this reason, it is wise to consult a health professional before using magnets for an extended period of time.)

FUTURE RESEARCH

Much debate surrounds EMF research results, which vary for a number of reasons. In the past, there has been much debate over the scientific findings. One major factor hindering epidemiological studies is the lack of an unexposed control group. (Everyone living in today's world experiences some EMF exposure.) The second factor involves specific aspects of exposure; the size of field and the length of time exposed. Parameters which constitute "exposure" must be set before consistent scientific results emerge.

Because the U.S. falls short of Sweden and Canada in providing solid government funding, varying study results between these and other countries will continue to differ. Hopefully, in the near future, a higher priority will be given to research for conclusive evidence of the effects of EMFs on the human body, despite the enormous challenges inherent in their design.

The public has justifiably become increasingly uneasy about electromagnetic fields. The public has a right to substantive answers!

MEASURING THE FIELD

Electromagnetic fields are measured in *milligauss* (mG), a unit measurement of a magnetic field. Although small, some people have been affected at a level of only one milligauss. The Swedish government indicates adverse health effects at a level of 2.0 milligauss.

A hand-held device known as a gauss meter measures the strength of the magnetic flux or magnetic field component of EMFs. It may be used to generally identify EMF "hot spots" in the home, or measure the field from electrical appliances in the home.

Another consideration to keep in mind is that the electrical appliances used in the home daily register sixty hertz or sixty cycles per second. Meanwhile, the human body is only "wired" to ideally receive maximum external input of thirty cycles per second (the same as naturally occurring frequencies of the earth) before it becomes unbalanced. That's an instant overload to the body's energetic system, which may have deleterious effects such as headaches, nausea, dizziness, allergies, rash, soft tissue soreness, or nervous system disorders which interfere with many normal body-mind processes.

New awareness, combined with some fairly simple guidelines, enables people to eliminate most unnecessary exposure to magnetic fields.

First, try to determine any existing danger to exposure by taking a careful look around your home or place of business. Make note of any obvious visual indicators: high-voltage power lines and the service drop where lines enter the home. These may need to be rerouted or re-designed. Observe sleeping areas and note the proximity of electrical products or appliances. Check out living and work areas. Determine any unnecessary electrical appliances currently turned on but not in use. For example, be sure to make note of fluorescent lighting both above your head and below your feet on lower floors. Undertake the arduous task of refusing the installation of a "smart" meter by your utility company. Having these meters removed may be more challenging, but it can be accomplished with perseverance and diligence. In the meantime, you can search out methods that lessen the RF effects.

Second, contact your local utility or professional EMF testing company to request that they measure the EMFs in your home or office. They should conduct a thorough audit and provide you with a written record. Instead, you may want to purchase your own gauss meter. Because field strengths change, you may want to use your own gauss meter to check more frequently, while traveling, or in the event of a move. Your local utility is unlikely to provide you with any health information.

While gauss meters prove quite reliable in testing silent, invisible EMFs, only Clinical Kinesiology can uncover an *individual* response to electromagnetic pollution. Begin to utilize Clinical Kinesiology testing as outlined in the self-testing portion of this chapter to determine EMF effect on each individual body.

Once the intensity of a magnetic field is determined by a gauss meter, or a weak muscle test confirmed, move away from the source or rearrange any appliance in use to increase the distance between yourself and the EMF source. Keep children away from EMF sources and never allow them to play directly under power-lines or near transformers. Reduce time spent in any EMF field by turning off computer monitors and unplugging other appliances when not in use; or run them (such as a dishwasher) when you are not at home.

"Prudent avoidance" of electromagnetic pollution is the technical term coined by Pittsburgh's Carnegie Mellon University researchers to describe a no-cost method of reducing exposure to EMFs. However, "prudent" avoidance for one person may prove totally unacceptable for another. When in doubt, seek out professional Clinical Kinesiology evaluation and holistic treatment through nutrition, acupuncture, homeopathy, and magnet therapy to monitor and rebalance the body's internal electrical system.

Drastically altering one's lifestyle by giving up the comfort and convenience of all electrical appliances still won't provide the complete answer.

However, gaining new awareness of the EMF problem and taking a few simple and effective steps to reduce exposure remains to render the body's utmost benefit.

ENVIRONMENTAL TESTING

Professional environmental surveyors like Michael Riversong of Qi Consulting, Cheyenne, Wyoming, and Environmental Kinesiologist, Ken Lesser of AdvancedLiving.com in Colorado can be contracted to go into homes and offices to conduct an environmental audit and recommend solutions. (See Resource Guide.) Some will even offer products designed to help rebalance excess EMF energy.

The nature of electromagnetic fields that these consultants evaluate invariably proves complex. Electromagnetic fields interact with one another. Not only that—they change with the amount of current, which is also constantly changing. (For example, air conditioners draw a large current in the summer causing EMFs to rise.) These complex interactions make determining the extent of exposure more difficult.

An electric current generates a magnetic field. Conversely, a magnetic field will generate an electric current. When current flows, an electromagnetic field results. Electric and magnetic fields normally exist together. However, most health studies associate the magnetic field with the more severe adverse health effects. Electric fields behave differently and also have different effects on the body. There is much more to learn about the electromagnetic effect.

Electric fields are not robust and can be easily shielded by walls or trees. Magnetic fields, on the other hand, can pass unimpeded through nearly everything—even lead.

As EMF consultant Michael Riversong reports, "Most people spend nearly a third of their lives in the bedroom. In fact, most don't even spend that much time in one spot at work."[22] Not surprisingly, most environmental testing concentrates on one specific room in the home—the bedroom. One quick, effective way to safeguard the bedroom from electromagnetic pollution involves turning off electrical power to any circuits near the bed.

During evaluations, Riversong routinely tests fluorescent lights at 90 milligauss or more. Without exception, the closer the proximity to the source of the electromagnetic pollution, the stronger the milligauss readings—and the further away, the weaker.

I have seen photographic evidence of EMF visibly lighting a fluorescent light bulb held by a man standing under transmission power lines. The resulting light is bright enough to read a book—powered only by invisible electromagnetic fields. The photograph is further evidence of the power of electric currents flowing through the air.

DANGER: MICROWAVES

The electromagnetic spectrum depicts the organization of electromagnetic fields based on their frequency (of oscillation). The spectrum is divided into regions including extra low frequency (ELF), very low frequency (VLF), radio frequency (RF), microwave, infrared, visible light, ultraviolet (UV), X-rays, and gamma rays.

Hertz (Hz) designates the frequency of electromagnetic radiation in cycles per second. Sixty hertz equals sixty cycles per second. The next higher frequency band is Kilo Hz (1,000), followed by Mega Hz (1,000,000) and Giga Hz (1 billion). An extremely low frequency ranges from zero to 3,000 cycles per second. As mentioned, the human body operates up to 30 cycles per second.

Although humans thrive in natural frequencies from the earth at zero to 30 Hz, the vast arrays of EMF frequencies now dominating the earth are human made. Frequencies which oscillate around a billion cycles per second, are designated as microwaves, a level considered extremely harmful.

Microwaves consist of extremely concentrated beams which may be pointed in specific directions. If they should happen to be concentrated through people's living rooms, they could prove quite harmful. Therefore, current guidelines for regulating microwaves include transmission only in "line of sight" and never through buildings. When microwaves fall out of these bounds, regulators should be notified.

The higher the frequency, up to infrared, the more dramatic effect microwaves have on certain individuals. "Microwaves can and do cook people's internal organs," Qi Consulting's Michael Riversong warns. However, he adds, "Fortunately, the level at which that happens is extremely high and very unlikely."[23] Few people are ever exposed to such a high level of microwaves.

Still, the dangers exist. The former Soviet Union was discovered to have been beaming extremely high intensity microwaves at the American embassy in Moscow for many decades. Columnist Jack Anderson broke the story in 1972, followed by further coverage by *The Boston Globe*. Far above safety standards, the Russians reportedly concentrated microwaves at the embassy twenty-four hours a day to partially de-activate bugging devices.[24]

In 1976, *The Boston Globe* reported that Ambassador Walter Stoessel had developed a rare blood disease similar to leukemia. Two of his predecessors also died of cancer. In addition, about a third of the Moscow staff showed abnormal white blood cell counts.[25] A health investigation of American embassy personnel around the world followed. However, no public result or finding was ever acknowledged.

Fortunately, few people will ever be exposed to such high levels of microwaves on a daily basis. Often, even these can be blocked. Simple experimental procedures utilizing aluminum foil have been effective in safely blocking microwaves at certain frequencies. However, more research and experimentation is needed before the effects of microwaves can be completely understood.

EMFS AT HOME

Professional surveys of electromagnetic pollution indicate certain home appliances and devices are more problematic than others. Can openers often measure as high as 1500 milligauss. Hairdryers emit about seven hundred milligauss and electric razors have been known to register as high as one thousand milligauss during testing. An EPA manual singled out hand-held electric hairdryers and electric razors as especially unsafe due to the daily use and length of exposure.[26]

"Smart" meters, which transmit strong bursts of EMF energy into your home and environment every few seconds, are a new concern. If you have a "smart" meter, your neighbors likely do as well, and you are all giving second-hand EMF pollution to each other. You will need to relentlessly pursue your local utility company to replace your meter with a safer analogue meter.

Cable TV is also suspected of leaking electromagnetic pollution. Many cable companies install amplifiers on certain cable parts which, from time to time, have been known to leak. Fortunately, Cable TV installations are usually far enough removed from sleeping areas as not to constitute major problems. Cable TV converter boxes may be another story, however. CATV converters and active broadcast satellite dishes (not to be confused with passive home satellite dishes) emit huge magnetic fields.

In today's world, nearly every family home includes at least one EMF polluting cellular phone and computer or laptop. Some additional "hot" electromagnetic fields to watch out for include microwave ovens, televisions, water bed heaters and electric blankets.

Wertheimer's study of electric blanket and water bed users proved that seven or eight hours of exposure while sleeping continually bombarded the body with an excessive dosage of electricity for that period, resulting in greater risks for illness or disease.[27]

Again, prudent avoidance of electrical appliances in operation suggests remaining three to five feet from the equipment to lessen the risk of exposure.

EMFS AT WORK: COMPUTERS

While modifications in the home may be fairly inexpensive and controllable, the workplace may prove otherwise. The length of exposure to home or office computers remains important. Some tips to follow in the workplace:

- Routinely get up and move about the office area every half hour.
- Attempt to stay at least twenty inches from any computer monitor screen.

Surveys indicate that a majority of the electromagnetic pollution generated from computers may be found emanating from the CRT's power supply. As a result, more EMFs may be emanating from the back or sides of the monitor than from the front. When operating a computer it's advisable to:

- Move the CRT power supply approximately five feet away from office chairs.
- Remain at least three feet from the backs and sides of coworker's computer monitors.

Based on their findings in epidemiological studies, the Swedish government implemented stricter requirements for its nation's sale of video monitors. The Swedish MPR II standard now prohibits monitors from emitting more than 2.5 milligauss at approximately twenty-one inches from the VDT surface. The MPR II has become the *de facto* standard in the computer industry worldwide.[28] The Swedish government is cited most often in studies of electromagnetic fields because, among world governments, they remain the pioneers in setting standards in the area of electromagnetic pollution.

The MRI

One of the most common medical diagnostic machines, the MRI, or magnetic resonance imaging device, may prove to be one of medicine's most dangerous in terms of electromagnetic pollution. Roughly 30 million MRI tests are done each year by a machine that produces the highest magnetic force humans have designed to date.

Magnetic Resonance Imaging machines may be helpful in evaluating critical situations using high levels of electromagnetic radiation. When the diagnostic need arises an MRI may be justified or even critical. However, the vast majority of these tests, in my opinion, aren't critical. Obtaining specific information at the risk of such close-range electromagnetic exposure to the body simply cannot be justified!

So far, few studies have been conducted and it's not likely that any forthcoming medical journals will report on any long-term health problems which developed as a result of people receiving MRIs. MRI systems are costly, often in the millions. To recoup the cost of these machines, MRI facilities must perform a great many tests. The old idea that modern medicine must be a money-making venture is regrettable. Hopefully, that mode of thinking will change in the future.

So, in critical cases—the MRI? Yes. However, take caution and weigh all the options before having the test done.

EMF ILLNESSES

What steps can you take if you suspect that you're being over exposed to electromagnetic pollution? According to Robert Becker, there is a growing population of people who are "highly allergic" to electromagnetic fields.[29] Becker cites that continued exposure may also lead to electromagnetic hyper-sensitivity syndrome, chronic-fatigue syndrome, SIDS (sudden infant death syndrome), and changes in preexisting diseases such as HIV, Alzheimer's disease, Parkinson's disease, cancer, and other mental illnesses.[30]

Many people complain of health problems that are non-specific in nature. They often brush aside symptoms that mysteriously come and go. With no single organic cause identifiable, medical doctors can't help. After numerous tests and examinations, most doctors finally conclude, "It's all in your head." That may be the clue to suspect an electromagnetic imbalance in the body.

Women, especially, suffer unique reactions affecting menstrual or hormonal cycles and thyroid function which can be traced to electromagnetic pollution. These women report a worsening of their symptoms related to higher rates of exposure. In general, people have varying levels of sensitivity depending on the overall strength of the immune system.

Multiple sensitivity syndrome often results from electromagnetic pollution compounded by exposures to other dangerous environmental or chemical substances called exotoxins. Environmental exposure, a precursor to multiple sensitivity syndrome, may involve severe reactions to any number of exotoxins including heavy metals such as mercury, cadmium, aluminum, arsenic or lead.

In Sweden, "electrosensitivity" is a medical diagnosis.

Symptoms of Electromagnetic Imbalances

NEUROLOGICAL	EMOTIONAL	HORMONAL	CARDIAC	GENERAL
Headaches/ migraines	Anxiety	Increased cortisol	Arrhythmia (irregular heart beat)	Nausea
Dizziness	Depression	Unbalanced thyroid	Tachycardia (rapid heart rate)	Skin rashes
Hearing disturbances	Irritability	Unbalanced male/ female hormones	High blood pressure	Worsening of diabetes
Visual disturbances	Anger			Mineral imbalance
Fatigue	Rage			Rapid aging
Tingling				
Numbness				
Disorientation				
Worsening of multiple sclerosis symptoms				
Trouble concentrating				
Diminished Cognition				

Other environmental dangers include chemical hydrocarbons, super-pesticides, herbicides, genetically modified organisms (GMOs), and drug residues which are urinated into the sewage system, and seep into our rivers, streams, and oceans. Thousands of new substances have been introduced into the environment over the last one hundred years with the advent of the petrochemical age. These toxins, along with electromagnetic sensitivities, may result in near total immune system breakdown for some individuals. From there, some people have no future resistance to any other chemicals or electromagnetic fields.

Many doctors haven't updated their education adequately enough to recognize the rising cases of environmental illnesses now in evidence. This cluster of unique symptoms can be puzzling and aggravating to its victims because most doctors aren't even aware they exist. Many times, without specific energetic testing, it's difficult to determine if one suffers from multiple sensitivity syndromes.

Deborah's Story

Many years ago, I had a patient named Deborah. Deborah was the receptionist at a local insurance office. She suffered multiple health problems over several months with no apparent organic cause. Her doctors couldn't put a finger on the precise cause of her illnesses.

Then, during a series of electric field measurements of her office, high levels of EMF pollution in excess of thirty volts per meter (a measurement of the amount of force in an electrical current) were found emanating from her electric typewriter, *while it was turned off*! The computers, Wi-Fi, satellites, and ever-present cellular and wireless phones that have replaced these typewriters in today's world pose even higher levels of pollution and pose an even greater risk of problems.

Deborah switched the typewriter "on" during testing, and the level mysteriously dropped to eleven volts per meter. Still ten times stronger than the human body's one-half to one volt per meter, the reading proved somewhat better than when the typewriter was turned off.

According to Qi Consulting's Michael Riversong, this phenomenon occurs many times with machines such as electric typewriters, which house an energy center called a transformer. A small black box radiating huge amounts of electromagnetic energy, half the transformer is energized, the other half is not. By definition, all transformers waste energy. The wasted half of the current then radiates out as an electromagnetic field.

In Deborah's case, Riversong recommended she plug the typewriter into an outlet strip, which enabled her to turn the typewriter on and off with her foot. This simple measure assured that the current would be contained to a safe area, rather than being diverted through the transformer to Deborah's body.

Other appliances, which often carry a transformer or power adapter, include computers, laptops, printers, and most electronic devices. Most have a thin cord attached to the back, leading to the transformer which is often plugged in next to a person's feet. Transformers such as these typically convert 110 volts A.C. to about 12 volts D.C. have excess electricity "spillage." The only good news? In such small transformers the electromagnetic field falls off within a foot or two.

Take caution. The next time you're in the office, look around your workspace, above your head and down at your feet. You may be surprised by what you find. Making a few simple alterations may go a long way in preventing exposure to electromagnetic pollution and serious illness in the long run.

CLEANING UP ELECTRO-MAGNETIC POLLUTION

Begin to look for ways to minimize exposure to electromagnetic fields that you can control at reasonable cost, effort and convenience. Several small instruments designed to balance and "clean up" electricity in a general area are now available to consumers.

A Comfort Technology device (a small EMF clearing device) was used by my patient, Carol, to protect her from harmful electromagnetic pollution in her television station office. For years, my patients, my staff and I have noticed the soothing and calming effects of various EMF-clearing devices while in my office. Based on professional evaluation of a number of different brands, Comfort Technology has been found to be the most effective set of EMF conditioning instruments, which reorganize electromagnetic fields in a way that neutralizes harmful EMF stress effects on the human body. Comfort Technology devices help to "clean the air" of disorganized EMF scatter radiation and make your living or work space more livable.

While there may be no simple way to influence the quantity of EMFs, environmental kinesiologist Kenneth Lesser believes one can influence the "quality" of the EMFs, thus changing the effect on the body. He illustrates the following example: "Imagine a friend arriving at a party in a bad mood desperately in need of cheering up. Essentially, these clearing devices put EMFs in a 'good mood.' The energy, just like that friend, becomes healthier for everyone to be around.[31] In return, a more energetic balance is retained within the body, and other more subtle health problems may begin to subside.

Given the pervasive and growing EMF exposure levels there are likely to be substantial numbers of adults and children suffering from a disruptive electromagnetic imbalance. These disruptions can manifest in different forms of stress, aches or pains, fatigue, foggy thinking, tension, restlessness and/or irritability. Fortunately, there are several EMF-clearing devices which all neutralize biological stress in humans arising from electro pollution. They can be used separately or together for added protection for people who are more sensitive and also for those who routinely sit in front of computer monitors for hours at a time.

The next step would be protecting your home and work environments. You may find benefit and protection by using an EMF unit designed to clear an entire house or office area. Comfort Technology devices are specifically designed for the users of computers, modem and Wi-Fi-routers, fax machines, cordless and electronic telephones, cellular phones, and other electronic equipment. Often, the stress relieving, healing effects are noticed in little more than three to five days. As more energetic balance is restored, other health problems may begin to subside. (See Product Guide in the Appendix at the end of the book.)

TESTING EMF-CLEARING DEVICES

With fluorescent lighting, wiring, or other invading appliances, EMF-clearing devices help combat electromagnetic pollution at a safe and economic level.

Clinical Kinesiology energetic testing can help determine which electrical appliances currently "over AMP" the body (along with designating the best room in which to place an EMF-clearing device). Conduct your own sample test utilizing a hand-held hairdryer in the following manner:

Step 1: First, plug in any hand-held hairdryer into a convenient electrical socket and turn it on.

Step 2: Holding the hairdryer, use Clinical Kinesiology energetic muscle testing to determine if the hairdryer's electromagnetic field weakens an indicator muscle.

Step 3: Turn off the hairdryer and plug in an EMF-clearing device into the same outlet as the hairdryer and wait five minutes to allow the clearing device time to activate.

Step 4: Retest the indicator muscle to determine the strength or weakness of the indicator muscle while the hairdryer remains in operation.

The arm test will result in the muscle being fully strong or noticeably stronger with the EMF-clearing device than in the unprotected state. If you find no difference, the EMF-clearing device is not working, or it wasn't given enough time to become activated.

ELECTROMAGNETIC POLLUTION TEST

External, as well as internal information, which the body coordinates, controls and evaluates may be "displayed" for diagnosis through Clinical Kinesiology muscle testing. To check the body for electromagnetic pollution, enlist the help of a partner/tester to perform specific tests as the individual being tested stands in close proximity to various appliances while they are in operation.

Because incompatible electrical outputs do affect the body, Clinical Kinesiology testing allows individuals to "read" this information, act upon it, and make needed health changes. Testing determines, quickly and easily, any incompatibility of electrical appliances with the electromagnetic body.

Before proceeding with any Clinical Kinesiology muscle test, be sure to first determine the strength of the test-subject's indicator arm muscle. (See Chapter 1 for instructions.) Following confirmation of the indicator muscle strength:

Step 1: Choose any electrical appliance such as a cellular phone, computer screen, television screen, microwave oven, hairdryer, electric razor, satellite dish, or fluorescent light.

Step 2: Have the test-subject stand approximately one foot from the appliance, which is turned on, and look at the item to be tested.

Step 3: Perform the muscle test.

Step 4: If the test subject's indicator muscle goes weak, the electrical appliance *is* incompatible with his or her body *at this distance*.

Perform the test at distances from close range to many feet away. At some point, the negative energetic effect on the body will begin to drop off, enabling the individual to eventually complete a strong muscle test. Without EMF protection, different individuals may need to keep their electrical appliances at varying distances to insure safe exposure to the electrical field.

Consistent overexposure to electromagnetic pollution may be suspect when symptoms reach a certain level of degeneration. The manifestations of EMF pollution can be subtle and varied. Progressive symptoms for which no solution can be found may result from a case of high level EMF exposure. Many times, after relocation to a new home or office some individuals quickly develop unusual illnesses or exacerbation of an ongoing problem. In that case, EMF pollution is often suspected. EMF exposure typically aggravates the weakest area of the body depending on the individual. For example, someone who uses a computer daily may have significant eyestrain that is much more pronounced than if he or she was simply reading a book. The eyestrain may be more severe and much harder to recover from. The same hours working at a computer versus reading a book will manifest differently simply because of the EMF factor.

One wonderful self-help measure is called "earthing." This is a process in which you go outside and touch the earth, lay on your lawn or in a meadow, walk barefoot, or sit with your shoes off, touching the earth's surface. Earthing or grounding helps you to attune to the earth's natural frequency (similar to your body's inherent chi'.) It is believed that earthing helps us dissipate excess electrical pollution into the earth, and relieve the load on our body. I like to simply be in a state of "unplugged." For me, unplugged is being outside with no electronics. Optimally, being "unplugged" is being miles from the electrical grid infrastructures.

While there are many ways to intervene on your own, you must see a trained natural health or Clinical Kinesiology practitioner when you are totally baffled about worsening symptoms and health problems or clearly see health deterioration connected to environmental changes in your life.

Gaining new awareness of your own electromagnetic body and its sensitivities prepares you to make subtle changes. If you accept the hazardous realities of this unseen new health threat, you will be motivated to take the steps you can to avoid it. Your reward will be improved physical and emotional function, and strengthened body energy.

In our exploration of electromagnetic pollution, we have examined a specific quality of energy relating to electrical cycles. Part III of this book is specifically devoted to the health of the male, female and child energetic systems, which interestingly enough, maintain their own individual body and life cycles. Chapter 10: *Premenstrual Syndrome* addresses solutions for women with pre-menstrual syndrome through natural balance of these unique energetic cycles.

CHAPTER 9 SUGGESTED READING

Becker, Robert, M.D. and Gary Selden. *The Body Electric: Electromagnetism and the Foundation of Life.* New York: William Morrow and Co, Inc., 1987.

———. *Cross Currents. The Perils of Electropollution, The Promise of Electro-Medicine.* Los Angeles: Jeremy P. Tarcher, Inc., 1990.

Brodeur, Paul. *The Great Power-Line Cover-Up: How the Utilities and the Government Are Trying to Hide the Cancer Hazards Posed by Electromagnetic Fields.* New York: Little, Brown and Company, 1993.

Eisenberg, David M.D. and Thomas Lee White. *Encounters With Qi, Exploring Chinese Energy.* New York: W.W. Norton and Company Ltd., 1995.

Gerber, Richard, M.D. *Vibrational Medicine: The #1 Handbook for Subtle-Energy Therapies.* Santa Fe, New Mexico: Bear and Co., 2001.

Gittleman, Ann Louise. *Zapped: Why Your Cell Phone Shouldn't Be Your Alarm Clock and 1,268 Ways to Outsmart the Hazards of Electronic Pollution.* New York: HarperCollins, 2010.

Payne, Buryl, Ph.D. *Magnetic Healing: Advanced Techniques for the Application of Magnetic Forces.* Twin Lakes, Wisc.: Lotus Press, 1997.

Pelletier, Kenneth. *Longevity: Fulfilling Our Biological Potential.* New York: Delacorte Press, 1981.

Pinsky, Mark A. *The EMF Book.* New York: Warner Books, 1995.

Tansley, David O. *Subtle Body Essence and Shadow.* New York: Thames and Hudson, Inc., 1984.

PART III

THE ENERGETIC SYSTEMS OF WOMEN, MEN AND CHILDREN

CHAPTER 10

Premenstrual Syndrome

As Lou Anne stooped to pick up the morning paper from her leaf-cluttered driveway, a wave of dizziness overtook her body. Weak and lightheaded, she tenuously made her way back into her house and immediately dialed her local woman's clinic.

For several months Lou Anne had coped quietly with her premenstrual symptoms (PMS), enduring the pain and hoping it would eventually subside. Now, the heavy periods and dizzy spells seemed to be worsening with no relief in sight. After the incident in the driveway she wondered if perhaps she'd waited too long.

Lou Anne fidgeted nervously in the clinic waiting area. Finally, a triage nurse beckoned her into a small, sterile room and questioned her briefly about her symptoms. Then the doctor arrived. Within minutes and with no examination and little consultation, a prescription for a synthetic progesterone hormone was thrust into Lou Anne's hand. "Take this for one year," the doctor ordered, "... after that, you'll probably need a hysterectomy. Come back and see us if you have any more problems."

Lou Anne left the clinic in tears.

Like Lou Anne, many women suffer both physical and psychological symptoms of PMS, yet have found few avenues of treatment offering more than chemical drugs or surgery for premenstrual problems.

This chapter seeks to alter perceptions of the standard accepted medical treatment of PMS. Instead of uncaring or uneducated physicians, unnecessary surgeries, synthetic hormone replacement therapy and tranquilizing medications, I seek to offer new hope and healing to women. I recommend safe and simple holistic methods such as Clinical Kinesiology energetic testing.

Readers will be urged to consider that the true "cure" for PMS can be achieved *only by treating the "total" body*. In evaluating previous treatment, assessing symptoms and therapies, Clinical Kinesiology diagnosis and treatment provides lasting improvement through rebalancing the body's organ and hormonal systems, allowing each to heal itself naturally.

This chapter further presents simple healing measures involving diet, nutrition, detoxification, and acupuncture which allow the female energetic body to develop increased energy and functionality. With implementation of simple suggestions, women can *rediscover* a menstrual cycle originally designed to be easy and effortless.

You will learn about little known organ relationships, such as the thyroid/uterus connection, which illustrate how these organs work in tandem to balance the entire female system; and how surgery on any part of the female anatomy, *always* compromises the rest of the system.

Included here is a PMS test which will allow you to identify symptoms and determine specific body imbalances through classifications of the four PMS Types.

Step-by-step Clinical Kinesiology self-testing will be presented to provide important clues to evaluating *current* organ imbalances. Finally, I will share some valuable advice on additional natural therapies such as herbs, nutrition, homeopathy, and acupuncture.

Lou Anne's Evaluation

Lou Anne angrily threw the prescription for synthetic progesterone in the trash. The same day, she underwent a Clinical Kinesiology evaluation which indicated that both her uterus and thyroid were out of balance and in dire need of treatment.

During treatment, other revelations presented themselves as part and parcel of Lou Anne's physical problems. They included sudden new remembrances of sexual abuse that had occurred many years before.

Acupuncture treatment rebalanced Lou Anne's uterus and thyroid, and specific homeopathic Neuro-emotional remedies dealt with the PMS on an emotional level. Through Clinical Kinesiology testing, Lou Anne's "true" problem slowly emerged as she began to see a clearer connection between her "total" body disorder (which included PMS), and the long-buried sexual abuse.

Sexual Abuse and PMS

Studying clinical case histories of a number of PMS patients, it is clear to me that women who experience a high degree of PMS are more likely to have suffered some type of sexual abuse in childhood. Any woman who suffers from PMS should question whether this issue applies in her case.

Though unapparent to the conscious mind, abuse victims often repress these experiences in the body—specifically, in the female organs. Because PMS manifests from both psychological and physical problems, many times the unconscious mind needs additional healing. With treatment, psychological or physical abuse may be brought to the surface and released. The good news? Most women can be helped to move beyond limiting or repressed thoughts affecting their physical well-being.

TOTAL HEALTH FOR THE TOTAL BODY

Clinical Kinesiology energetic testing uses the body as a simple feedback system to confirm, "Yes, a problem exists in the uterus, or glandular system." However, in relation to PMS or other menstrual disorders, the body is really saying *"PMS is a total body problem."* Recognizing PMS symptoms may be the first indication that the female energetic system is not totally in balance.

The problem of an imbalanced system didn't start yesterday—many individual factors have been at play for years to cause this situation. However, once the primary imbalance is understood through Clinical Kinesiology evaluation, one can move into the specifics of attitude, diet, lifestyle and the need for supplements or treatment.

Upon learning about "total" body imbalances, some women may feel rather uneasy, bewildered and somewhat frightened, "Gee, I thought I had PMS," they say. "Now, I've discovered I have a liver imbalance, a dysfunctional uterus or an unexpressed emotional trauma that has stifled an organ."

All health problems, including both physical and emotional, stem from "total" body problems.

That's why it's important to support all organs and glands in obtaining their most normal function.

Rest assured! *The discovery of that organ/energy imbalance is the important thing.* It's better to make early discoveries and begin treating and rebalancing the organ or gland, than to dwell in confusion and uncertainty about the causes of PMS.

Surgery Is Not the Answer

In Lou Anne's case, even though her doctor gave her a prescription for hormones he obviously didn't believe in his own treatment. Otherwise, a hysterectomy would never have been mentioned until much later. Or, is it possible that Lou Anne's condition was something her doctor had seen with so many other women that he simply systematically programmed Lou Anne for a hysterectomy in the same fashion?

Once surgery is performed on one part of the female system, the synergy of the female organs becomes so out of balance that, many times, the problems compound until another surgery may be required ... and another. This downward cycle affects so many women.

The underlying symptoms that initially lead most women to undergo surgery for female disorders are the first warnings of a serious imbalance in the "total" body. Whether someone experiences PMS, other menstrual disorders, complications from tubal ligation, endometriosis, or hysterectomy—virtually all these conditions stem from imbalances in the body's glandular system and uterus. Undoubtedly, the uterus is not functioning correctly and its communications to various other organs and glands have broken down.

Naively, surgeons think, "Remove the uterus ... remove the problem." *Instead, all they succeed in doing is taking out the focus of the worst symptoms.* So, yes, there may be some relief at first, but often only partial relief. Many women continue to suffer the same symptoms, and just as many mood swings, as before their surgeries. Some women develop worse problems, but may not realize where they originated.

Organs In Tandem

Organs that control body functions in the female energetic system work in tandem with one another to maintain homeostasis in many ways.

The hypothalamus, controller of many body functions, is located in the brain about mid-forehead, half-way back in the skull. Directly in the center of the head, the hypothalamus lies close to the pituitary gland. From this proximity, it sends messages to the pituitary, which in turn, communicates with the adrenals, thyroid, ovaries, and uterus.

The uterus acts as a "target" organ for many different hormones. In fact, the uterus does produce small amounts of the hormones estrogen and testosterone. Following a surgery, such as a hysterectomy, the uterus cannot transmit the normal hormonal messages needed to be sent to other organs—and that "short circuitry" sets the stage for an imbalance in the body.

Uterine hormones act as messengers which return to the thyroid and serve as a feedback system to help balance the thyroid. The thyroid and uterus also work in tandem this way. So for many thyroid problems, uterine treatment may be required and vice versa.

Removal of a symptomatic organ, such as the uterus, simply means the true problem has yet to be resolved. The remaining imbalance will resurface at a later time, *as new symptoms; most likely hip, leg, or foot pain.* The uterus may be gone, but the total body imbalances go uncured.

One example which underscores the uterus/thyroid relationship involves women who previously had overactive thyroid glands removed or radiated. These women frequently develop uterine problems of one sort or another, and are directed to have a hysterectomy.

Traditionally, if one organ becomes unnaturally disturbed, the remaining organs usually exhibit more and more problems. Often, surgeons then want to remove the second organ ... and so on. This downward cycle happens so often with the uterus affecting the thyroid.

HORMONES FOR THE TOTAL BODY

The body was designed to maintain a complete balance of health—its own personal software system instructs the female energetic system to produce hormones, build up the uterine lining to prepare for upcoming hormonal changes, and anticipate many other functions. The body was originally created to produce all female hormones in the correct balance. Should an imbalance upset the female system, that delicate equilibrium must be rebalanced and maintained as naturally as possible. The standard allopathic medical approach recommends that if a woman becomes low in this or that hormone "... simply supplement her with the extra hormone."

The body needs the most natural conditions possible to produce needed hormones on its own and to carry out functions correctly *without unnatural chemical supplementation*. Obviously, there will be a few exceptions to this rule; however, reliance on the body's own natural hormonal system should remain the optimal goal for most women.

Many times, hormonal imbalances trigger PMS and other menstrual disorders. Stress constitutes a major factor. Anyone who suffers extreme stress puts added pressure on the adrenal glands to continually pump out more and more adrenalin.

Stress affects the whole endocrine or glandular system, which works together as one. The hypothalamus, pituitary, thyroid, adrenals, ovaries, and uterus represent various endocrine organs and glands that coordinate together to maintain perfect balance in the body. Each one has a part to play. Researchers have only touched the tip of the iceberg in comprehending the observable pathways by which the body's glands and organs communicate. Known hormone messages travel from the pituitary to the thyroid to the ovary. Numerous other hormonal messages can be traced, although many have yet to be discovered.

Observing the body's software system, one can see how each hormone relates to another, or how one stimulates the production of the other. These interactions merely provide the beginning clues to uncovering instances of hormonal communication breakdown. Understanding how wrong messages are sent becomes the impetus for helping the body's glandular systems begin normalizing.

Messenger Hormones

The formation of any hormone requires that a "messenger" hormone first be produced. For example, imagine mailing someone an invitation to a party. The invitation states all the information needed to guarantee a response from a prospective guest. When that guest receives the invitation, he or she naturally responds, often by buying a gift, bringing a dessert, or dressing in a certain manner.

Messenger hormones elicit similar responses in the body. In response to instructions, they produce more of one specific hormone, stop production, or change the chemical content of a needed hormone. Once a messenger hormone delivers its message, it circulates on through the blood and travels to the liver, where its molecular components are broken down and recycled.

Many times a day, the liver must reconjugate or recycle hormone messages. In order to prevent hormone messages from being continuously delivered to the same organs twenty-four hours a day, the liver must stop and start. In this way, the liver employs a system of checks and balances to maintain proper functioning in the body.

Another function allows the liver to save and recycle a large number of the components from each messenger hormone to be utilized again and again. For example, if the thyroid has been running full speed for a certain amount of time, and the body software determines, "It's time to let the thyroid slow down," the pituitary will then produce a messenger hormone that travels to the thyroid and delivers the word, "Slow down for awhile."

The body's complicated hormone circuitry can become broken down in any number of ways. The most common way hormone activity becomes unbalanced and counterproductive involves liver function. A congested or dysfunctional liver cannot break down or recycle the messenger hormones. Messages prevented from getting through may then "short circuit" the thyroid/uterus connection—resulting not only in a continuation, but an escalation of PMS symptoms.

The same message begins circulating over and over, like a dull needle caught in the groove of a broken record. Although the correct, message may have been sent, the liver may be too busy or congested to handle the workload. The messenger hormone then has no alternative but to return to the original organ and deliver the same message *repeatedly*—when, in fact, the body doesn't really need or understand that particular order. The message ultimately ends up taking the body out of balance.

Estrogen and Progesterone

Two of the most important hormones that become out of balance, in relation to PMS or menstrual disorders, are estrogen and progesterone. Once again, *the body knows* how to regulate estrogen and progesterone if supplied the correct tools—proper diet, lifestyle and environmental factors. When diet, lifestyle and environmental factors are monitored, organs of the female energetic system such as the ovaries, uterus and thyroid will be less dysfunctional. However, if PMS still occurs, the organs may need further evaluation and treatment. Ultimately, the cases of health-conscious women will be more manageable in the long run than those of women who live a less healthy lifestyle.

In addition to nutrients, diet change and adjustments, acupuncture may be used to rebalance the energy of the ovaries, uterus and thyroid, allowing them to take over and regulate estrogen and progesterone levels more adequately. When that *doesn't* happen, women may become prone to mood swings during their menstrual cycle, stemming from imbalances of estrogen and progesterone hormones.

The level of progesterone affects the level of estrogen and vice versa. If the body is low or high in one form or the other, the related hormone also becomes unbalanced. Too much estrogen may lead to feelings of anxiety, while depression results from the production of too much progesterone. However, simply because someone becomes anxious or depressed, prescribing a synthetic hormone to balance the situation is not the answer! In fact, synthetic hormone supplementation often results in the opposite effect.

Other imbalances of the estrogen hormones may trigger certain types of hypoglycemic reactions. Estrogen naturally lowers blood sugar, while progesterone raises it again. Often, with high levels of estrogen, women begin to experience hypoglycemia or intense food cravings. When this imbalance occurs, many doctors wrongly prescribe even more estrogen. In my experience, the real probability is that the patient needs more progesterone.

Natural Progesterone

Natural progesterone cream or tincture, produced from the wild yam root of South America, rebalances natural hormone levels and may be effectively used by women who want to avoid synthetic hormones. The cream provides a good alternative for women with PMS, difficult periods, pre-menopausal symptoms or as a preventive therapy for early signs of osteoporosis. Women who experience any or all of these symptoms benefit from this pure and natural progesterone cream, which is quite different from synthetic hormone replacement therapy.

Recommended usage of wild yam root cream is 1/4 or 1/2 teaspoon rubbed directly into the skin. Most times, the body fully absorbs and accepts the cream as if it was any natural progesterone. As with any natural treatment, each individual body determines whether or not the wild yam root cream is appropriate through Clinical Kinesiology testing. Before using any supplementation, be sure to test the product in the energetic field of the body to be sure of compatibility.

Although one patient, Dina, felt comfortable using the wild yam root cream, during Clinical Kinesiology testing her body indicated that it was unacceptable for her. Eventually, following successful treatment and rebalancing of Dina's liver, she may be able to use the cream. Until that time, however, she must seek a different route.

Estrogen Replacement Therapy

Synthetic estrogen replacement is continually touted to masses of women by their doctors. "Let's just try it for a while and see how it works," is the tact most medical doctors take. The results may be disastrous, however.

For years, Alice lived a healthy lifestyle, adhered to a basic organic diet, maintained a regular exercise schedule and had preventive checkups. Nearing age fifty, she gradually began noticing recurring hot flashes and other vague symptoms of menopause. Her medical doctor immediately prescribed an estrogen replacement drug. Within a year, Alice developed breast cancer. Today, Alice believes she can offer no other explanation for her cancer than the introduction of synthetic estrogen into her body. After years and years of a pure, healthy lifestyle, she felt that her body simply could not tolerate the strong, unnatural hormone.

Alice's story is not related with the intent to frighten but to warn, especially when millions of women could be potentially affected in the same way.

Ask questions! How do synthetic hormones effect the body? Will the drugs react as expected? What will the side effects be? These are pointed questions every woman needs to discuss with a doctor.

Natural Estrogen

Recently, new clinical studies have suggested that a German estrogen replacement product called Remifemin™ may be helpful for PMS and/or menopausal symptoms. The product contains black cohosh root. According to studies, Remifemin™ compared to synthetic estrogen has proven quite effective without unnatural side effects or other risks.[1] More information on Remifemin™ may be obtained from your natural healthcare practitioner or at your local healthfood store. By supporting the body's natural functions with proper diet and lifestyle, nutrients, acupuncture and gentle adjustments, the body can learn to self-regulate at a higher level and produce more or less of needed natural estrogen or progesterone hormones to correctly balance itself. Ultimately, successful treatment proves much more complex than figuring out whether a woman's going to use an unnatural, synthetic hormone.

OTHER UNNATURAL HORMONES AND PMS

Artificial hormones in general aren't something that most women have been made aware of mainly due to the extremely effective advertising of the American Dairy Association, Beef Council, and Beef and Poultry Boards.

Women who aren't careful about the food they buy are more likely to ingest a great deal of meat and poultry (including eggs) that contain artificial hormones.

In the course of pursuing a healthier diet, Martha decided to discontinue serving beef to her family. Unbeknownst to her, the supermarket at which she shopped sold chicken containing numerous synthetic hormones. As the family proceeded with their new found "healthier" diet, Martha's nine-year-old son, Eric, slowly began developing breasts. There was no doubt in my mind that Eric's problem stemmed from the artificial estrogen hormone in the supermarket chicken.

A well-known artificial hormone, DES, can still be found in meats in residual form. DES has contaminated the land. When ingested by cattle it shows up in beef products. Traces of DES can be found in the breast milk of women who eat beef. If you're an American and you eat beef, you too have DES in your system.

DES triggers a hormone overload in the body that inflames the entire system. So, anyone who tends to inflame or swell with PMS symptoms would do well to eat little red meat—or stick to naturally grown or organic products. Artificial hormones are the last thing you want to be feeding your body.

Meat, poultry, and eggs are not the only products which contain artificial hormones. Many dairy farmers have openly admitted to using Bovine Growth Formula, the first reported mass use of a genetically engineered product in the American food chain. The hormone is now used by more than 7 percent of dairy farmers.

Monsanto, the corporation that manufactures Bovine Growth Hormone and leads the market in genetically modified organisms (GMOs), sharply opposes labeling milk products containing the drug, claiming it's impossible to tell drug-induced milk from natural milk. More recently, Monsanto has contributed millions of dollars in opposition to labeling GMO foods of all kinds, including produce, boxed, canned and otherwise. Vermont and Maine became the first states to mandate labeling of dairy products from animals treated with Bovine Growth Formula. Because the drug boosts production, the economic rewards are luring more and more farmers to try it.

It's important to learn about such health hazards before they reach your body. Ensure your safety by becoming aware of standard practices so that you can make informed choices about the foods you eat.

PMS TYPES

Total body health is dynamically tied to the health of the female system. Perhaps premenstrual anxiety, bloating, depression, and cravings classify you among the hundreds of thousands of women who suffer monthly from Premenstrual Syndrome. Often, the body provides clues that help pinpoint problem areas before they become full-blown menstrual disorders.

The following overview of the four PMS types, as researched by Dr. Guy Abraham, former Clinical Professor of Obstetrics and Gynecology at UCLA, provide classic examples of recognizable total body imbalances manifested as premenstrual syndrome.[2]

Type A — Anxiety

Emotional and psychological well-being are often affected by more than just attitudes. Growing and continuing stressors in today's society affect current generations of women more than ever before. New hope for women who suffer from extreme anxiety during PMS comes with testing, diagnosis, and treatment with Clinical Kinesiology.

Type A PMS disorders manifest in fearfulness, excessive worry, edginess, insecurity, vulnerability or mood swings. Often, women with Type A PMS may exhibit persecution complexes.

Francine, for example, experiences a typical Type A-Anxiety form of PMS. During PMS, Francine often misinterprets statements from well-meaning friends or coworkers. If her boss asks to meet with her in his office, she suddenly becomes fearful. Her mind races, "Will I be fired?" At other times of the month, she realizes that routine office meetings are necessary only for simple discussions or clarification of office problems.

Francine's Type A PMS also affects her long-term relationship with her fiancé, Bill. Once a month, she becomes extremely insecure about their future together. Francine often finds herself obsessively and repeatedly calling Bill on the telephone—simply to reassure herself that he's alone at home—only to hang up! Francine also exhibits the personalities of "different people" at different times of the month.

The first question that must be raised regarding women with Type A PMS? "Is there an organ or glandular issue, or possibly a neuro-chemical imbalance in the brain?" Upon Clinical Kinesiology testing, specific homeopathic or neuro-emotional remedies or amino acid therapies may provide help in rebalancing emotional and physical imbalances in the body and brain.

Help for TYPE A

Type A's should consistently be aware of eating the kinds of foods which help promote a calm, happy atmosphere within the body.

One basic diet-related problem stems from excess salt intake. One teaspoon of salt results in the body retaining roughly five pounds of fluid. It takes that much water to absorb the salt that has been consumed. Salt also causes water retention throughout the whole body, including the nervous system and brain. The brain literally swells, causing intense anxiety and other types of mood swings in Type A women prior to their menstrual periods.

Women, such as Francine, who suffer from Type A PMS are also more likely than others to be overly stressed. Many times, Type A PMS symptoms may be alleviated by taking such minerals as chromium, zinc, and especially B vitamins. In nearly every aspect of PMS, B vitamin shortages come into play.

Everyone needs B vitamins, due to the daily stress that often depletes them as fast as they're taken. B_6 helps alleviate PMS symptoms; however, always be sure to take B vitamins in a balanced complement, as can be found in such products as B-Complex™ by Nutri-West®; or check with your local health food store. Taking B_6 vitamins alone, for example, may cause the body to become deficient in B_{12}. It is best to take B-Complex™ as a basic helper for stress and add extra B_6 or B_{12} if necessary.

Type C — Craving

Many women notice unusual cravings a week to ten days prior to their period. Women who fit the classic persona of Type C PMS often experience compulsive sweet or sugar cravings and a tendency to hypoglycemia, which are magnified premenstrually. Many times these cravings are a result of the body becoming more responsive to its own insulin during this time. The body may actually deplete its own insulin so quickly that increased amounts of blood sugar surge into the cells resulting in hypoglycemic conditions and the cravings that follow.

Once Type Cs succumb to sugar cravings, the body chemistry is thrown off balance, blood sugar levels lower and headaches often result.

Julie typifies a woman who experiences a Type-C Craving PMS disorder. Extremely pale,

Julie's skin appears dry, exhibiting a yellow to pallor tint. During her first consultation, Julie informed me that she existed on candy. Beyond the craving stage, Julie had become truly addicted to a high sugar intake.

Coffee with sugar, soda pop, and candy were the "staples" Julie relied on for quick energy. Unfortunately, on this diet Julie was literally "burning out" her body. At PMS time, Julie's cravings were so heightened that she regularly bought bags of candy and carried them with her, keeping one at her desk, and one in her car, while continually gorging on sugar.

Many Type C women like Julie exhibit low hemoglobin levels. From all indications she does not take any chlorophyll or minerals, which are necessary sources of Vitamin A, iron and magnesium, and which regulate and build healthy body function.

Unfortunately, Julie decided not to make the necessary diet changes. She did, however, take one recommendation—a pancreas supplement to strengthen her pancreas and help balance her blood sugar. Electing to continue with her favorite diet probably means Julie will be prone to continuing PMS, difficult menopause, osteoporosis and adult onset diabetes. All these problems may be avoided if Type Cs control sugar cravings and refuse to allow taste buds to overrule logic and common sense.

Help for Type C

In a nutshell, when sugar cravings come, the worst thing a Type C can do is eat sugar. Most of the time the cravings simply lead women astray and actually indicate the need for some type of nutrient that has been excluded from the diet.

Research indicates that most women crave sugar or chocolate at PMS time. Sugar cravings also signal a deficiency in chromium or zinc. Excessive sugar intake expends the body's stores of chromium and zinc because sugar is a refined carbohydrate and doesn't have any supplies of its own. Simply restricting sugar and processed foods, along with eating more whole grains, contributes a great deal to warding off cravings during PMS time.

Magnesium has also proven to be an important mineral in controlling water retention and cravings. Chocolate cravings usually indicate a lack of magnesium in the body. We've all been told we need much more calcium; however, interestingly enough, the body contains more protective mechanisms to retain calcium than it does magnesium. Magnesium is truly the "forgotten" mineral.

How can Type C women provide more magnesium in their diet? Any "green" food contains a great deal of magnesium. In chemistry class you may remember studying diagrams of a benzene ring structure—a stable, six-sided hexagon.

A chlorophyll molecule is composed of the same benzene ring structure as the hemoglobin in the blood. The only difference? The center of the chlorophyll molecule consists of magnesium while the center atom of hemoglobin contains iron.

Wise Mother Nature consistently tries to match iron with chlorophyll. Dark green foods such as kale, spinach, mustard greens, beet greens, sprouts, wheatgrass and wheatgrass juice provide the body a good supply of magnesium and iron. Upon eating the dark green food, the body instantly says, "Let's extract the magnesium out of the chlorophyll molecule and use it for something else. Then, we'll replace it with iron, and build some more hemoglobin."

In *The Wheatgrass Book*, author Ann Wigmore cites a study done in 1936 in which scientists J.H. Hughs and A. L. Latner of the University of Liverpool increased the speed of hemoglobin regeneration by fifty percent in research animals by feeding them chlorophyll extracted from green plants.[3] Wigmore cites numerous experiments on animals and humans which show chlorophyll as effective in protective oxygenation and treatment in deficiencies of the blood.

Sometimes women experience excess bleeding during their menstrual periods or transition to menopause. With a greater loss of blood, more magnesium, iron and hemoglobin are needed. In essence, all women need more green in their diets.

Type H — Hyperhydration

Out of a crowd, I can often pick women with inflammatory reactions along with PMS and menstrual disorders. Their condition often worsens around the age of forty, with some women developing noticeably blotchy red cheeks and blotchy areas around the throat and thyroid area. These women also report a general feeling of puffiness and complain of being swollen most of the time.

The tendency for hyperhydation or water retention is just that— a swelling of the body tissues. Often these Type H women are referred to as "swellers" or "inflamers." Physiologically, their bodies tend to swell or inflame more than others. Other Type H symptoms include sore, tight muscles, stiffness, and water retention.

Whenever a slight physical problem develops, it always feels much worse to an "inflamer." They experience daily swelling, premenstrual swelling, or they sustain an injury which lingers for a much longer period of time. Food sensitivities have proven to be a co-factor in most Type H women, especially those who get stiff and swell for no apparent reason.

Jeannette represents a classic case of a woman suffering from Type H PMS. Nearly eighty pounds overweight, Jeannette feels that a great deal of her excess weight results from fluid retention during her period. At PMS time, Jeannette's been known to gain ten to twelve pounds seemingly overnight.

She often complains of painful, swollen ankles. Jeanette's shoes become too tight for her feet, and the rings on her fingers immovable. In addition to this generally bloated feeling throughout the body, all her joints also become stiff.

During Jeannette's Clinical Kinesiology examinations, her hyperhydration problem became quite obvious. Significant indentations appeared as my thumb pressed into her tissue. This *pitting edema* was most pronounced in Jeannette's legs and feet. As a result, any prolonged standing further complicated her joint pain and swelling.

Through Clinical Kinesiology, Jeannette's food sensitivity evaluation uncovered extreme sensitivities to wheat and dairy foods. Once the sensitivities were indicated, an herbal detoxification was recommended to cleanse further impurities from Jeannette's system and begin the rebalancing.

Help for Type H

Figuring out foods to which Type H's are most sensitive, and restricting these foods from the diet, halts the process of inflammation in the body. Pinpointing food sensitivities may be done quickly and easily with Clinical Kinesiology testing.

Generally, women with Type H PMS should avoid salt (even refined sea salt) or other food sensitivity items which stimulate the inflammatory process. Be sure to read labels and avoid prepared soups and processed foods (including dairy foods) which contain extremely high levels of sodium. Celtic Sea Salt, which is totally unrefined and contains a natural, complete balance of ninety-three minerals, does not have these adverse effects. (See the product guide in the Appendix of the book.)

Women experiencing type H symptoms also need to avoid caffeine. Along with coffee, soda pop and certain teas, most of the popular brands of ibuprofen (under various names on the market) also contain caffeine. These drugs further inflame the body and interfere with hormone production.

B-vitamins, magnesium and natural diuretics can be safely taken by Type H women until the body is rebalanced. Some foods and herbal supplements which *temporarily* may be used include dandelion, parsley, alfalfa, fennel seed, shave grass, celery, uva ursi, potassium, and B_6. These are good natural diuretics; however, they are not meant to be used long-term.

Type H healing regimens should also include a daily dose of flaxseed oil, which remains a healthy diet choice for women who experience a great deal of swelling or hyperhydration. Natural, cold-pressed flaxseed oil simply puts out the "fire" in the body. Imagine the flaxseed oil as a little fire hose dousing the body and calming down any extra heat or swelling.

I take a teaspoon or two of flaxseed oil every day at home. Quite fragile, the refrigerated oil must never be heated; however, it can be used in salad dressings or marinades if that's preferable to drinking it straight down. Pure flaxseed oil itself proves more effective than processed capsules. Always be sure to check for the date on the bottle. It's easy to store in the refrigerator or freeze it for later use. Containing the best complement of Omega 3, 6 and 9 fatty acids, flaxseed oil provides the most healthful oils (even better than fish oils) ever needed in the diet. The oil also contains Vitamin E and serves as an antioxidant. However, just think of it as nature's little firefighter in the body!

Obviously, Type H women should refrain from smoking. In addition to the extra heat from the inflammation, smoking simply adds heat and fire into the body. As a result, oxygen is depleted from the cells. Wherever a cigarette burns, it's consuming oxygen in the air and in body tissues.

Smoke that enters the body, coming into contact with delicate tissues, simply oxidizes or "rusts" the body. So, by stopping smoking, eating non-irritating foods, the use of flaxseed oil, B vitamins and magnesium in the diet, Type H women will go a long way in quelling the hyperhydration of PMS.

Type D — Depression

Extremely volatile emotions can be observed in women with Type D PMS or menstrual disorders. Many times, these emotions represent intensified reactions to everyday occurrences that normally wouldn't be bothersome in the least.

The most severe cases of Type D PMS may involve prolonged depression, self-inflicted injury or suicidal tendencies. Additional symptoms include irritability, forgetfulness, insomnia, or lethargy.

What happens to the hormones during menstruation that leads to depression? Progesterone and estrogen balances become tipped, and the resulting imbalance causes the progesterone overload to lead to depression. Women who suffer from this form of depression do not have enough estrogen to counterbalance the progesterone, so the body often needs help in producing more estrogen.

Occasionally with depression, the possibility of excess lead in the body may also be a contributing factor. Two ways of confirming excess lead poisoning are through Clinical Kinesiology muscle testing, as well as hair analysis (trace mineral analysis of the hair). Hair analysis performed by a laboratory provides measurable readings of low, normal, or high mineral concentrations inside the cells of the body. Consult a natural health practitioner for guidance in scheduling this laboratory procedure.

Andrea, an example of Type D PMS, found herself in a complex situation. Previously diagnosed with Candida, along with fear, anxiety and depression, Andrea exhibited a tendency for premenstrual violence. The mother of four small children, she routinely became extremely depressed and virtually "out of control" during her PMS time each month.

One morning, Andrea's anger became so violent that she broke several things around the house. Further driven by uncontrollable emotions, she physically "attacked" her washing machine, which wasn't working correctly. Eventually, after many destructive episodes of Type D PMS, she became so concerned that she sent her four children away for six months for fear she would become abusive during her bouts with depression.

Clinical Kinesiology testing ultimately revealed that Andrea lacked progesterone and needed complete rebalancing of her hormonal system. With additional progesterone from the wild yam root, along with successful treatment of her Candida, Andrea eventually overcame her Type D PMS. Her children returned home and she resumed teaching piano lessons in her neighborhood.

Help for Type D
Type D PMS women need to avoid sugar and other refined carbohydrates, or strong stimulants such as coffee, soda pop and alcohol which trigger "pick me up, let me down" reactions. During depression time, rely on simple fruits and vegetables and whole grains, while avoiding any intense spices to maintain calm in the system. In addition, soy products, pumpkin seeds, and almonds prove beneficial.

Supplements which help alleviate Type D symptoms include B and E vitamins, magnesium, zinc, and amino acids as evaluated by Clinical Kinesiology testing. The amino acids Tyrosine, L-Phenylalanine and L-Glutamine are especially useful for depression, as well as liquid Choline or Choline tablets. Valerian and passiflora, in herbal tincture form, tablet or combination homeopathics may be used as relaxants, as well as various brands of calming teas such a chamo-mile. In addition, homeopathic seratonin can be obtained from many health practitioners. Homeopathic Anti-Depression Drops are available from Mountain States Health Products. Ask your health practitioner for more information.

For all PMS Types, solving underlying PMS problems through Clinical Kinesiology means evaluating certain organs and glands, treating with acupuncture, or adding nutritional support. Evaluating diet and the need for additional vitamins and supplements serve to balance the body and allow women to function normally with fewer symptoms of anxiety, craving, hyperhydration and depression.

THE LIVER: YOUR BODY'S VACUUM CLEANER

A major contributing factor in hormonal imbalances stems from the condition of the liver. For example, think of your age today and then consider that you've been using the same liver/vacuum cleaner all these years—without ever changing the bag! Obviously, if you never attended to your ordinary vacuum cleaner you wouldn't get much carpet cleaned and you would risk polluting the air each time you switched it on.

Daily, the liver serves as a vacuum cleaner for the blood. Today's unhealthy diets, pollution, chemicals and lifestyle factors affect the liver more so than ever before. Changing those factors which you can control, like changing your diet and doing occasional internal cleansing for your liver and other organs (see description of the "liver flush" which follows), can help heal your liver along with your PMS symptoms.

Adult acne constitutes a problem that women encounter prior to or during their monthly period. Again, most acne problems stem from an overburdened liver. Call it dermatitis, excema, or whatever you want—the liver is overburdened and excreting poisons out through the skin. If acne occurs regularly during the menstrual cycle, obviously the liver is excreting certain toxins that it hasn't been able to deal with effectively.

Diet and lifestyle hold the keys to controlling adult acne and other aspects of health. However, it's extremely difficult to monitor everything breathed in the air, drunk in the water, or eaten from the land. The more carefully you plan your diet and manage your lifestyle, the better your chances of protecting your liver.

Yes! Your liver/vacuum needs a rest! Allowing the liver to function correctly by completing its hormone recycling job means giving your liver/vacuum a rest from the constant onslaught of toxic input which ultimately drags down total body function. With a few, simple changes, you can obtain lasting relief from a myriad of problems— PMS being only one.

Internal Cleansing

In many European countries, the idea of a "spring tonic" or fast has become a tradition. I once employed a woman, Elena, from Finland, who remarked that every home in her native country contained a sauna. Elena recalled wonderful memories of the saunas that she had used since childhood.

Young-looking and vibrant, Elena remarried later in life and gave birth to a baby at the age of forty, although by outward appearances she looked to be only about twenty-eight years old. Elena continued working until the final day before delivering her healthy baby.

We can learn new ways of internal cleansing which our European friends have practiced for centuries. And we can take important cleansing steps right now for future benefit. Anyone who suffers from PMS should routinely cleanse the liver. One of the simplest liver cleansers available is dandelion root, in capsule or tincture form. An additional cleanser, milk thistle, makes these two in combination a powerful liver cleanser.

The Liver Flush

One effective liver flush involves fasting from solid food and drinking only large quantities of organic apple juice or fresh-pressed apple cider for a period of three days. Women who tend to be hypoglycemic may want to dilute the juice and also eat something light each time the juice is drunk.

Besides flushing out accumulated toxins in the liver, the malic acid found in apple juice helps dissolve or soften any gallstones that may be present in the gallbladder, providing a two-fold benefit.

Anyone with suspected or confirmed gallbladder problems may also use the apple juice for longer than the three-day period. However, don't do this without guidance. Try it for three to seven days along with a light diet of organic produce, and the benefits will prove significant.

Another popular liver flush involves juicing half a grapefruit, a whole orange, and half a lemon. Toss the fruit juice into a blender along with six to eight ounces of water. Add up to two cloves of garlic, or for those who may need to be sociable during the day, a ginger substitute is recommended in place of garlic. (Quite woody, raw ginger must be cut into small pieces before blending into any mixture.) Then, add a good quality olive oil, such as extra virgin— the purest and least processed. The goal requires starting with a small amount of oil and working up to near 1/4-1/2 cup by the end of the flush.

Finally, mix all these wonderful ingredients together in the blender until the drink is smooth and frothy. Discard any small fibers from the ginger root that need to be separated. Drink the entire amount first thing in the morning once a day for seven days. You'll notice terrific results and obtain a much cleaner liver.

> ### The Liver Flush
>
> 1 orange
> 1/2 grapefruit
> 1/2 lemon
> 6-8 oz of water
> 2-4-6 oz pure olive oil (gradually increase daily)
> 2 tablespoons cut raw ginger root or garlic

Most people do not encounter significant problems using the liver flush. However, the higher the level of toxicity in the body, the more likely the individual may experience discomfort ranging from mild nausea to gagging or vomiting. These are indicators that the body is toxic and needs some type of cleansing. Individuals who experience problems should discontinue the liver flush and work at a milder type of cleansing such as Dandelion root or Milk thistle combination capsules, tinctures or various detoxifying teas. If the liver flush is done in conjunction with a fast be cautious when reintegrating food into your system. Eat only easily digestible foods such as raw or steamed vegetables, a light vegetable soup or fresh juices. For questions or further guidance concerning detoxification, consult your natural healthcare practitioner.

Fasting

Fasting proves effective for many women; however, it is difficult for most. The bottom line? Women who aren't psychologically ready to try a fast do have other cleansing alternatives. A good, light cleansing diet of fruits, vegetables and whole grains also works well. For those who do want a serious fast, I recommend reading the classics on the subject: *The Master Cleanser* by Stanley Burroughs, *Juicing for Life* by Cherie Calbom and Maureen Keane, and *Fasting and Eating for Health* by Dr. Joel Furhman. (See Recommended Reading for this chapter.)

Dr. Furhman states on the first page of his book:

> Although fasting has been around as a therapeutic approach for thousands of years, only now is the medical profession studying the broad-reaching restorative properties of the fast…the medically supervised fast is the safest and most effective treatment for many dangerous but common illnesses.[4]

HERBAL REMEDIES FOR PMS

Throughout history, women have relied on herbs for a variety of female problems. Black cohosh root, originally a Native American root, has been used successfully to quell menstrual cramps gently and naturally. It may also be used for women entering menopause who suffer from hot flashes. This herb proves so helpful due to its effect on the thyroid. (Again, we see the interplay of uterus and thyroid, an important balancing act for control of PMS symptoms.) But, do not use the black cohosh root each month while ignoring the underlying conditions resulting in the cramps. Do use the herb (which proves much safer than a chemical drug) *while at the same time figuring out what is really going on in the body*. See your natural healthcare professional.

Another effective herb for balancing the entire hormonal system is the chasteberry. Especially helpful for the pituitary gland, chasteberry communicates with the rest of the endocrine and glandular systems.

In addition, another Native American herb, squaw vine, along with red raspberry may be helpful in balancing the uterus. Squaw vine is especially useful in balancing levels of progesterone, while cramp bark rounds out the list of helpful herbs that provide health for the female system in general.

Evening primrose oil, borage oil, black currant seed oil, lecithin and others have long been recommended supplemental oils for women with PMS. Taken in capsule form, the oil helps prevent diarrhea, headaches, and skin eruptions during menstruation.

ON THE PRIMROSE PATH TO HEALTH

No matter which PMS symptom complex, category or type of symptom you suffer, recognize it as the first indicator that somewhere, something may be out of balance in your female energetic system— your diet, your hormonal or glandular system, acupuncture meridians, or your emotions which involve the neurotransmitters of the brain. Perhaps these remain the untold reasons why PMS has been no primrose path for you.

The following Clinical Kinesiology self-testing steps and PMS questionnaire provide the simplest solution in initially determining what area of the body is out of balance. The next step involves seeking out a trained natural health practitioner who is able to naturally treat underlying imbalances.

Testing the Female Energetic System

The following self-testing instructions may serve as a guide for further examination, for seeking more knowledge or as a preliminary check of your current health status.

Before proceeding with any Clinical Kinesiology testing, refer to Chapter One for instructions on performing the preliminary Indicator Muscle test. Following determination of base-line strength of the Indicator arm, proceed with further testing.

Hypothalamus Test

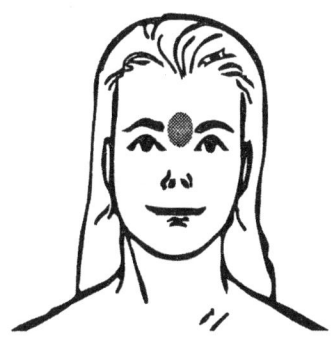

Any test of the female energetic system should begin with testing the hypothalamus. This small part of the brain serves as the master controller of all other glands and organs and directs many body regulating functions.

If out of balance, the hypothalamus may trigger erratic hunger and thirst patterns, wakefulness and sleep patterns, emotional disturbances, mood swings, memory and depression.

Test the hypothalamus by having the test-subject place the index finger directly at the bridge of the nose on the mid-line of the forehead, in the space between the eyebrows. The tester then performs the Clinical Kinesiology muscle test on the subject's opposite arm.

> Hypothalamus TL + Muscle test + Strong arm = Hypothalamus balance.
>
> Hypothalamus TL + Muscle test + Weak arm = Imbalance of Hypothalamus.

PMS QUESTIONNAIRE: DETERMINE YOUR PMS TYPE*

Menstrual Symptom Questionnaire

Grading of Symptoms

1. none
2. mild-present but does not interfere with activities
3. moderate-present and interferes with activities but not disabling
4. severe disabling (unable to function)

Grade Your Symptoms for Last Menstrual Cycle Only

	Symptoms	Week After Period	Week Before Period
PMT-A	Nervous tension		
	Mood swings		
	Irritability		
	Anxiety		
		Total _____	Total _____
PMT-H	Weight gain		
	Swelling of extremities		
	Breast tenderness		
	Abdominal bloating		
		Total _____	Total _____
PMT-C	Headache		
	Craving for sweets		
	Increased appetite		
	Heart pounding		
	Fatigue		
	Dizziness or fainting		
		Total _____	Total _____
PMT-D	Depression		
	Forgetfulness		
	Crying		
	Confusion		
	Insomnia		
		Total _____	Total _____
Total MSQ Score		_____	_____

*Adapted From: Abraham G.E.: "Nutritional Factors in the Etiology of Premenstrual Tension Syndromes." *Journal of Reproductive Medicine* 28: pp. 446-464, 1983. Used with permission. All rights reserved.

Should the test indicate the hypothalamus is out of balance, consult a Clinical Kinesiology or natural health practitioner who should be able to help rebuild and strengthen the hypothalamus function through acupuncture, nutrition, or other natural methods.

Thyroid Test

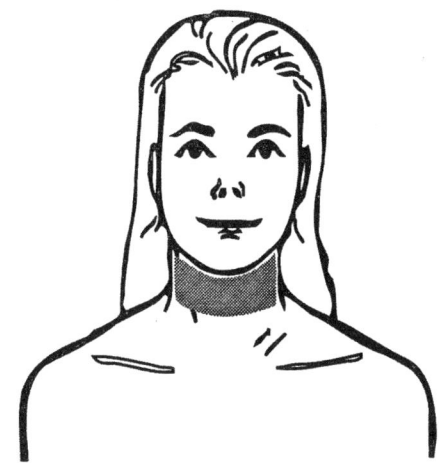

When testing the female energetic system for PMS it's first necessary to check the most relevant organs. The thyroid also plays a key role in balancing the female energetic system.

Problems with fluctuations or flow of the menstrual cycle usually indicate a thyroid malfunction. In order to test the thyroid balance, therapy localize over the thyroid by having the test-subject place an open hand over the front side of the throat, while simultaneously muscle testing the strength of the subject's opposite arm.

Thyroid TL + Muscle test + Strong arm = Thyroid balance.

Thyroid TL + Muscle test + Weak arm = Thyroid imbalance.

Follow up with a Clinical Kinesiologist, acupuncture, nutritional support and other treatment can strengthen the thyroid and change the imbalance.

Uterus Test

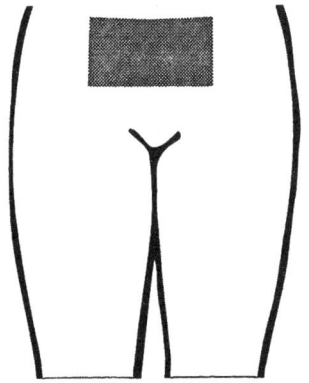

It's a good idea for any woman with female energetic problems to therapy localize over the uterus. To perform this test, the test-subject places the palm of the hand over the lower abdomen approximately three inches below the navel, while the tester checks the strength of the subject's opposite arm. Anyone who has experienced menstrual cramps or labor pains should have little problem locating the uterus.

Uterus TL + Muscle test + Strong arm = Uterus balance.

Uterus TL + Muscle test + Weak arm = Uterus imbalance.

Once again, a weak muscle test confirms that the uterus is energetically imbalanced. The test does not necessarily mean a fibroid tumor or any type of pathology or disease is present; simply, that a uterus imbalance has been detected and can be treated with natural measures.

Ovary Test

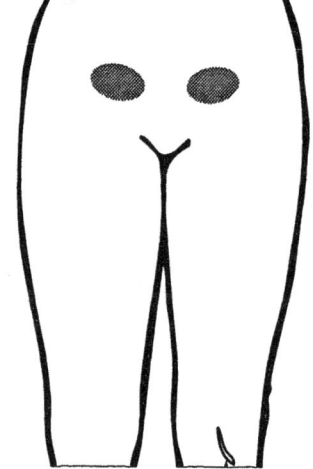

Following a surgical procedure, some women retain only one ovary. Unfortunately, many times that ovary becomes out of balance. In this case, ovary supplements or glandulars may help strengthen the ovaries. It's difficult to therapy localize over the ovaries because they are so small, so try to be precise.

To locate the ovaries, place both hands on the waist. Slide hands in a downward V until thumbs reach the pointed bones of the hip with the fingers touching the pubic bone. Approximately midway along that V-line you will find the ovaries.

Ovary TL + Muscle test + Strong arm = Ovary balance.

Ovary TL -f Muscle test + Weak arm = Ovary imbalance.

If an imbalance is found, consult a Clinical Kinesiologist or an alternative healthcare practitioner.

Pituitary Test

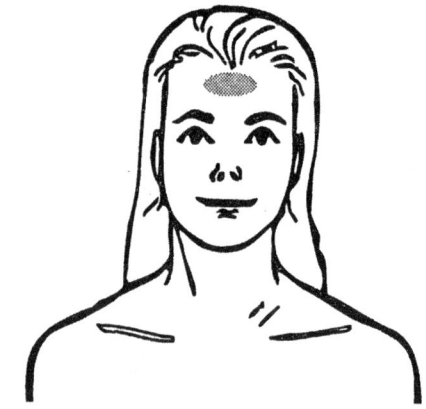

The pituitary may be tested by placing the hand two to two and one-half inches above the hypothalamus in the center of the forehead.

Pituitary TL + Muscle test + Strong arm = Pituitary balance.

Pituitary TL + Muscle test + Weak arm = Pituitary or hormonal imbalance. Consult a Clinical Kinesiologist.

THE CHOICE IS YOURS

The goal of any treatment for PMS remains rebalancing the system in a way that enables body cycles to work well and effortlessly for the remainder of a woman's menstruation. Doing this may require acupuncture, additional nutrients, diet changes, detoxification measures or gentle chiropractic adjustments. Many self-help measures may also be implemented as far as lifestyle, exercise, or resolving emotional trauma or stress from abuse in the past. In all cases, any woman with PMS will improve simply by eating a healthier diet.

Don't leave underlying "total" body imbalances untouched by simply treating localized symptoms. Give your body what it needs naturally and simply. It will heal itself and you will finally achieve a real solution to your problems with PMS.

Conquering Premenstrual Syndrome is an important prerequisite to a healthy transition to menopause. As the body continues through its natural balance of life cycles, finding healthful solutions to menopause remains a woman's most important goal. Chapter 11, *Menopause*, gives women new hope and new options for meeting the challenges that lie ahead.

CHAPTER 10 SUGGESTED READING

Aguilar, Nona. *The New No Pill, No Risk Birth Control*. New York: Macmillan, 1985.

Burroughs, Stanley. *The Master Cleanser*, Original Ed., Auburn, Calif.: Snowball Publishing, 2012.

Calbom, Cherie and John Calbom. *Juicing, Fasting, and Detoxing for Life: Unleash the Healing Power of Fresh Juices and Cleansing Diets*. Garden City Park, N.Y.: Hachette Book Group USA, 2008.

Ford, Gillian. *What's Wrong With My Hormones?* Newcastle, Calif.: Desmond Ford Publications, 1992.

Fuhrman, Joel, M.D. *Fasting and Eating for Health: a Medical Doctor's Program for Conquering Disease*. New York: St. Martin's Press, 1995.

Lark, Susan, M.D. *PMS: Self-Help Book: A Woman's Guide*. Berkeley, Calif.: Celestial Arts, 1984.

Lark, Susan, M.D. *Menstrual Cramps*, Revised Ed. Berkeley, Calif.: Celestial Arts, 1995

Mendelsohn, Robert S., M.D. *Male Practice: How Doctors Manipulate Women*. Chicago: Contemporary Books, Inc., 1981.

Meyerowitz, Steve. *Juice Fasting and Detoxification: Use the Healing Power of Fresh Juice to Feel Young and Look Great, 6th Ed.* Great Barrington, Mass.: Sproutman Publications, 1999.

Norsigian, Judy and The Boston Women's Health Book Collective. *Our Bodies, Ourselves, Touchstone Ed.* New York: Simon and Schuster eBook, 2011.

Ojeda, Linda. *Exclusively Female: A Nutrition Guide for Better Menstrual Health*. San Bernadino, Calif.: Borgo Press, 1985.

Reichenberg-Ullman, Judyth, N.D. *Whole Woman Homeopathy: The Comprehensive Guide to Treating PMS, Menopause, Cystitis, and Other Problems—Naturally and Effectively*. Roseville, Calif.: Prima Publishing. 2000.

Wade, Carlson. *Carlson Wade's PMS Book*. New Canaan, Conn.: Keats Publishing, Inc., 1984.

Wigmore, Ann. *The Wheatgrass Book*. Garden City Park, N.Y.: Avery Publishing, 1985.

CHAPTER 11
Menopause

Sixty-year-old Vyana lives atop a 10,000 foot mountain range in Kashmir, among a village of native tribal people known as the Hunza. In Hunzaland, elderly women are revered, possess great social value and remain the center of attention in the family. All her life, Vyana lived simply, toiling tirelessly in her village orchards, gardens and fields. Despite her years, she never experienced menopausal symptoms. J.I. Rodale's classic book, *The Healthy Hunzas*, documents the amazing physical and mental strength Hunza women demonstrate in progressing through natural life transitions such as menstrual cycles, childbirth and menopause.[1]

How different the health and longevity of women in our society would be if they were embraced with the same love and respect for aged persons that Vyana received in the Hunza village. Until that acceptance is given, natural health processes such as menopause will continue to be a subject of dread (an occasion for anxiety, depression or pain and embarrassment) which subverts the happy, healthy longevity—not only of women, but of the cultures they live in.

SIMPLE AND EASY MENOPAUSE

Viewing menopause and other turning points in life as the simple and natural "passages" they were designed to be may require a new sense of purposefulness for many women. Giving this healthy transition the high priority it deserves means finding new ways of diminishing energy-stress and new ways of increasing the female body's adaptability, to better accommodate all body cycles throughout life's natural changes.

This chapter recommends that as with PMS, women readdress "total" body function through improving their diet and lifestyle, and by limiting daily stress. These vital modifications will lessen the chances that future imbalances will disrupt health before, during and after menopause.

Essential prerequisites to a smooth transition to menopause include:

- monitoring symptoms
- counteracting stress depletion of hormones
- increasing awareness of biochemical changes
- and maintaining healthy organ connections.

This chapter encourages women to avoid the chain reaction consequences of synthetic hormones while discovering new therapies which help counteract the outliving of the natural hormones which are meant to function throughout a woman's entire lifespan.

Additional recommendations include the avoidance of unnecessary surgeries, such as hysterectomies, tubal ligations and other invasive procedures, and the use of natural treatments for rebalancing little known organ systems, such as the thyroid/uterus connection.

Finally, this chapter offers new hope for women. Information about their specific health concerns is available with simple self-testing procedures utilizing Clinical Kinesiology testing, diet, herbs, homeopathy, acupuncture and gentle chiropractic. As women begin to trace the true origins of imbalances they take a major step forward on the path to health.

MARY'S STORY

Forty-two-year-old Mary woke up unexpectedly from a sound sleep, her hair, nightgown and sheets soaked with perspiration. Already uneasy about a business presentation the next day, Mary shuddered to think what would happen if she experienced one of her dreaded "hot flashes" in front of co-workers and clients. (Just the week before, she'd made an unplanned exit from work because of extreme cramping from a heavy menstrual period that wasn't due for another two weeks.)

Confused, extremely weak, tired, and suddenly chilled, Mary quickly changed into a fresh nightgown, took a few sips of water and fell back into a restless sleep.

The next day, however, with all her other attempts at healing failed, Mary chose a new path—one that would lead her to the true cause of her problem along with a natural solution.

Mary's initial Clinical Kinesiology evaluation clearly pointed to an energetic imbalance in her uterus, along with her thyroid. Surprisingly, at her young age, she exhibited the same type of energy imbalance as many older menopausal women.

Acupuncture treatment immediately helped rebalance both her thyroid and uterus. Testing also determined additional nutrients Mary needed to help counteract future problems. After weeks of hot flashes and heavy bleeding, Mary's symptoms completely stopped within three days of her first treatment. All subsequent menstrual periods resumed with regularity and no further complications.

The good news? Mary is going to avoid premature menopause, prescriptions for synthetic hormones, a hysterectomy, or any other drastic treatment as long as she continues with diet and lifestyle changes that promote good health. By rebalancing her uterus and thyroid, Mary was able to heal her female energetic system and her pre-menopausal symptoms ceased.

During treatment, Mary discovered how easy it was to maintain "total" body health, provided the body is given the helpful nudges it needs. She came to appreciate how her body, as the master of so many complex functions, was designed purposefully to function correctly throughout her entire lifespan—including menopause.

Why would it be any other way? Why would the female body be designed to out-live the important hormones (particularly estrogen and progesterone) that it needs to support life? I see two major causes for the deleterious effects of natural menopause. First, *many women's hormonal systems were significantly out of balance prior to the onset of menopause*, and second, *many do not accommodate the natural changes, such as menopause, that do occur*. Both of these causes are tied into one thing—lifestyle.

More than any other aspect, a woman's lifestyle determines the overall well-being of her body and its organ/energy systems. Monitoring diet, exercise, stress, and environmental factors are paramount in the healthy progression through natural menopause.

THE BODY CHANGES

Typically, between the ages of forty and fifty, a natural slowing down of hormonal output by the ovaries begins to occur. This includes a lessening of production of both estrogen and progesterone. One viewpoint, which differs from most of the others, centers on the theory that progesterone production slows down first.

Initial signs of progesterone slowdown usually develop a few years before menstruation ceases. According to medical definition, the actual onset of menopause is indicated when menstruation ceases. However, the progressive changeover in the body actually takes several years, including a premenopausal and postmenopausal stage. The progesterone slowdown theory hints that before a woman begins to notice any other symptoms, numerous "brown spots" or "age spots" appear, and increased skin dryness, wrinkling, and other symptoms develop.

Often, allopathic medical approaches narrowly classify all premenopausal symptoms as stemming from lack of estrogen. Most alternative paths, including Clinical Kinesiology, propose a more holistic approach to the body. Clinical Kinesiology supports many new ideas, most of which are not typically what women are used to reading in mainstream medical journals. As you approach decisions about menopause, keep in mind the dichotomy in thought and practice between different diagnostic methods and modes of treatment which may eventually compromise your health.

Premature Menopause

More than likely, menopause occurs earlier and earlier due to imbalances in diet, lifestyle, and pre-existing imbalances in our bodies. While not always widely discussed, you might recall or have a sense of when a grandmother or mother experienced the onset of menopause.

You may also know women in their late thirties and forties who are currently experiencing pre-menopausal symptoms. It may even be happening to you.

Women who previously may have suffered from PMS generally experience a more difficult menopause. They experience an earlier age of onset, more severity of symptoms, and more general discomfort. Again, due to pre-existing imbalances in the body, these women may also exhibit more problematic emotional changes at menopause.

In today's fast-paced world, women's body functions are slowing down and wearing out too early from many factors—stress being only one. In the 1960s, the average age for menopause was fifty-five. Today, treatment is often required by quite a few women in their forties. At age forty-two, forty-four, or forty-five many of these women begin to experience symptoms and changes.

Allopathic medicine lists some causes for premature menopause as stemming from viral infections, inherited chromosomal abnormalities, defects in gonadotrophic secretion (a hormone from the brain that tells other hormones to be stimulated), auto-immune disorders such as Lupus, or enzyme defects in the body, excessive smoking or cancer. These precursors all constitute strains on the body.

The use of birth control pills has also proven to be a significant factor in the onset of premature menopause. Why? Birth control pills consist of a steroid based drug. All hormones contain a steroid base. However, the steroids in the body which form the building blocks for hormones are completely natural. In chemical drugs, the steroids are synthetically made and unnatural.

During the late 1960s and early 1970s, many high school girls complained of irregular periods, only to have their doctors prescribe birth control pills. "Taking birth control pills helps maintain regular cycles," was the popular thought as doctors wrote prescription after prescription. It remains a common practice today.

Synthetic hormones have dramatic effects on young women's bodies. The pills unnaturally force the body to alter its physiology, no longer allowing it to function normally. Wheels are set in motion that throw off the delicate balance of hormones, the repercussions of which these young women may not see for many years.

Other factors which precipitate premenopausal symptoms include fibroid tumors, endometriosis, uterine cancer, and extreme stress.

These traditional medical disorders, which cause lack of ovulation, may lead to premature or difficult menopause increasing the incidence of irregular menstrual patterns and erratic bleeding.

Women who prematurely experience progesterone slowdown should search out the true underlying causes for their disorder and treat them—helping to arrest premenopausal symptoms before they become more serious.

Rebalancing the hormonal system is strongly recommended should illness or trauma prematurely stop the menstrual cycle. Some women experiencing premature menopausal symptoms may be tempted to say, "Oh good … no more periods!" However, at ages under fifty, it remains vitally important to keep menstrual cycles functioning as planned by the body's normal physiology. This proves much better for the body in the long run. That way, the system continues to produce the needed hormones, avoiding additional menopausal symptoms, such as osteoporosis and further imbalances in the body.

Emotional and Physical Trauma

Emotional and physical traumas also cause cessations of menstrual periods, which may not be "true" menopause. Linda, a female patient, experienced an abrupt cessation of her menstrual periods in her thirties following the breakup of a long-term relationship.

During her Clinical Kinesiology evaluation, the muscle testing signaled the priority problem as stemming from her pituitary gland. Following treatment of Linda's pituitary with acupuncture, nutrients, and glandular supplements, her monthly periods came back like clockwork.

Two other women, Monica and Sheryl, required treatment after being severely injured in car accidents. Although outwardly recovered for many months, neither woman had resumed her menstrual periods. Again, Clinical Kinesiology evaluation uncovered imbalances in the pituitary glands of both women. Treatment resulted in their periods returning in a normal, natural cycle.

Without treatment of the pituitary and restoration of energy to other imbalanced organs, these women may have been incorrectly classified as typical cases of "premature" menopause. Most importantly, their problems were treated and resolved.

HORMONES, GLANDS AND MENOPAUSE

As hormones cycle in a natural rhythm, they regulate the body's glandular system, which maintains the menstrual cycle essentially on schedule each month.

Often the first symptoms of menopause include hot flashes and night sweats. These stem from imbalances in the thyroid and hypothalamus, the temperature regulating systems of the body. In addition, women may experience fatigue, depression, irritability, and insomnia.

Little is written about the thyroid in most of today's popular books. Much more is written about the hypothalamus. However, Clinical Kinesiology research indicates that the thyroid is the more important organ in healing menopausal problems.

One traditional idea regarding menopause suggests that with a lack of ovulation, the pituitary continues to attempt to stimulate the follicle in the ovary through a follicle-stimulating and a leutinizing hormone, which cause the follicles to ripen and develop at least one egg. Researchers blame the pituitary for attempting to force the ovary to ovulate. Resulting high levels of follicle-stimulating hormones and leutinizing hormones then appear in the blood. Due to the fact that the ovaries have diminished or ceased production of their own hormones (once needed in large amounts) a resulting imbalance of low estrogen and progesterone levels occurs, again resulting in cessation of menstruation.

Along with the primary hormonal system, a secondary source for the manufacture of all hormones exists in the adrenal glands. In addition to estrogen and progesterone, a woman's adrenals also produce testosterone throughout her life. Conversely, men make estrogen in extremely small amounts. Of course, a great deal more remains to be learned about hormone interaction. Researchers have only scratched the surface in describing the job these important messengers hold in a healthy body.

Risks of Synthetic Hormones

The hormonal system comprises many different glands in the body. For it to function effectively requires a number of "pieces and parts," including "messenger hormones" which circulate in the body systematically couriering messages from point A to point B and back again. When women ingest synthetic hormones involving human-made attempts to re-create nature, the whole message communication system can be disrupted.

In introducing synthetic hormones into the body, there's always a chain reaction. Imagine a pool table laden with colorful pool balls. The player takes a shot—and all the balls break in different directions, scattering and hitting one another. Although the person may be aiming correctly, still, an unexpected or opposite reaction occurs.

In hormone research, experimenters neglect to ask, "Might there be something missing in the equation that the body needs to correctly decode this hormone's message?" Take, for example, the "message" of a human-made birth control pill which travels to the ovary. This seems to be modern medicine's attempt to fool the body. Often, synthetic chemicals such as birth control pills cause unnatural reactions and often toxic consequences. Possible side effects of birth control pills include nausea, vomiting and weight gain. They may also increase a woman's chances of cardiovascular disease, breast cancer, and cervical dysplasia (a precancerous cervical condition.) Was something extra added to the hormone message inadvertently commanding an unplanned change in the body? *Doctors don't know.* One thing is sure. Synthetic hormones may dramatically change body physiology rather than augment or heal it.

Gentle, Natural Treatment

Normalizing body functions and recommending appropriate therapies enable hormonal messages from the pituitary to trigger the ovary to produce needed estrogen, which stimulates the menstrual cycle.

If an ovary is incapable of producing any longer, medical practitioners should not get out the whip, crack it and demand, "You have to perform!" No, treatment should always be handled in a more gentle, natural way.

The body may accept the help and continue the needed function, or it may say, "Thanks for the extra ginseng or vitamin E; however, I'm not going to use it for that purpose." The body is so wise. It's best to allow it options and choices.

Each woman's genetics and physiology, body imbalances or past traumas will direct the time of menopause. Early menopause is undoubtedly due to some type of body imbalance. Solving the imbalance or remedying the effects of the physical trauma is the important step. As a consequence, if menopause is postponed that means the body's natural pattern warranted a later onset. Menopause coming early is a symptom. The underlying imbalance is the cause. Once the cause is addressed, the symptom may change or it may not. Therefore, women shouldn't necessarily prolong menstrual periods and postpone the onset of menopause strictly in regards to age, but rather for health! Allowing the body to continue its normal functions for the maximum amount of time proves far healthier for most women.

MENOPAUSE: THE ENERGY CONNECTION

The body organs only contain a certain amount of expendable energy. Should the heart require healing, or a biochemical process need changing, energy must be immediately diverted to the needed area. If one area of the body cries out for help, the body probably has the energy to aid in healing. However, if five other areas vie for attention at the same time, none will receive much help. Healing menopausal symptoms, therefore, requires that women relieve the body of as much energy stress as possible.

Obviously serious illnesses such as cancer put a tremendous strain on the body's energy reserves. In many cases, the body prioritizes, saying, "I cannot deal with the irritation to my lungs or the cancer in my body *and* go through a menstrual cycle." The body may then put the menstrual cycle on hold, dealing first with its most pressing problem.

Often, women may notice that major losses in the family or other devastating or disruptive experiences result in missed periods. Again, the body may not have enough energy to proceed through a whole menstrual cycle *and* cope with a loss or devastating episode. This provides another clear indication of the body's hormonal regulation system.

Heart Symptoms And Menopause

Numbness and tingling, arm pain or chest pain may occur at menopause in relation to imbalances in the Heart Meridian—all related to the heart under stress. Associated problems in post-menopausal women include increased heart disease.

Researchers say that estrogen prevents heart disease. Indeed, natural estrogen produced in the body does afford women extra protection over their lifespan. Following menopause, however, less estrogen production may result in an increase in heart disease.

A unique relationship between the uterus, thyroid and heart is observed in more and more women. A great deal of women on thyroid medications also experience increased heart problems. As yet, it's unclear whether the dysfunctional thyroid affects the heart, if the drug is the precipitating factor, or both. One thing is for sure; a most definite feedback system exists between the heart and thyroid.

Maintaining proper blood pressure during menopause remains vitally important to all the organ/energy systems. One caveat: treat them naturally. The organs must not be allowed to remain dysfunctional, without help, or be given four or five chemical drugs to further tax the body. Instead, find constructive treatment, rebalance and heal.

Bladder Symptoms

Increased urinary frequency and incontinence remain common problems related to menopause. Although the bladder and kidney both connect to individual meridians, the kidney more often needs treatment than the bladder.

Sometimes women experience a "dropping" bladder or uterus. This may occur as time progresses and uterine muscle tissue becomes weak from insufficient energy in the area.

In recent years, vaginal mesh transplants have gained in popularity. These are synthetic, sling-shaped pieces of mesh that are surgically placed transvaginally (first passed through the vagina before being implanted). They are generally prescribed to women who suffer from conditions caused by weak pelvic floor muscles, including incontinence and pelvic organ prolapse. Complications associated with the transvaginal mesh surgery include perforation of the bladder, bowel or blood vessels, erosion of the mesh into other parts of the body, pain, infection (sometimes fatal), increased urinary incontinence, painful intercourse, vaginal bleeding, vaginal shrinkage, and many others. As lawsuits for product defects and problematic surgical procedures increased exponentially, on July 13, 2011 the Food and Drug Administration (FDA) issued a public safety warning about potential risks and possible side effects involved with the transvaginal mesh procedure.

Before being enticed to have a surgery using mesh, or a surgery that would remove one of your vitally important organs, please exhaust all natural therapy options.

Performing Kegel exercises, a methodology named after Dr. Arnold Kegel, which has been recommended for decades, strengthens the pelvic floor and vaginal muscles. In addition to performing the basic calisthenics, Kegel weights offer a more strenuous routine and build muscle tone more effectively. Small, individual weights are placed inside the vagina in order to provide resistance against the contracting vaginal muscles. These weights are readily available from numerous online vendors.

Acupuncture, Chiropractic treatment, and other energy balancing techniques may also be helpful to restore energetic balance to your pelvic floor.

Tia's Story

Tia loved to run and play with her two small children in their neighborhood park. One afternoon as she tossed a red rubber ball to her son, Evan, she experienced an uncomfortable feeling within her lower abdomen, as if something had dropped inside. Her symptoms advanced to the point where her cervix noticeably began to protrude. Because of a dropping uterus, Tia was advised to undergo a hysterectomy.

Tia reluctantly consented to the surgery, only to discover a few months later, that her bladder had begun to drop! Obviously, the hysterectomy did little to change the situation. By now, Tia was beside herself. "What else can I do?" she cried in my office. "I don't want to have surgery again. Now, I have a new problem!"

Following Clinical Kinesiology testing, I used acupuncture, recommended specific nutrients, and made a few adjustments to Tia's spine. Her dropping bladder receded and the muscle tissue sufficiently restrengthened to support her bladder. Additionally, I recommended Tia take superoxide dismutase, a supplement designed to attack scar tissue.

Tia's story illustrates how easy it is, through natural methods, to change most situations, no matter how progressed.

Back and Hip Pain

During menstrual periods some women experience pain or cramping in the lower abdomen, back or both. Interestingly, the back may not hurt at any other time of the month, but the pain may flare up during the menstrual period. This type of pain, located in the lower body, again clearly illustrates the relationship between the uterus and referred pain areas close to the uterus. The lower back represents one such referred pain area and the hip another. These external pains, that seemingly have no other connection with the menstrual period, are actually referred pains from the female organs.

HYSTERECTOMIES: THE UTERUS/THYROID CONNECTION

Within one year, I treated Sonia and Eleanor for hip pain associated with hysterectomies they had received twenty years previous. As I worked with them I again pondered, "Why do so many women agree to such surgery?" Sadly, most base their decision for surgery on a desire to alleviate heavy menstrual bleeding, fibroid tumors, endometriosis, or other ongoing symptoms for which their doctors tell them there is no other cure.

For many women, however, hysterectomies prove devastating. Think about it. Part of the body is removed! And afterward, many women, like Sonia and Eleanor, find that the surgery didn't solve their problems after all. *It merely removed the focus of the worst symptoms.*

Surgeons removing a uterus don't really fix the energetic problem related to it. The uterus just happens to be the most symptomatic part. Meanwhile, the problem needs to be traced through the entire body system just as an electrician will search out the reason for a blackout in your home, or a car mechanic will test out the electrical system of your car. Only then can you expect to rebalance and "rewire" the energy needed to maintain the health of a symptomatic organ.

The body's electrical system runs like the compact car I drove while attending Chiropractic college in Portland, Oregon. A mysterious malfunction kept making the car's battery go dead. I immediately had the battery tested, along with the entire electrical system, and the mechanic assured me everything was fine. As a precaution, however, the mechanic recommended that I buy a new battery anyway. I did, and the car still wouldn't run. New battery cables? Negative results. Whenever the car was left sitting in a temperature below twenty degrees, it simply wouldn't start—even with a new battery and cables.

Finally, two mechanics, one new battery and new cables later—the solution! The car's "starter" had been the culprit all along and the cold temperatures merely provided added stress. I could have installed a new battery every day, yet, until the real electrical problem was uncovered, the car refused to function correctly.

The acupuncture system within the human body works exactly on the same premise as the electrical system of a car. A simple "short" someplace in the body's system may render the meridian unable to hold a charge. Until the basis for the "glitch" in the body's electrical system is discovered, the true problem remains unsolved.

Removing the end organ that ties into that electrical system renders the system unbalanced and unhappy. In addition, an energy spill-over may then occur. The spill-over of unbalanced energy may now affect the thyroid, causing new problems that weren't noticeable before—such as difficulties with temperature regulation or metabolism.

In case after case, more organ correlations can be drawn. As the connections are explored, an interesting pattern repeats itself. In my experience, hysterectomies send the body into an energy "black-out," if you will.

We've all seen the effects of a power outage followed by a return to normal: lights flash, digital clocks blink, alarms ring, and we have to go around and reset everything that was thrown off by the power outage. The same thing happens in the body. Not only *doesn't* the hysterectomy solve the imbalance; now, energy that normally flows from the meridian to the uterus has no place to go. Consequently, the removal of the uterus forces the energy to be diverted. This excess energy over-AMPs the thyroid, throws it out of proper function and, in a chain reaction, the thyroid then affects the heart.

What happens when there's no one around to re-balance or "reset" your body's electrical system? Serious organ/energy imbalances take a period of years to manifest in disease or disorders.

At this time, research money is very limited to evaluate further and document energetic healing and non-invasive diagnostic methods, such as Clinical Kinesiology. Sadly, until then, women will continue to be told that surgery is the only answer.

Menopausal Chain Reactions

I treat *absent* uteruses and *present* ones. In actuality, I'm treating the electrical system that connects to the uterus. Researchers have recently discovered that the uterus does indeed produce hormones.

A hormone message delivered to the thyroid might say, "The uterus is balanced and happy now and you, thyroid, can continue functioning as you are." Or, "The uterus isn't quite happy and you need to change your function." All hormones serve as messengers in your body telling glands and organs alike how to interact more harmoniously with each others. Make a drastic change in the body and you will experience repercussions. Whether the change involves something as serious as a hysterectomy, the removal of an ovary or something as seemingly routine as a tubal ligation, doctors are tampering with nature. Sara's case sadly demonstrates the menopausal chain reaction which can follow such tampering.

Many years ago, Sara consented to surgery to remove an ovary. Following the ovary removal, and I believe, quite uncoincidentally, two years later, a tubal pregnancy occurred requiring another surgery. The result was premature menopause in her thirties. Sara, now sixty-five, has developed serious bleeding. Her doctors, typically, have recommended a hysterectomy.

TUBAL LIGATIONS

Women considering any surgery on the female organs should be cautious, especially regarding tubal ligations. Often, following this type of surgery, the female system becomes extremely out of balance. Menstrual periods also become more difficult.

Fortunately, doctors do recommend fewer hysterectomies these days. Quite possibly, many of them are gaining some understanding of how seriously the body can be traumatized. Most medical doctors, however, still have little or no knowledge of the body's energetic system.

Acupuncture meridians are disturbed by tubal ligation surgery. Somewhere, something *changes* in the complex system of hormone communication. Damage occurs to the fallopian tubes which often results in the uterus becoming out of balance.

Research is unavailable to pinpoint the exact cause of the imbalance; however, the energetics that control the organ/meridian system (including the hormonal system) are disturbed. Like a house with too many appliances plugged into the electrical outlets, the body's circuitry becomes overloaded and it's electrical system (like the house's circuit breaker) flips off and shuts down.

Any time one experiences a major disruption or change in the body, it most likely triggers another organ imbalance as a result. It may not happen the next day. In fact, it may be months or even years later that questionable symptoms appear. At first you may not think, "Gee, ... *this* problem relates back to when I had *that* surgery." But many times it does.

RELIEF FOR MENOPAUSAL SYMPTOMS

Connecting all the pieces of the menopausal health puzzle includes recognizing and dealing with emotional changes and mood swings, together with physical symptoms. Awareness that such mind-body imbalances may be largely nutritional and stem from obtaining the right balance of vitamins, minerals, and amino acids provides an important first step. Supplementing the building blocks of neurotransmitters in the brain better regulates mood and helps allay physical symptoms.

Diet

A basic, healthy diet should be the core of your regimen. Eating fresh fruit, vegetables, grains, and drinking clear, pure water will do much to aid the functioning of the body. Many women feel like a weight has been lifted as they buoy up with more health and energy.

Evening primrose and black currant oil provide essential fatty acids which provide the necessary building blocks for a balanced hormonal system. Essential fatty acids also help the digestive process, enhance skin texture and moisture, and assist in joint lubrication. Both oils are commonly found in capsule form and are taken orally.

Flaxseed oil, another highly recommended oil, helps alleviate menopausal symptoms in the same way. In the cold-pressed liquid form, flaxseed oil taken orally helps lubricate the body and its tissues. It also fights inflammation by stopping excess build-up of irritating toxins and chemicals. Additionally, flaxseed oil naturally lowers the blood fat level in lessening the chance of arteriosclerosis following menopause. Coconut oil shares many of these attributes.

Foods and supplements high in calcium and magnesium, including dandelion greens, also supply needed nutrients during menopause. Current popular journals recommend twice as much, or even three times as much, calcium to magnesium. I believe there is a greater need to focus on the magnesium. Balanced multiple-mineral supplements provide overall support; additional specific minerals may be added at the body's "request."

Unfortunately, many women need to be reminded about diet because it's the one thing most tend to overlook. Healthy plants require good soil, sunlight and additional nutrients. Healthy pets thrive on the best quality food that can be found. Do the same for yourself and you'll set the groundwork for a much healthier menopause.

Glandular Supplements

Specific glandular formulas, based on protomorphogen therapy (tissue-derived concentrates which operate at a tissue specific level) originated in the early 1900s. Dr. Royal Lee was one of the first holistic practitioners to see the need for adding a glandular substance to help build and rebuild an imbalanced organ or gland.

For example, if an ovary tests weak, specifically designed glandular supplements may be used which support the ovary. If the uterus proves out of balance, another supplement formulated especially for the uterus may be beneficial. In cases involving a missing uterus, ovary or other organ, practitioners may use the corresponding glandular to provide additional support to the body. One mechanism for this support is that the glandular substance will provide a complement of all nutrients that this gland or organ requires.

The best quality glandulars contain organ tissue from livestock grown in New Zealand, an area still environmentally unpolluted. Another source is livestock raised on organic pastures. Although I'm a vegetarian, I do take glandulars to help build tissue in organs or glands that specifically need extra energy. The bovine glandular tissue of the uterus may contain some of the same hormones that I believe the uterus produces.

As mentioned, a present as well as an absent uterus may be treated with glandulars. With a missing uterus, the needed hormones and the glandular supplement can help the body to compensate. Glandular supplements for all the major glands and organs, including the heart, kidney, lung, may be found for sale in most holistic practitioners' offices. I recommend the Core-Level™ brand from Nutri-West®, formulated by Dr. Alan Beardall, the originator of Clinical Kinesiology muscle testing. Dr. Beardall experimented until he isolated the nutritional components which help balance a particular organ or gland. He then formulated a synergistic complement. Each glandular contains at least fifteen ingredients that include vitamins, minerals, amino acids, and herbs, and whole food substances (such as almond meal), making this brand quite different from most glandulars on the market. Core Level Uterus™ by Nutri-West is an excellent choice. (See Product Guide.)

Vitamins and Supplements For Menopause

The aging process (the wrinkling process included) may be characterized by the loss of oxygen from body tissues. As normal hormone production decreases, the body's oxidation process increases. Along with glandulars, the multi-vitamins, minerals (including potassium) and antioxidants such as selenium all work to strengthen the hormones. Germanium serves as an effective antioxidant mineral to help build immune system and tissue strength.

The wild yam root (a source of natural progesterone) also proves helpful for many women in giving a "kick-start" to a sluggish hormonal system. B-complex and vitamin C are also highly recommended for this same reason.

Each woman may be tested with Clinical Kinesiology to specifically determine what her uterus, thyroid or pituitary needs. It's important to know specifically which vitamins and minerals work best for you.

Herbal Teas and Tinctures

Licorice taken in herbal teas and tinctures proves quite effective for alleviating menopausal symptoms. It may be used as a uterine tonic to help the body make estrogen, counteract the effects of stress, and as an anti-inflammatory agent and detoxifying herb. Licorice is well known in Chinese medicine for its properties as a balancing agent. The root itself may even be chewed in some cases.

Raspberry and squaw vine may also be used to balance the female system at any time of life. Squaw vine, a Native American herb, helps the body make its own progesterone. Other tinctures, such as helonias root or false unicorn root, are also effective in balancing the uterus.

In addition, blue cohosh root and black cohosh root, (including the natural German estrogen replacement product, Remifemin™) taken in supplement form also help the uterus maintain proper balance. I suggest black cohosh for women who complain of hip pain—referred from the uterus. Even when no menopausal symptoms are present, black cohosh works well to strengthen and tone the uterus in many stages of life.

As mentioned previously, often when the uterus tests out of balance there is a thyroid connection. In order to rebalance the thyroid, women may use an herb called bladderwrack. Bladderwrack has a double identity in health food stores. It's used as an herb, under the name "bladderwrack," and in another aisle "bladderwrack" is known as "seaweed" or kelp.

HCL

Just as nausea normally accompanies the first trimester of pregnancy, it's also a menopausal symptom. Why? Because of continual fluctuations in the hormonal system. Balancing the hormones aids all the other glands in interacting better. Provide them the healthy diets and nutrients such as HCL (hydrochloric acid), and its likely symptoms of nausea will fade out.

Menopausal women, as most older people, tend not to produce sufficient quantities of hydrochloric acid in their stomachs. Hydrochloric acid tablets aid in proper digestion for menopausal women. However, some gastro-intestinal symptoms or distress may be early indications of a larger problem. Through individual testing with Clinical Kinesiology, we can investigate the need to help the digestive system and all other systems work better.

CLINICAL KINESIOLOGY TESTING

Through Clinical Kinesiology testing, you may glean as much information as possible regarding the body's reactions to different stimuli...whether it's food, medication, nutritional supplements or natural progesterone.

For example, on every woman I've tested, synthetic progesterone such as Upjohn's Provera®, renders the indicator muscle *consistently* weak. Synthetic estrogen, such as Wyeth-Ayerst's Premarin® doesn't always result in weak muscle tests; however, remember that the medication is only being tested at the current moment in time. Often, the *prolonged use* of a synthetic drug such as estrogen may later manifest problems or create imbalances in the body.

Every woman, no matter what her age or how advanced her menopausal symptoms, needs to build progress toward natural healing. Part of that progress may involve scheduling treatment with a local natural health practitioner. While self-testing may be used to gain familiarity with the female energetic system, it should not be used in lieu of professional treatment.

Testing the Female Energetic System

The following self-testing instructions may serve as a guide for further examination, for seeking more knowledge or as a preliminary check of your current health status.

Before proceeding with any Clinical Kinesiology testing refer to Chapter One for instructions on performing the Indicator Muscle Test. Once confirmation of a strong arm is determined, proceed as follows:

Hypothalamus Test

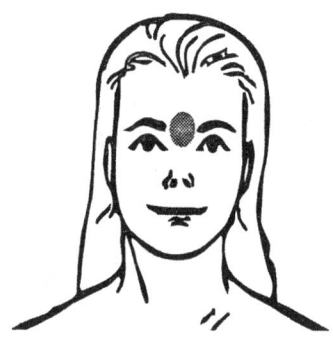

Any test of the female energetic system should begin with testing the hypothalamus. This small "organ" in the brain serves as the controller of other glands and organs and directs many body-regulating functions.

If out of balance, the hypothalamus may trigger erratic hunger and thirst patterns, wakefulness and sleep patterns, emotional disturbances, mood swings, and depression.

Test the hypothalamus by having the test-subject place the index finger directly at the bridge of the nose on the mid-line of the forehead, in the space between the eyebrows. The tester then performs the Clinical Kinesiology muscle test on the subject's opposite arm.

> Hypothalamus TL + Muscle test + Strong arm = Hypothalamus balance.
>
> Hypothalamus TL + Muscle test + Weak arm = Imbalance of Hypothalamus.

Should the test indicate the hypothalamus is out of balance, consult a Clinical Kinesiology or natural health practitioner who should be able to help rebuild and strengthen the hypothalamus function through acupuncture, nutrition, or other natural methods.

Thyroid Test

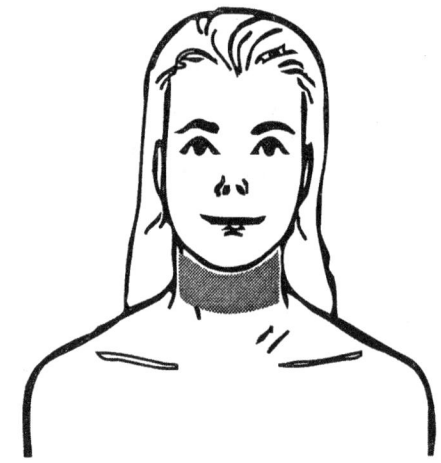

When testing the female energetic system for menopausal symptoms, it's first necessary to check the most relevant organs. The thyroid also plays a key role in balancing the female energetic system.

Problems with fluctuations or flow of the menstrual cycle or symptoms of approaching menopause, including hot flashes, usually indicate a thyroid malfunction. In order to test the thyroid balance, therapy localize over the thyroid by having the test-subject place an open hand over the front side of the throat, while you simultaneously muscle test the strength of the subject's opposite arm.

> Thyroid TL + Muscle test + Strong arm = Thyroid balance.
>
> Thyroid TL + Muscle test + Weak arm = Thyroid imbalance.

Follow up with a Clinical Kinesiologist, acupuncture, nutritional support and other treatment can strengthen the thyroid and change the imbalance.

Uterus Test

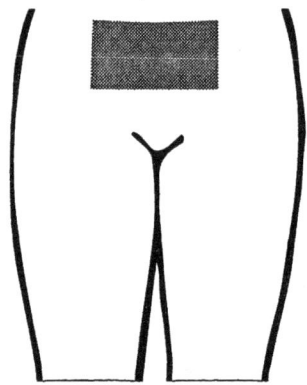

It's a good idea for any woman with female energetic problems to therapy localize over the uterus. To perform this test, the test-subject places the palm of the hand over the lower abdomen approximately three inches below the navel, while the tester checks the strength of the subject's opposite arm. Anyone who has experienced menstrual cramps or labor pains should have little problem locating the uterus.

> Uterus TL + Muscle test + Strong arm = Uterus balance.
>
> Uterus TL + Muscle test + Weak arm = Uterus imbalance.

Once again, a weak muscle test confirms that the uterus is energetically imbalanced. The test does not necessarily mean a fibroid tumor or any type of pathology or disease is present, simply that a uterus imbalance has been detected and you should consult your natural healthcare practitioner.

Ovary Test

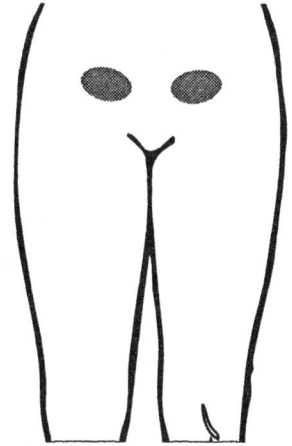

A post-menopausal woman should experience good overall health. Even after menopause, a healthy ovary should test strong, not weak. However, following a surgical procedure, some women retain only one ovary and, unfortunately, many times that ovary becomes out of balance. Whether a woman has both or only one ovary, if the test is weak, ovary supplements or glandulars may help strengthen the ovaries before, during or after menopause. It's difficult to therapy localize over the ovaries because they are so small, so be precise.

To locate the ovaries, place both hands on the waist. Slide hands in a downward V until thumbs reach the pointed bones of the hip with the fingers touching the pubic bone. Approximately midway along that V-line you will find the ovaries.

> Ovary TL + Muscle test + Strong arm = Ovary balance.
>
> Ovary TL + Muscle test + Weak arm = Ovary imbalance.

If you locate an ovarian imbalance, check with your natural healthcare practitioner for guidance and treatment.

Pituitary Test

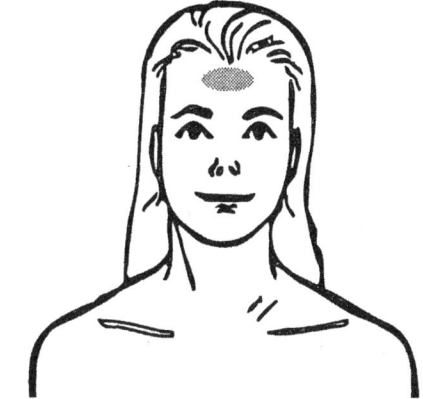

The pituitary may be tested by placing the hand two to two and one-half inches above the hypothalamus in the center of the forehead.

> Pituitary TL + Muscle test + Strong arm = Pituitary balance.
>
> Pituitary TL + Muscle test + Weak arm = Pituitary or hormonal imbalance.
>
> Consult a Clinical Kinesiologist.

All of the organs in the female energetic system relate to one another. Treatment often requires strengthening the pituitary, hypothalamus, thyroid, ovary, and uterus.

Troublesome menopause may stem from a lack of self-esteem, a stressful job, difficult family relations, insufficient exercise, or unhealthy eating habits. Every factor of environment, diet, and lifestyle impacts your life. Begin to benefit from reevaluating those factors more often as you explore Clinical Kinesiology diagnosis and natural treatment on your path to new healing for natural menopause.

While each individual proves different, women and men need to be appraised of each other's health concerns in order for both to reach a deeper understanding and fuller support of one another. Chapter 12, *The Male Energetic System*, is specifically devoted to optimal health for the male energetic system and educates male and female readers on steps to maintain overall health throughout life.

CHAPTER 11 SUGGESTED READING

Ford, Gillian. *What's Wrong With My Hormones?* Newcastle, Calif.: Desmond Ford Publications, 1992.

Hufnael, V.G. and S.K. Golan. *No More Hysterectomies.* New York: Penguin Books, 1989.

Lark, Susan M.D. *The Menopause Self Help Book.* Berkeley, Calif: Celestial Arts, 2000.

Laux, Marcus, N.D. and Christine Conrad. *Natural Woman, Natural Menopause.* New York: HarperCollins, 1998.

Lee, John R., M.D. and Virginia Hopkins. *What Your Doctor May Not Tell You About Menopause: The Breakthrough Book on Natural Hormone Balance.* New York: Warner Books, 2004.

Perry, Susan and Katherine O'Hanlan, M.D. *Natural Menopause: The Complete Guide to a Woman's Most Misunderstood Passage.* New York: Addison-Wesley, 1992.

Rodale, J.I. *The Healthy Hunzas.* Emmaus, Penn.: Rodale Press, 1948.

Weed, Susan S. *New Menopausal Years: The Wise Woman Way, Alternative Approaches for Women 30-90.* Woodstock, New York: Ash Tree Publishing, 2002.

Wolfe, Honora Lee. *Menopause: A Second Spring.* Boulder, Colo.: Blue Poppy Press, 1992.

Wood, Lawrence C. M.D., F.A.C.P. et al. *Your Thyroid, A Home Reference.* New York: Ballantine, 2006.

CHAPTER 12

The Male Energetic System

Two-day-old Michael slept peacefully, snuggling deep into his mother's arms. Suddenly, a pair of dutiful hands scooped up the new baby boy. "Just standard procedure," the nurse assured his mother.

Minutes later, an orderly wheeled baby Michael into a brightly lit operating room. Stripped of his warm gown and soft diaper, doctors strapped Michael's legs and arms onto a molded plastic board, much like a child's infant carrier.

The baby's eyelashes slowly began to flutter open as the doctor expertly affixed a stainless steel metal device to the little boy's penis. A sharp scalpel methodically spun around, surgically cutting the foreskin from Michael's body.

Instantly, tiny Michael began to scream.

THE STAGES/THE AGES OF MAN

From the first moments of life, men face increased susceptibility to cardiovascular disease, cancer, lung problems, liver ailments, and diabetes. Often, their reluctance to treatment results in higher rates of early illness and death. On average, men live seven years less than women.

While many new health issues for adult men are recently coming to light, I believe the key to maintaining healthy function begins at birth. For clarity, this chapter addresses health issues affecting the male energetic system organized by specific age categories.

Complete alternative healthcare of the male body begins with birth to age twenty (Stage One), and covers early issues such as circumcision, hyperactivity, bedwetting, and hernias.

Stage Two, early adulthood issues, involves the maintenance of a healthy and functioning genitourinary system. Topics in this stage range from hair loss, impotence, infertility and depression, to complications from vasectomy.

Middle and older age male concerns will be covered in Stage Three. Here we will explore general vitality, diet and stress-related disorders, digestion, and prostate problems.

Preventive measures include simple exercises, nutritional recommendations, suggested herbal and homeopathic remedies and Clinical Kinesiology self-testing procedures, which round out the care of the male energetic system.

STAGE ONE: BIRTH – TWENTY YEARS

Circumcision

Early parental choices often result in far-reaching consequences on the body and health of the male infant. Many times, these procedures set the stage for practices that affect men's health through adulthood, middle age and eventually old age.

Circumcision poses one issue which may have life-long effects significant to males. As many parents address the question of whether or not to circumcise a male child, many negatives should be weighed.

During my early student nursing career, I worked in labor, delivery and post-partum areas of the hospital. I was often required to be present and assist during circumcisions. In my opinion, the procedure is inhumane, harsh and difficult. First of all, circumcision is performed with no anesthetic of any type, and usually no parental presence or contact. During the procedure, the baby boys scream as if they are being injured—which they are.

Natural pain relieving measures, such as numbing the region with ice, could be undertaken during circumcision; however, the typical harsh tact remains, "It just takes a minute! It will be over with and then the baby forgets it." However, anyone who has witnessed circumcision would disagree with doctors who insist, "There is no pain," or, "Circumcision doesn't hurt."

Circumcision must be considered in light of the psychological trauma it may cause newborns. If not complete trauma, it may signal the beginning or seed of psychological trauma that may affect some men throughout life. How can one justify a circumcision which represents a defenseless little person being aggressively and unkindly treated in his first hours. How does one explain such unexpected pain? Many psychologists concur that often our earliest experiences do guide and mold individuals in later life. Personality, behavior, emotional patterns of responding and reacting may all be negatively influenced by this practice.

In some cases, circumcision may be done out of religious and cultural tradition, passed down through generations, stemming from the concept of "permanent cleanliness." In olden days, conditions were often unhygienic and circumcision seemed to provide a method for assuring cleanliness. We now know that this was flawed thinking from a biological perspective. Smegma is produced under the foreskin and serves as a natural lubricant, and contains lysozyme, a naturally occurring antibacterial enzyme. Some Jewish and Muslim families are reconsidering this tradition.

The most natural approach is to leave the little boy's genitalia intact, provide regular bathing, adequate diaper changings, and not retracting your infant's foreskin, which may cause premature tearing. Circumcision unquestionably causes pain and emotional trauma. If an uncircumcised adult male elects to undergo circumcision, this should be his own personal decision.

Male Emotional Health

Although naturally inborn differences exist between males and females, our culture often promotes these differences in specific ways which may manifest problems for males—particularly the social pressure on boys to follow certain occupations and conform to a model of male superiority.

Oftentimes, in grade school, one child may be compared with a room full of children. Other children may be reading at a certain level, retaining information and sitting quietly until called on. When a child does not fit this mold, he may be labeled as a learning disabled or an Attention Deficit Hyperactivity Disorder (ADHD) child.

Visible signs of ADHD are more noticeable among school age boys between first and third grades. Complicated and controversial to diagnose, hyperactive children usually lack self control, are inattentive, overly talkative, exhibit nervous mannerisms, impulsivity, and sometimes excessive irritability.

Hyperactivity may stem from sensitivities to foods, chemical additives and preservatives, excessive sugar intake, heavy metal toxicity and/or an imbalance of the hypothalamus.

Jamie's Story

"The principal will see you now," smiled the administrative assistant. Mrs. Edwards had been summoned by the school principal and a district psychologist after her seven-year-old son, Jamie, had been warned following several outbursts of disruptive behavior.

"We believe your son may have an attention deficit hyperactivity disorder," the psychologist began.

"Jamie?" Mrs. Edwards' flushed. "But, he's a smart boy."

"Mrs. Edwards," the principal continued, "Jamie exhibits an above average level of intelligence. We simply don't want to see that potential go unrewarded." Mrs. Edwards nodded.

The psychologist snapped close his briefcase. "We suggest you put your son on Ritalin ... if you want him to remain in school. Of course," he smiled, "the choice is entirely up to you."

At first, Jamie's mother was determined to follow an all natural treatment plan. Following Clinical Kinesiology evaluation and treatment of Jamie's hypothalamus with acupuncture, his anxiety calmed and family and school conflicts lessened. His attention span lengthened and previous sleep problems resolved.

Then suddenly, at Christmas, Jamie's mother started him on Ritalin. "I want him to be sitting down in January, taking notes, and paying attention," she said determinedly. "It will be better for everyone."

Ultimately, Jamie's mother ended up giving her son a drug. She had broken down due to the pressure school authorities were placing on her.

Will the drug enable Jamie to get to the root of the problem and heal his hyperactivity? No. With Ritalin, Jamie risks continued imbalance, possible addiction, and later withdrawal from the drug on which his body has become dependent. Unfortunately, medical researchers not only urge pediatricians to use Ritalin with ADHD children, but lately are recommending that doctors increase dosages from twice a day to three times a day to further relax the child.

Along with other side effects, Ritalin acts as a stimulant in adults. In many areas, parent's groups have formed to warn other parents, teachers, and the public of the Ritalin risk factors, including Ritalin withdrawal which triggers higher risks of suicide.

Help for Hyperactivity

Often, chemical imbalances in the brains of children with ADHD, such as Jamie, stem from nutritional deficiency, digestive disorders and the mother's diet while the child was in utero. The main factor in each indicates an energetic imbalance of the hypothalamus, which results in improper functioning of hunger and thirst patterns, wakefulness and sleep patterns, memory, moods, concentration and hormonal functions.

Hyperactive children often benefit from a Nutri-West® glandular, Total Brain™, which includes nutrients necessary for brain health. Such a comprehensive, nutritional supplement for this part of the brain may be helpful. Rather than using tranquilizing drugs, which merely cover up symptoms, natural supplements provide nutrients that the body utilizes to help balance itself. In addition, chemical drugs always alter or change the normal physiology of the body, while the inherent problem continues to degenerate below the surface.

Alternative therapies include totally natural treatments such as amino acid therapy, nutrients for the hypothalamus, a calming diet which excludes sugar, caffeine, food additives, and other stimulants. Supplemental vitamins needed may include niacin, Vitamin C, magnesium and zinc.

In addition, a diet high in complex carbohydrates, including whole grains, vegetables and legumes may be especially beneficial. Following these guidelines within a context of love and acceptance promises a good response for children who once exhibited hyperactivity problems.

I am not alone in asserting that "hyperactivity" is likely an inappropriate diagnostic term. Often I believe that the child is either suffering from "Physical Activity Deficiency" or "Sugar and Excitotoxin Overdose." Dr. Benjamin Feingold's (1899-1982) groundbreaking work spanning an era from the 1960s until his death is still relevant today. He demonstrated unequivocally that food additives including food colorings, preservatives, especially BHA and BHT, functions as excitotoxins and overstimulate the nervous system. More current corroboration exists, yet the pharmaceutical and education industries promote drug intervention as the only venue for help.

Bedwetting

Another emotional issue that affects many young school age boys (and girls) involves involuntary bedwetting during the night. Although bedwetting may indicate deeper, underlying problems, it may also stem from emotional stress, small or weakened bladders, over-consumption of liquids, heredity, or other behavioral issues.

Many children report that during sound sleep they often do not have an awareness of the need to urinate; therefore, don't wake up. However, bedwetting may serve as a psychological method of controlling or manipulating parents. Often, a bedwetting child may be feeling too constricted or regulated without understanding why. Subconsciously these children may think, "I'll show them! I'm going to make some work." Bedwetting remains an area that the child alone can control.

In other cases when children who previously had no bedwetting problem experience stress, trauma, or a change in their lives, bedwetting may suddenly occur. One young boy, Roger, never had a problem until he reached the age of thirteen. Then, suddenly, the bedwetting started. In Roger's case the emotional component does seem to have played a major role.

Bedwetting may also be linked to hypoglycemia, diabetes, urinary tract infections and food sensitivities. The biggest food factor to suspect in bedwetting stems from allergies to dairy foods.

One simple remedy for a bedwetting child may involve avoiding milk for several weeks. Milk contains tryptophan, which works as a relaxant. While some parents use milk to help a child obtain deeper sleep, many bedwetters have been found to be milk allergic. Upon elimination of milk, bedwetting may no longer be an issue.

Following Clinical Kinesiology evaluation, treatment for bedwetting often requires stimulation of acupuncture points on the Kidney Meridian and, occasionally, the Bladder Meridian. In diagnosing bedwetting problems, the kidney proves predominant in controlling more functions, which means it usually requires more help.

The bladder remains the stronger of the two organs. However, treating the kidney automatically helps the bladder. Other times, the bladder needs specific treatment, depending on the results of Clinical Kinesiology testing.

Helpful supplements include amino acids, magnesium, calcium, B-complex and a high quality multi-vitamin. Herbal recommendations include horsetail, St. John's wort, cornsilk, and lemon balm before bed. In addition, some parents find berberis, a homeopathic remedy, to be helpful.

Hernias

Some young boys are prone to develop hernias, which result from bulging of tissue through a weakened area of the abdominal wall. Hernias may also involve an organ or some portion of the intestinal tract.

Usually, Clinical Kinesiology testing indicates that inguinal or lower abdominal hernias relate to an imbalanced Kidney meridian. The muscles of the abdomen prove initially weak due to kidney stress. Hernias may be treated naturally without surgery following Clinical Kinesiology evaluation.

At the age of five, Benjamin developed a hernia in his lower abdomen. His doctor recommended immediate surgery to repair it. Two weeks after Benjamin underwent the surgery his mother discovered another hernia two inches above the previous one.

During Clinical Kinesiology testing, little Ben's kidney responded weak and his evaluation further indicated many nutritional deficiencies and hidden emotional imbalances. During a full year of treatment, Ben's hernia did recede; however, he continued to suffer from a myriad of emotional problems involved with his kidney.

Surgically fixing Benjamin's hernia did not attend to his deeper problem of the imbalanced kidneys. Continuing on the same path, Ben would merely keep repairing and repairing. Hernia surgery may temporarily patch up the problem, but it doesn't heal the underlying reason for the hernia.

Specific nutritional remedies for hernias include Core-Level™ Kidney™, various Kidney/Bladder herbals or tinctures including stinging nettle, goldenrod, horsetail, shavegrass, uva ursi, and juniper. Homeopathic remedies which may be used for the kidney are Renal Drops from Professional Health Products, or belladonna, lobelia, and atropine.

STAGE TWO: YOUNG MEN AGE 20 – 40

Teen Guidance

During male teenage years, important individual decisions that affect the rest of a young man's life begin to be made. Questions such as smoking, drinking, taking risks, or involvement in situations that may have long-term emotional, social and health consequences often carry a price. While parents should offer prior guidance and teaching, most times the final decisions rest on the free will of the male teen.

Unlike early Native American cultures which guided their young boys and men, our culture's response to the young male remains fairly amorphous. As a result, many teen males simply roll along with what the other kids are doing.

Young men need the opportunity and guidance to be able to choose a wise, healthy lifestyle. Without cultural care and attention to guide them, many young men often find it difficult to make the transition to manhood. Such "lostness" often leads to a high rate of teenage suicide, which has been increasing over the last several years. Young men ponder, "Where am I? What am I supposed to be doing? What are my values? What's the value of my health? My life?"

Teenage boys who make a commitment to being healthy can successfully walk that path and go forward. *But, they will not be walking the commonly tread path.* They will constantly have to fight the social compulsion to do what the rest of the crowd is doing. With regards to diet, for example, it is difficult in this fast food world—to say no! However, if parents can impart, "This is the healthful way to eat and live. This is *my* diet plan," and carry that through, young men will have strong role models to follow, and hence an easier time. When tempted, they can say, "I eat this way, simply and healthily!" Consequently, their peers will know where they stand from the beginning. No further explanations will be needed.

Boys who grow into adulthood without the information and role-modeling to make healthy decisions may eventually be faced with more serious underlying health issues. Patterns of neglect or abuse become set. What happens to men who aren't taught to pay attention to their bodies, listen to symptoms or have health checks? From age twenty to forty, signals being sent from the body may be saying, "Hey, I need help! I'm not quite balanced. Everything isn't functioning perfectly any longer."

Young men in this age category begin to notice definitive health glitches. Glandular and hormonal systems may not be functioning correctly. Organs may be breaking down due to energetic stressors. Often, this age group of men complain, "I just don't have the energy I used to have." or, "When I was younger I could do such and so, now, I'm too tired."

Hair Loss

One sign that the body may be out of balance is male pattern baldness. Hair loss, male pattern balding, hair thinning—many words describe this issue of concern to over thirty-three million American men.

According to the American Hair Loss Council, two out of every three men face balding by the age of fifty. Expensive hair loss clinics, scalp treatments, transplants, and the drug Monoxodil don't fix the problem. They really aren't addressing the bottom line of what's energetically gone wrong in the body.

While some hair loss can be traced to genetic abnormalities, in other cases diet seems to be the underlying cause. Dr. Paavo Airola, author of *Stop Hair Loss* cites countries such as Japan, China and Italy as cultures that exhibit little hair loss among men. Their diets of fruits, vegetables and grains, including seaweed, which is rarely eaten in U.S. culture, are linked to decreased hair loss.[1]

Healthy alternatives to cosmetic treatment for hair loss do exist. Clinical Kinesiology evaluation may identify one or more weak organs or systems that may contribute to hair loss. The kidney, liver, heart and thyroid are pinpointed most often. Most of the time, the primary organ imbalance involves the liver.

Tom was often complimented on his thick, black shiny hair. Suddenly at age thirty-eight, he began developing a large bald spot a couple of inches in diameter on one side of his head. When Clinical Kinesiology testing indicated an imbalance of his liver and thyroid, both were treated with acupuncture and specific nutrients. Tom's hair began growing back almost immediately.

In another case, Stan, a middle-aged man with thinning hair, experienced two serious episodes of stress involving an impending divorce and the death of a friend. Suddenly, his hair began falling out in handfuls. In Stan's case, the Clinical Kinesiology test determined that his kidney was the culprit.

As noted, hair loss may stem from a number of different organ weaknesses, or a combination of more than one. During Clinical Kinesiology testing of actual bald areas, the individual touches the scalp or area of concern. Then, the Clinical Kinesiology test may be performed to determine which organ is involved.

Many times, hair loss and other negative health factors stem from the cumulative effects of prescription drugs, poor nutrition, hormonal changes, or physical and emotional stress. It's that same old pattern of emotional stuffing—men holding in emotions which in turn stagnate the energy of an organ.

Additional remedies for hair loss include supplementing with antioxidant vitamins A, C, E, and biotin (which promotes both growth and strengthening), along with the mineral, silica, rich in the herb, horsetail.

Depression

An increasing number of men in the twenty to forty age group experience serious depression. The first question to ask regarding depression is: What's going on in these men's diets? Are they, like the hyperactive child, consuming sugar, coffee, artificial sweeteners, soda pop?

Along with hyperactivity, depression often stems from underlying imbalances in the hypothalamus and associated organs which may be confirmed through Clinical Kinesiology testing. Treatment involves acupuncture and supplementation with Core-Level™ Total Brain™, by Nutri-West® or other brain glandulars. Homeopathic drops may also be used for depression and anxiety, including specific Anxiety Drops, Anti-Depression Drops, and Neuro-Calming Drops by Mountain States Health Products. (See Product Guide.) In addition, homeopathic drops are available for insomnia, also a symptom of depression.

While homeopathics and nutritional supplements may be used as helpful assistants, emotional health stems from lifestyle and body balance. Help is readily available; however, many men desperately need to learn how to balance their obsession for work with a healthier, stress-reduced lifestyle.

Scott, a courier for a huge Colorado aerospace company, reported for work one morning. Without notice, his boss informed him, "You're going to Washington, D.C." An envelope was thrust into his hand with orders, "You are not to sleep while this is in your possession." No hotel room. No sleeping on the plane. Scott was warned not to let the top secret document out of his sight until he delivered it. Scott routinely made cross-country trips several times a month, at all hours of the night. It wasn't surprising that Scott developed increasing anxiety and depression after a year on the job.

Logic should tell Scott's company and its employees that something needs to be drastically reorganized, or a more healthful plan implemented to keep important people healthier longer.

In *The 7 Habits of Highly Effective People,* Stephen Covey relates the old fable of the goose that laid the golden egg. As the story goes: A farmer discovers a magic goose capable of laying golden eggs. Unsatisfied, the greedy farmer kills the goose to get all the golden eggs at once. Covey admonishes those businesses who continue to kill the goose—the good employee—simply to get the golden eggs.[2]

When the body balks, men are told, "Don't pay attention ... just keep on going." The body then wears down and men succumb to stress, depression, cardiovascular disease, stomach upsets, or cancer, and they die at much younger ages than their female counterparts.

The irony of it all? In fifty years, will anyone remember all the blood, sweat and tears that men have shed as a result of the pressures of their jobs?

Ulcers

The first symptoms of an ulcer involve an irritated stomach, or gastritis. The stomach simply doesn't feel good. "Stressed executive" often equals stomach pain. "Ah," the man complains, "I think I've got an ulcer." He schedules a visit with a doctor who may or may not recommend an upper gastrointestinal examination to confirm the problem. More than likely, the doctor recommends a pill or antacid drink to coat the stomach. Unfortunately, the antacid also slows down digestion, and guarantees that the man will no longer absorb any minerals out of his food. While it may placate the body into thinking the stomach feels better for a little while, what's really needed is *more acid* ... for digestion.

Few doctors test to evaluate, "Is there enough stomach acid? Too little? Is digestion functioning properly?" No, the stomach may be slightly upset, so the first thing doctors prescribe is an antacid.

Many men (as well as women) require extra hydrochloric acid, the natural acid produced in the stomach, to aid digestion. Otherwise, poorly or slow digesting food may become an irritant to the stomach lining. Taking antacids compound the problem, leading to an endless cycle that can quickly develop into an ulcer. *From my own personal case studies tested with Clinical Kinesiology, most of the people who develop an ulcer are the ones who have been taking antacids for a long period of time.*

Every now and then medical journals publish a new study that touts, "OK, now we've really figured out the cause of ulcers. It's a bacteria in the stomach. We'll call it helicobacter pylori." However, if the stomach contains enough hydrochloric acid *bacteria couldn't grow in the system in the first place.*

Do not attempt to stop your stomach from making acid. Many people (doctors included) are unaware that stomach acid remains a critically important factor in digestion and immunity. Strong stomach acid kills bacteria and prevents illness. It's supposed to be there.

My Clinical Kinesiology practice includes a specific test to determine if enough Hydrochloric acid exists in the stomach. Refer to the end of the chapter for self-testing procedures.

If you have an active ulcer, postpone the use of hydrochloric acid until the ulcer has healed. You will likely find relief by moderating your diet, and listening to your body for feedback about your dietary choices. Moderate, easily-digested foods will be most tolerated. This is the time to avoid jalapenos! Healing your stomach or intestinal lining may be facilitated by using aloe vera gel, the amino acid glutamine, mangosteen (as Xango® juice), gum mastic, or deglycyrrhizinated licorice, cat's claw herb, or probiotics. Choosing 2 or 3 of these items will be helpful. Avoid the licorice if you have high blood pressure. Use your Clinical Kinesiology skills to select your remedies.

Hiatal Hernia

What are the main reasons so many men don't make enough hydrochloric acid? Excessive stress, overeating or eating too fast, and/or not relaxing over an enjoyable meal are several contributing factors. A hiatal hernia is another.

An umbrella-shaped muscle, the diaphragm separates the thoracic cavity which holds the heart and lungs from the abdominal cavity, containing the intestinal tract. The diaphragm also includes an opening through which the esophagus connects with the stomach. This area is called the hiatus.

Pressure on the stomach often pushes it against the diaphragm. Then, the stomach may begin protruding through the hiatal opening into the esophagus triggering a condition known as a hiatal hernia. As a result, the hiatus can no longer prevent stomach contents—including strong acids—from moving upwards.

Symptoms of a hiatal hernia include a full feeling, heartburn and possible chest pain. Men who suspect this condition should specifically avoid overeating, spicy and fried foods, coffee, carbonated drinks and alcohol. To lower the risk for hiatal hernia, more fiber should be added to the diet in small meals throughout the day. Also avoiding drinking liquids during meals to allow for better digestion.

Physical manipulation of the stomach by a trained practitioner may release pressure on the hiatus. In addition, specific reflex and acupoints may be stimulated to help rebalance the process and retain function. Additionally, the stomach meridian may also need rebalancing.

Relief for hiatal hernia may be obtained through extra hydrochloric acid, supplemental digestive enzymes, vitamin B complex, liquid chlorophyll and aloe vera juice.

Burping, Belching, Bloating

In addition to hiatal hernias, many men suffer from burping, belching, and bloating, or a gassy overly-full feeling, after eating. If this condition lingers for an abnormally long period of time, it's probably an indication that the meal hasn't been properly digested. Again, additional hydrochloric acid may be needed.

People who experience diarrhea or vomiting also benefit from extra HCL. A female patient, Renee, suffered from diarrhea for a full year before obtaining treatment. She began to take two hydrochloric acid tablets after each meal, and the diarrhea went away. So, many aspects of digestion may be affected.

A gentian herb, known as herbal bitters, may also stimulate the body to make more hydrochloric acid. Bitters can be found in most health food stores. Also, apple cider vinegar and other fermented foods, such as sauerkraut and miso, prove to be important digestive aids which inspire helpful bacteria to grow.

Hemorrhoids

Men are especially susceptible to hemorrhoids—enlarged or varicose veins in the lining of the rectum. Men commonly require more treatment for bleeding, protruding tissues, itching, mucosal discharge, discomfort and pain than do women. Because of embarrassment, fewer men seek help for hemorrhoids resulting in a progression of symptoms and discomfort. Although women are also prone to hemorrhoids, men generally practice dietary and lifestyle factors which more often predispose them to hemorrhoids. Lifestyle factors which lead to hemorrhoids include excess caffeine intake—including coffee and soda pop—which irritates the kidneys. Improper digestion of proteins leading to constipation is another factor that promotes hemorrhoids. Constipation also means added back pressure which compounds distention of internal and external veins.

As with hernias, hemorrhoids most often occur in response to imbalances of the Kidney Meridian, which energy flows directly through the rectal area. Along with stroke, heart attack, and other vein problems, hemorrhoids may also be related to Heart and Circulation/Sex Meridians.

In general, recommendations for treatment include a high fiber diet including whole grains, vegetables, nuts, grains, and seeds. (This diet greatly diminishes the risk of chronic constipation.) In addition, good quantities of fluids (juices and pure water), along with a daily teaspoon of organic flaxseed or other healthful oil also help reduce the inflammation of hemorrhoids. Vitamin C with bioflavinoids, vitamin A, beta-carotene, B-complex and zinc are also beneficial. For immediate relief, sitz baths and Epsom salts baths reduce pressure and inflammation of hemorrhoids.

Treatment may also include stimulation of acupuncture points on the Kidney Meridians, specific kidney nutrients, homeopathic remedies for inflammation or specific herbal formulas for hemorrhoids. Also, rubbing the crown of the head is often helpful.

A.J.'s Story

A.J. developed a coffee-caused hemorrhoid problem at the age of thirty-five. The more incessantly he drank coffee, the more stressed his Kidney Meridian became. A.J. even underwent surgery to repair the damaged tissue; however, he continued to experience constipation and other kidney-related ailments.

Once he was finally able to give up coffee he began using a magnesium/oxygen supplement called OXY-OXC to ease his constipation. Without the coffee he managed to avoid irritating his kidneys any further and the hemorrhoids began to heal.

Men's Diets

Diet remains the root of so many male health problems. Men in the twenty to forty-year-old age group routinely pay less attention to their diets than women do. When looking at broad generalizations and parameters, it's fairly appropriate to say that men don't often take a great deal of responsibility in diet decision-making or family meal planning. The question that more men need to address is, "Am I eating this because it's good for my body, or simply because it appeals to my tastebuds?" Many men are easy targets of the fast-food world. Under pressure in the job, driving here and there, busy men may only have a short time for lunch. They want something quick, and don't want to have to cook it! Thus, some men eat on the job or while they drive to the next appointment. This need for "convenience" lures them into fast-food chains more than any other group. That in itself is an occupational hazard!

It's well documented that fast foods contain more high-fat/high-salt content and overcooked fats (believed to be carcinogenic) than other foods. As of late, many fast-food restaurants have amended their menus to include healthier items; however, from what I see of men in regards to their health and diet when they come in for treatment, most of them don't seem to be ordering those healthier items.

Men would do well to start bringing their own healthy lunches to work, possibly leftovers from the previous night's dinner or some healthy, wholesome foods. Frequenting a salad bar or other more naturally-orientated type of restaurant or health food store can make a big difference.

Infertility

The basic level of diet and health has also been linked to today's steadily increasing infertility rates among both males and females. Infertility remains an emotionally charged issue. Fifty percent of the time, the reason a couple cannot conceive has been traced to the man. Often it's hard for men to admit, "Maybe there's infertility because something is out of balance in my body."

In *The Wisdom of Amish Folk Medicine* by Patrick Quillin, Ph.D., R.D. reported that folk medicine from this German sect suggests that both men and women should consume a daily tablespoon of carrot seed oil and wheat germ oil. This oil is concentrated in vitamin E, which does help the reproductive system and process.[3]

The Amish also recommend that men consume large amounts of alfalfa sprouts, which provide minerals, enzymes and other concentrated nutrients. Various other remedies include eating pumpkin seeds or taking a daily zinc supplement. Additional vitamin B_{12} up to 6,000 micrograms is also beneficial. Other recommendations include adding vitamin C or the amino acid L-Arginine to the diet.

A healthy diet does have a significant impact on the male reproductive system. With a poor diet today, a man's body has a difficult time simply struggling with its own health. When asked to deal with reproduction, it doesn't have the strength or stamina to produce the right balance of substances necessary to procreate.

The Pottenger Study

Dr. Francis Pottenger conducted a pioneering study of dietary effects on cat mortality in the 1940s.[4] Pottenger fed one group of cats devitalized, dry, commercially produced cat food. Another group was fed an all-natural, raw meat diet along with a tiny bit of vegetable matter, similar to the diet of a cat in the wild. Pottenger then studied the cats for several generations. The results of the experiments indicated that the synthetically fed cats produced a significantly lower number of second-generation kittens with lower birth weights than the naturally fed cats. The longevity of the adult cats was also shorter with the synthetic diet; their infant-mortality rate was significantly higher than that of the cats fed the natural diet. After only three generations of eating synthetically produced foods, all of the cats died out. The naturally fed cats on the healthy diet maintained the same birthrate throughout the three generations.

Among the findings, Dr. Pottenger concluded that the diet of the parents genetically altered the offspring. Genetically weakened offspring result in a decline of strength and less aptitude for healthy procreation. Applying these findings to human males, the extrapolation is that infertility may stem from the current diet and from diet patterns passed down genetically through an individual's parents.

A study in the British Medical Journal which evaluated sixty-one studies from 1938 to 1991 reported that sperm counts had dropped fifty percent over fifty years. The study cited lifestyle factors, diet, the use of prescription drugs (Tagamet® is specifically documented), toxic chemicals, and even synthetic clothing as primary causes for lowered sperm count.[5]

Bitter Herbs

Herbs that combat infertility include saw palmetto which helps increase sperm count and sperm motility, burdock, ginseng, licorice root, hawthorn, ginkgo, gentian, sarsaparilla, mugwort, yarrow, wild yam and goldenseal. Bitter herbs, such as gentian, mugwort, yarrow and goldenseal are listed in *The Male Herbal* by James Green, who discusses the importance of using bitter flavors in a healthy culture.[6]

People in the U.S. culture avoid bitter tastes, however. Many addict themselves to beer, coffee and chocolate as a result of few opportunities given to eat bitter foods. In these cases, sugar is added to the mix, making the bitter unhealthy.

Green correlates the bitters with the Chinese Five Element Theory, stating that bitter herbs are specifically beneficial to the Fire Element containing the Heart Meridian or cardiovascular system, and the Circulation/Sex Meridian, which regulates hormonal production in the body.

Further treatment for infertility as a result of imbalances in the male glands and organs may require acupuncture, and nutrients for building up the tissue and health of the testicles and prostate, specifically.

Vasectomy

While infertility poses problems affecting men and women equally, family planning has long been an issue relegated to women. Then, in the 1970s a new surgical procedure promised men more control, more responsibility in family planning and birth control. Millions of men rushed to have vasectomies performed. Today, however, important new health issues are coming to light regarding vasectomies that need to be addressed for men.

Doug's Story

Doug and Veronica both agreed that he would undergo a vasectomy after the birth of their third child. The fairly painless procedure took only minutes and Doug went home from the clinic feeling fine.

About a year and a half later, however, Doug began to notice extreme weakness and obvious weight loss. As the months went by, he began to feel sicker and sicker. Friends and acquaintances were shocked at Doug's decline in health. His wife became alarmed to the point where she felt he must be suffering from a serious undiagnosed cancer.

Together, Doug and his wife consulted doctor after doctor. None could pinpoint the problem. Eventually, he became so concerned that he put himself on the Gerson Cancer therapy program.[7] He detoxified his body, ate a macrobiotic diet, but nothing worked. Doug was dying and no one knew why.

Finally, Doug visited a female colleague of mine who suggested that Doug may have become allergic to the sperm build-up in his body as a result of his vasectomy several years before. She urged him to have the vasectomy reversed, which he did. At once, Doug's immune system recovered and he began to get well.

Dangers of Vasectomy

The safety of vasectomy has yet to be determined. First of all, vasectomy is surgery, and complications and the risk of side effects exist with any surgery.

In a normal male, sperm is continually being made in the body. With vasectomy, the body retains the sperm, which now has no normal route out of the body. In turn, the sperm may now build up in the system. Seminal fluid build-up may then prompt the body to begin manufacturing antibodies against its own sperm. Reacting as though the sperm isn't a friendly or normal function or tissue, the antibodies cause some men to become quite ill. Such a chain of events may lead to environmental illness, immune system disorder, and serious autoimmune problems.

Men who have undergone vasectomy may also be more vulnerable to impotence in later years. Although impossible to predict, it is something that also needs to be monitored closely. Again, vasectomy should not be undertaken lightly. Every man needs to weigh the potential risks and problems that could develop before undertaking this or any other surgery.

Natural Treatment for Vasectomy Scars

In cases where scar tissue develops, treatment includes concentrating a large, soft laser on the scar, which helps diminish any further perineal scarring. In addition, rubbing vitamin E oil over vasectomy scar tissue nightly, allowing the oil to soak in, is helpful especially where there's been an incision. Castor oil packs are also useful when heated a bit.

Acupuncture may also be used directly on the surgical incision or any other large cut that's healed. The nutrient superoxide dismutase may also be used to combat the formation of scar tissue.

DETOXIFICATION: FOR ALL MEN

The most common men's health problems involve the male genitourinary system. Disorders include impotence, complications from vasectomy, enlarged prostate, prostatitis and prostate cancer. As these growing health concerns are imperative to the complete health of the male body, they must be readily addressed.

With many types of male infertility or other health problems, one of the first things a man needs to do is detoxify his "total" body. Various helpful cleansing methods and flushes exist, for which men may want to refer back to the women's chapter on PMS.

Toxicity takes so many forms. Food sensitivity, metal toxicity, mercury fillings, lead poisoning, or occupational hazards which expose workers to various toxins on a daily basis need to be addressed. Men who labor in heavy industry, in mechanical trades, in chemical labs, or near asbestos, or in plants where chemicals are used on the job need to be aware of the risks.

Traditionally, men are exposed to more chemical hazards than women. There are homeopathic remedies to purge toxic chemicals out of the system. Another remedy, Metal-Xeno by Mountain States Health Products is good for purging heavy metals. (Refer to the product guide at the end of this book). Clinical Kinesiology testing may be used to test for particular heavy metal toxicity and to see which homeopathic remedy works the best.

Although many health problems have a basis in toxicity, it's only one piece of the puzzle. Detoxification specifically helps promote the highest level of health and longevity possible. On a daily basis, it's a protective measure also.

My male clients ask, "Should I detoxify for one month, six months, a year?" I tell them there is no magic number: "You must detoxify until your body is clean." Some preparatory work in detoxification includes drinking huge quantities of fresh, pure water.

The liver remains one of the most important organs that benefits from detoxification. Dandelion root and milk thistle herbs prove to be powerful, simple steps that can be taken to ease the way into a longer, more specific detoxification plan. Since detoxification principles and pathways are similar for men and women, you may want to refer to Chapter 10, *Premenstrual Syndrome*, for more information and specific cleansing procedures.

Saul's Story

Saul was a man deeply in need of detoxification. One Friday afternoon he hobbled into my office hoping to get some relief from severe knee pain before playing in a weekend golf tournament. In addition to his painful knees, Saul's Clinical Kinesiology test indicated prostate problems.

For three or four successive Friday afternoons, Saul's treatment entailed stimulation of acupuncture points on his Liver Meridian along with herbal supplements. As always, he jovially looked forward to his upcoming golfing weekend. Each week, as Saul slid off the treatment table he'd casually remark, "Gotta go ... I have to pick up a case of beer for the cookout before tomorrow's game."

"Hmmm," I began thinking, "Saul drinks beer after each treatment and comes back still complaining about his knee and prostate. We're not getting anywhere here."

Finally, I suggested that Saul attempt a few weeks without drinking beer to reestablish balance of his liver and allow us to work more effectively on his prostate, since treatment of these two go hand in hand.

Saul never came back. Ultimately, that was his decision to make. Each person's response is influenced by his own priorities. Only Saul could decide what was truly important as far as his own individual health and well-being.

STAGE THREE: AGES 40 AND OVER

Impotence

Impotence currently affects over ten million men in the United States. Although it is not solely a problem of men over forty, it will be considered here because it has been traced to prolonged usage of prescription drugs, high blood pressure, arteriosclerosis, prostatitis, diabetes, Multiple Sclerosis and Parkinson's disease—problems found more often in the older man. In cases where impotence becomes a factor in infertility, I consistently find a strong link to imbalances of the Kidney Meridian.

An estimated eighty percent of impotence may also be related to emotional or psychological imbalances, including low self-esteem, performance anxiety, and depression.

Following Clinical Kinesiology evaluation, stimulation of Kidney Meridian acupoints, specific herbal remedies for impotence may include: yohimbe, ginkgo biloba, muira puama, saw palmetto and ginseng.

Prostate

An important centrally located organ in the male energetic system is the prostate gland. Endocrine dependent, the glandular system must be working effectively to keep the prostate gland functioning well.

Proper prostate function begins with the hypothalamus, which represents the part of the brain that controls the pituitary gland. In turn, the pituitary regulates other glands and sends messages to the thyroid. The chain of command is: hypothalamus to pituitary to thyroid to prostate ... etc.

The size of a walnut, the prostate secretes a milky protein fluid that is discharged into the urethra during the emission of semen. This fluid then mixes with the semen to transport the sperm out of the body. Generally, the prostate has a thick, muscular wall. During enlargement of the prostate, a hypertrophy or thickening of the prostate wall causes it to become much larger than usual.

By age fifty, nearly thirty percent of men may begin to notice problems with urination due to prostate imbalances. Because the prostate surrounds the lower bladder and upper urethra, symptoms of prostate enlargement involve more frequent urination, a slowing or change in force of urine stream, incontinence or dribbling.

Medical doctors often perform a "transurethral prostatectomy" (TURP) procedure which temporarily relieves symptoms of an enlarged prostate. An electrified blade "scores" out the central part of the prostate and the obstructing tissue is removed in an attempt to make a larger space for the passing of urine through the urethra. This procedure is traumatic and not necessarily successful. Complications can include sexual dysfunction and scarring of the urethra causing recurrent blockage. Men who've gone through it once often end up having it done again. And, again.

Imagine a prostate with tissue out of balance, added pressure from constipation, insufficient circulation in the pelvis, and nutritional deficiencies. It all adds up to prostate problems.

The prostate gland does not have its own acupuncture meridian. Rather, it shares energy with the Liver Meridian, which traverses both sides of the body, with two halves crossing over in the mid-pelvic area.

As one views the male and female body anatomically, the organs are basically the same. Both male and female have a single organ in the midline of the body—the prostate in males and the uterus in females are analogous or comparable organs. Each of these organs shares the Liver Meridian with the liver.

The prostate is also a gland which makes hormones. (In my opinion, many of those hormones have yet to be discovered.) A relationship in women (mentioned in the Premenstrual Syndrome and Menopause chapters) exists between the thyroid and the uterus. Although more clinical research is needed, I believe a corresponding relationship is also likely to exist between the thyroid and the prostate in men. Because the uterus and prostate are analogous organs—same location, same hookup to the meridian system and the nerves—it's logical to assume the same relationship exists in both sexes. Helping a man's thyroid likely helps his prostate.

Lyle, an eighty-year-old patient, has had two surgeries to reduce the enlargement of his prostate. Prior to the surgery, he had been on thyroid medication for many years. In my opinion, the thyroid weakness contributed to his prostate problems to some degree.

Lyle now takes an herbal/vitamin-based nutrient with good success. In fact, on his last medical evaluation, his ultrasound showed no increase in the enlargement of his prostate gland.

One mineral especially helpful for the prostate is zinc. Men typically need more zinc than women. Acne or other skin lesions can be traced to a zinc deficiency.

Signs of a zinc deficiency include white dots on the fingernails, low resistance to infection and immunity problems.

Prostatitis

The *Male Herbal* contends that," Men push their worries into their prostate."[8] Indeed, a common prostate problem is prostatitis, caused by inflammation or infection of the prostate, which may be irritated by cold, dampness, prolonged sitting, excess alcohol, caffeine, or hot spices.

Symptoms of prostatitis include difficulty in urination including frequency or urgency, muscosal discharge from the urethra, along with a burning sensation. Severe symptoms may involve pain and tenderness, pressure or throbbing in the rectal area, fever, chills, and general fatigue. Prostatitis may occur due to bacteria in the urine or auto-immune disorders stemming from a lack of zinc, vitamin C, and specific enzymes which thwart infection.

Although huge doses of antibiotics remain the standard medical treatment for prostatitis, simple, natural measures work just as well, and do not lead to other problems from the medication. For many cases of prostatitis, goldenseal herb proves wonderfully healing. The herb echinacea works as an immune system builder for prostate infections and inflammations, along with pipsissewa, uva ursi, and horsetail.

Saw palmetto remains a good preventive herb for enlarged prostate and prostate infection. Men who are suffering from any prostate problems should begin taking saw palmetto on a daily basis for an indefinite period of time. This herb specifically nourishes the prostate and increases its health and resistance to disease. Saw palmetto is available in capsule or tincture form, along with combinations of other nutrients.

Prostate Cancer

Since around 1995, the second leading cause of death in men (following skin cancer) was prostate cancer.

Aside from non-melanoma skin cancer, prostate cancer is the most common cancer among men in the United States. It is also one of the leading causes of cancer death among men of all races ... In 2010 (the most recent year numbers are available)—196,038 men in the United States were diagnosed with prostate cancer.*† 28,560 men in the United States died from prostate cancer.*†

*Incidence counts cover about 97% of the U.S. population; death counts cover about 100% of the U.S. population. Use caution when comparing incidence and death counts.

†Source: U.S. Cancer Statistics Working Group. United States Cancer Statistics: 1999–2010 Incidence and Mortality Web-based Report. Atlanta (GA): Department of Health and Human Services, Centers for Disease Control and Prevention, and National Cancer Institute; 2013. [9]

How do men develop prostate cancer? It's not a condition that suddenly sneaks up and appears one day. With few detectable physical symptoms, prostate cancer stems from an energetic imbalance and improper function, poor nutrition, poor circulation, and genetic and hormonal factors which disallow prostate health. Healthy prostates do not develop cancer. They must first become unhealthy, be debilitated and function improperly to allow cancer to take hold in the body.

Poor diet has been linked as one major cause of prostate disease. Anyone with prostate problems should avoid caffeine, alcohol, spicy foods, tobacco, high-fat, high-carbohydrate foods. Also, avoid prolonged sitting. Such periods of inactivity result in a weakening of muscles of the pelvic floor, which proves harmful for the prostate. Poor nutrition, poor circulation and electromagnetic imbalances which go unaddressed lay the groundwork for the types of serious imbalances which support cancer. In early stages, the prostate may contain only a few cancer cells. Normalizing any prostate problem early, and getting that organ as functional as possible, protects from cancer developing or taking hold. The job of a healthy immune system is to purge cancer cells out of the body.

Natural methods do exist to rebalance the prostate gland and return it to normal function. The book *Third Opinion* by John M. Fink provides options to standard chemotherapy or radiation treatment. The author offers a listing of holistic health cancer clinics all over the world including the Hoxsey Cancer Clinics.[10] The late Harry Hoxsey, N.D. developed successful alternative cancer treatments still used today.

Preventive therapy remains the key to a healthy prostate. Don't risk being examined at a local health fair at age fifty-five and being told, "Your prostate feels abnormal." Instead, from ages twenty to forty concentrate on maintaining a healthy diet, exercise, stress-free lifestyle, and preventive therapies, including Clinical Kinesiology testing to assure that the organs and energetic balance of the prostate remains healthy for life.

Healing the Prostate

Healing the prostate often requires treatment of the Liver Meridian, which may be strengthened by acupuncture, along with specific vitamin and herbal supplements. B-complex, vitamins C, D, E and garlic are crucial to prostate health. Essential fatty acids, including flaxseed oil which contains a good balance of Omega 3, 6, and 9, also foster good hormonal balance.

For its antibacterial and cleansing effects, men need more of the mineral zinc, found in high concentrations in seminal fluid. As semen leaves the body, the zinc concentration in the body becomes depleted. Calcium, copper, iron, potassium, magnesium, selenium, silicon, and sulphur are also recommended.

The prostate may also be strengthened with Oregon grape, echinacea, uva ursi, couch grass, saw palmetto, pipsissewa, cornsilk, marshmallow, comfrey, horsetail, hydrangea root. Also, milk thistle, dandelion root or a combination of the two. In addition, beets and beet greens and juice, carrots and carrot juice are natural cleansers.

Besides the herb saw palmetto, the Core-Level™ Prostate™ by Nutri-West®, Palmetto-Plus™ by Biotics®, as well as other male glandular supplements are also available for the prostate. A sometimes difficult-to-find herb known as flowering willow herb, from an old European treatment for prostate enlargement, is common in Europe and thought to be wonderful for the prostate.

Exercises for the Prostate

The following three-part Kegel exercise has been used by many men to stimulate circulation, restrengthen the pelvic floor and rebalance the prostate.

Exercise Position: Lying down on your back, raise the pubococcygeal muscle or PC muscle, (which runs from the pubic bone to the coccyx) by raising the lower back and the back of the pelvis off the ground.

- Attempt to contract the PC muscle up into the body for a slow, clenched count of three and then relax. Or,

- Rapidly clench and relax the PC muscle as quickly as you can. Or,
- Push or bear down with the PC muscle using moderate pressure for a count of three, and then relax.

Begin with only a few repetitions daily and build up as you build muscle strength.

Massage

While the simple exercises above strengthen the pelvic floor muscles, men may also massage the deep muscles around the perineum in the lower abdomen between the scrotum and rectum with the thumb or forefinger.

This massage may be done regularly as a preventive measure; however, it is not recommended during cases of prostatitis as it may spread the infection. In combination with massage, I suggest use of a natural progesterone cream, or wild yam root to augment the healing.

Sitz Baths

Another method of relieving pressure around the prostate involves taking hot and cold sitz baths. Alternating hot and cold water baths, similar to applying a hot and then a cold pack, affects the prostate and can be helpful.

One source suggests using a plastic basting syringe to insert the water into the rectum, which is in close proximity to the prostate. Be sure to first test the hot water on the skin so it doesn't burn delicate tissues.

Kegel exercises, massage, and sitz baths are some of the easiest self-help remedies to heal the prostate. Also, be sure to check the Liver Meridian, apply acupressure, and work on any tender points that may be found. Or, once acupuncture points are treated professionally, follow up by rubbing those points on your own. You can use these simple procedures to strengthen weak organ systems and thus achieve added vitality and the ability to ward off specific diseases.

SELF-TESTING THE MALE ENERGETIC SYSTEM

Prostate Test

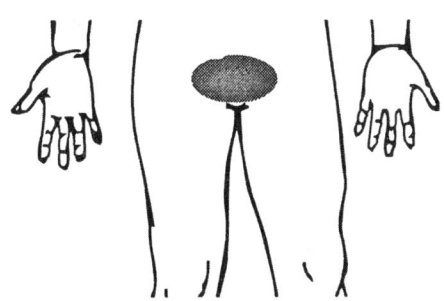

Following self-evaluation of prostate symptoms, utilize the aid of a partner/tester to follow up with a Clinical Kinesiology therapy localization over the prostate area.

Before performing any Clinical Kinesiology muscle test, a preliminary Indicator arm muscle test should be completed. See Chapter 1 for instructions.

Following confirmation of a strong Indicator muscle, the Prostate test may be done by having the test-subject place one hand over the lower front abdomen. (Since this area is also near the bladder, any bladder problem may also present a positive test.) As the person being tested touches the area, the tester performs the muscle test on the test-subject's opposite Indicator arm:

> Prostate TL + Muscle test + Strong arm = no current prostate or bladder imbalance.
>
> Prostate TL + Muscle test + Weak arm = possible prostate or bladder imbalance.
>
> Seek guidance or further testing from a natural health practitioner.

If you're unsure of the prostate test results, obtain a good quality saw palmetto herb in capsule or tincture. If therapy localization over the prostate rendered the indicator muscle weak, retest while holding the herb over the same area.

Prostate TL with Saw Palmetto + Muscle test + Strong arm = Prostate needs supplementation with the herb. Bladder problem has been ruled out as the primary issue.

As always, any positive self-test including symptoms should be followed up with professional evaluation by a natural practitioner or other physician.

Hypothalamus Test

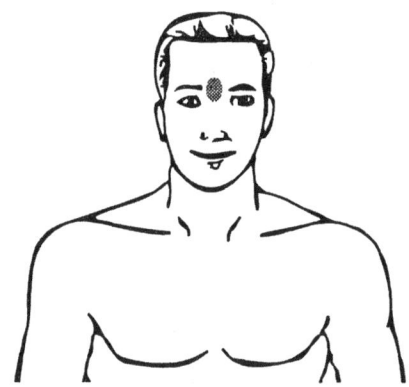

Depression, hyperactivity, and impotence may be pinpointed by self-testing the hypothalamus.

Use two fingertips (the index and third finger) which cover a larger area than one finger. Place them mid-line on the forehead between the eyebrows and over the hypothalamus and perform the Clinical Kinesiology muscle test.

Hypothalamus TL + Muscle test + Strong arm = no current imbalance.

Hypothalamus TL + Muscle test + Weak arm = imbalance of hypothalamus.

Consult a trained natural health practitioner for further testing and treatment recommendations.

Hydrochloric Acid Test

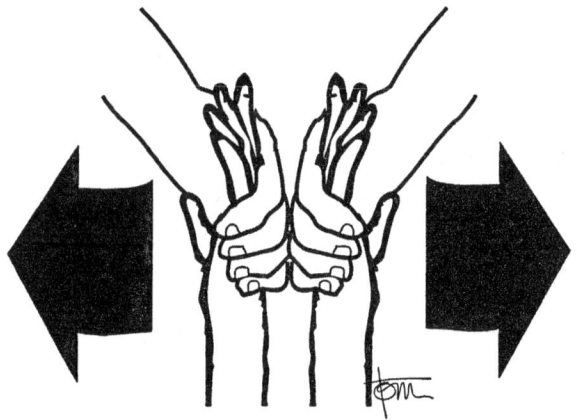

To evaluate the need for additional hydrochloric acid/HCL or to check for less than optimal digestion, perform a bi-lateral, pectoralis major muscle-strength test. This test is best done lying flat on the back. It's difficult to obtain an accurate test while standing.

Once the test-subject is lying down, ask him or her to place the back sides of the hands and wrists together, with the elbows straight. Instruct the person being tested to hold the arms perpendicular to the body or at a ninety degree angle. While the person being tested attempts to maintain the backs of the hands together, the tester firmly tries to pull the hands apart, or separate them.

The pectoralis major is the group of muscles being used to control the hands. Any hydrochloric acid deficiency may be pinpointed in this way.

> HCL Pectoralis major test + Muscle test + No hand separation = no HCL supplementation needed.
>
> HCL Pectoralis major test + Muscle test + Hand separation = need for HCL supplementation.*
>
> *As a double check, place a bottle of HCL on the stomach after an initial weak muscle test. Retest with the HCL in the energetic system of the body. If the hands remain closed with the HCL, it's confirmation that the stomach requires more hydrochloric acid for digestion.

Dr. George Goodheart originated the pectoralis major test during the formulation of Applied Kinesiology.

Along with hydrochloric acid, a number of digestive enzymes may also be tested in the energetic system to further pinpoint one or more combinations of supplements.

FATHERHOOD

Not all men experience fatherhood, but for those who do, it may be their greatest achievement and their proudest triumph. Nearly all fathers take great pride in passing on their names, beliefs, practices, and hopefully only the best of their personal traits. The responsibility of fathers may be different from that of mothers, but it is no less special a bond, nor any less sacred a role.

The miracle of parenthood often brings out the best in people, both women and men. Motherhood has traditionally been associated with gentle nurturing characteristics, while fatherhood has been more closely identified with disciplining and coaching. In some families, these traditional roles are still evident, but often in today's society, parents are relishing *all* aspects of child rearing, rather than being fixed in specific gender roles. In today's world, fathers may no longer be just the bread winners, but instead may be active participants in all aspects of raising their children. Just as mothers, fathers are called to be loving, nurturing, encouraging and playful.

Stay-at-home dads are more common in today's world. These days, along with teaching their children to build tree houses, play ball, or ride bikes, as well as the important lesson that scraped knees are not only okay, but badges of courage. Dads are modeling how important forgiveness, kindness, and love are. Some dads are even the main "teachers" in homes where parents have opted to home-school their children.

There is no doubt that the relationship between father and son is one of the most special bonds. Dads teach their sons how to be *men*, passing on lessons of strength, perseverance, bravery and hard work. In today's world, parents—fathers *and* mothers—are teaching these same lessons to their daughters. These "hands-on dads" are helping to create future generations that have strong characters, kind and respectful natures, and the ability to think critically.

Trillo is a father determined to help his children start off on the right foot. He is one member of a family that I have treated for four generations, including his grandmother, mother, siblings, and now his wife and children. Here is what he had to say about this aspect of fatherhood:

> The sights, smells, and overall feeling of *home*, complete with mommy and daddy lovingly caring for them, are the first things to greet our children in this world, and believe me, it shapes them. My wife and I have four children, all born in our home, all caught by dad. We were well

trained and educated about this life-event (notice I didn't say "medical emergency"), and we were confident doing what came naturally. Maybe homebirth is for you, maybe not, but learn about your options. You just might find it beautiful after all.

I have many patients, including Nate and his wife Melinda, who chose homebirth for their families. Here is what Nate had to say about his experience.

It was important to both my wife and me that we share the experience of parenthood as equally as possible, including the time during pregnancy and labor. We chose to have homebirths for all three of our children. I was the main support to my wife, acting as the nurse, as well as the birthing coach, and supportive husband. It's hard to put into words the magnificent awe I felt witnessing and actively participating in the delivery of each of my children. The overall feeling of wholeness and joy can only be described as miraculous and holy. Many fathers-to-be may be fearful or uncomfortable about homebirth. Having a midwife involved throughout the pregnancy and birth is a great comfort. We learned so much from our midwife, and are so grateful to her. The most important thing for dads to do is be supportive and active in the process and the decision making. It's been nearly five years since our youngest child was born. I'm now sharing home-schooling responsibilities with my wife, and I am able to stay home with my kids three days each week. The bond that was created in the first moments after each of my children was born—I was the first to hold each of them—grows stronger each day.

As you will read in the next chapter, fathers play an important role in all aspects of parenthood, even before conception. Nate and Melinda took time to prepare themselves emotionally, physically, and mentally before they became pregnant with their first child. Nate made sure that his diet was filled with healthy fruits and vegetables, and was extremely careful to avoid GMO foods. He also actively researched and educated himself about both pregnancy and the labor process in order to create a safe, comfortable and blissful homebirth scenario for his wife and growing family.

CHAPTER 12 SUGGESTED READING

Airola, Paavo, M.D. *Stop Hair Loss.* Sherwood. Ore.: Health Plus Publishers, 1994.

Biddulph, Steve. *Manhood.* London, Ebury Press, 2004.

———. *Raising Boys: Why Boys Are Different—and How to Help Them Become Happy and Well-Balanced Men, 2nd Ed.* Berkeley, Calif.: Celestial Arts, 2008.

Biser, Sam. *Save Your Prostate: Unproven Methods to Try When Regular Advice Gets You Nowhere.* Charlottesville, Va.: University of Natural Healing, Inc., 1993.

Blank, Martin, PhD. *Overpowered: The Dangers of Electromagnetic Radiation (EMF) and What You Can Do About It.* New York: Seven Stories Press, 2014.

Chaitow, Leon D.O., N.D. *Prostate Problems: Safe Alternatives Without Drugs.* Wellingborough England: Thorsons Publishers Ltd., 1998.

Covey, Stephen R. *The 7 Habits of Highly Effective People: Powerful Lessons in Personal Change, 25th Anniversary Ed.* New York: Simon and Schuster, 2013.

Feingold, Ben, M.D. *Why Your Child Is Hyperactive: The Bestselling Book on How ADHD is*

Caused by Artificial Food Flavors and Colors. New York: Random House, 1985.

Flatto, Edwin M.D. *Super Potency at Any Age.* New York: Instant Improvement Inc., 1991.

Fink, John M. *Third Option.* Garden City Park, New York: Avery Publishing. 1992

Gerson, Max, M.D. *The Gerson Therapy: The Proven Nutritional Program for Cancer and Other Illnesses, Revised and Updated Ed.* New York: Kensington Publishing Corp., 2006.

Gladstar, Rosemary. *Herbal Remedies for Men's Health (Rosemary Gladstar's Herbal Remedies).* Pownal, Vermont: Storey Publishing, LLC, 1999.

Green, James. *The Male Herbal: The Definitive Health Care Book for Men and Boys, 2nd Ed.* Berkeley, Calif.: The Crossing Press, 2007.

Ivker, Robert. *Thriving: The Holistic Guide to Optimal Health for Men.* New York: Three Rivers Press, 1998.

Lewis, Robert, *Raising a Modern-Day Knight: A Father's Role in Guiding His Son to Authentic Manhood,* Carol Stream, Ill. Tyndale House Publishers, 1997.

Murray, Michael T. N.D. *Male Sexual Vitality.* Rocklin, Calif.: Prima Publishing, 1994.

Pollock, William, Ph.D., *Real Boys: Rescuing Our Sons from the Myths of Boyhood,* New York: Henry Holt and Company, 1998.

Quillin, Patrick, Ph.D., R.D. *The Wisdom of Amish Folk Medicine.* North Canton, Ohio: The Leader Co, Inc., 1993.

CHAPTER 13

Optimizing Your Children's Health

Rejoice! The birth of your precious newborn is a joyous miracle! What a relief that he or she is safely delivered! Participating in the birthing process in any capacity (i.e., as mom, dad, midwife, obstetrician, nurse, birth coach, doula, sibling, extended family member, or other supportive person) reaffirms to us that each life is infinitely magnificent. At the moment of birth, an exuberant, yet quietly soft joy fills the room, captivating everyone present. I have experienced this joy numerous times, as I was present at several hospital births as a registered nurse, and several other births since then.

HAPPY BIRTHING DAY

Sharon, one of Dr. Burt Espy's patients, created her own birth plan for a hospital birth. She opted to have her obstetrician and nurses officiate, and for Dr. Espy and myself to be in attendance as her holistic support team. Sharon's husband also had an active role. He touched her arm or shoulder lovingly, maintained eye contact, coached her to push, and remained emotionally present with her. Her parents and sister were supportive observers. Sharon was an extremely calm birthing mom. Designing her own birth plan gave her peace and bolstered her inner strength.

My friends Kay and Jimmie asked me to be present at the birthing of their first child. Kay rode a bicycle throughout her pregnancy, even riding it to her prenatal visits. One evening, with the hope of inducing labor, she decided to take an extra long bike ride with Jimmie, since she was two weeks past her due date. Her strategy worked and she began labor the next day. Kay's birth plan included having a homebirth with an experienced midwife. She wanted me to be present and to assist the midwife, largely by fetching needed items. I was honored and pleased to help, and came soon after receiving their call at 6:00 A.M. They had been laboring for about four-six hours.

Rasa—Kay and Jimmie's newborn—appeared at about 10:30 A.M. She was the picture of health, and was given high APGAR scores (assesses newborns based on five criteria: appearance/complexion, pulse rate, reflex irritability, activity, and respiratory effort) by her midwife. The family and I have all maintained an enduring friendship. As an adult, Rasa served a brief informal "internship" in my office, which solidified her decision to become a Naturopathic Doctor (N.D.). She has subsequently given birth to her own son at home.

Another heartwarming homebirth experience occurred in Portland, Oregon while I was still in

Chiropractic College. Marcee, the birth mother (I was a classmate of her father) designed her own birth plan, and asked me to be her birthing coach. As I worked closely with Marcee's midwife and received instructions from her, Marcee's birthing experience was smooth and safe. I especially enjoyed the ambiance and family involvement of these homebirth experiences.

Baby Says "Now!"

For the birth of their second child, James, Kay and Jimmie had a working relationship with their trusted midwife, and felt confident that their birthing plan was in order. I was again invited to be present and was in route from Portland to Albuquerque to attend his birth. But James interrupted his parents' birthing plans. One evening, a short time prior to her due date, Kay felt the urge to relieve herself in the bathroom. Moments later she yelled out to Jimmie, "Call the midwife!" Before he finished finding the number and dialing, Kay said, "Jimmie, hang up the phone and come here! Now!"

James was delivered by his dad on the bathroom floor. Ultimately, they had a moment to call the midwife, who arrived soon afterward. My job, when I got there eventually, was to entertain big sister, Rasa, to allow Kay and Jimmie undistracted time with little James. Over the three week period that I stayed, Rasa and I gave mom and dad several small breaks, for rest, showers, and meals. She and I would sit together on the couch and hold her new little brother, and Rasa naturally learned how to be gentle and caring with little James. Rasa loved being the big sister because she felt included and that she contributed to his caregiving and nurturance. Because Rasa was encouraged to play an active role in interacting with her brother, she did not experience anxiety, frustration or jealousy as may happen in some families.

The most abrupt and precipitous of my birthing experiences occurred when I was the unofficial (and unexpected) "midwife" at the birth of one of my nephews, Max. He must have been anxious to arrive, as I caught him in the back seat of a car, parked in the emergency driveway of the closest hospital (not the chosen hospital). When the E.R. crew appeared, they clamped his umbilical cord, then cut it, wrapped him in a towel from the car, and ran with him to the newborn nursery. I instinctively ran after them, feeling that my nephew had been abducted by strangers. The staff surely saw me as an intruder, but they didn't even have the parents' names, and I did not let that little bundle of joy out of my sight, staying at my post, a few feet from the baby, until I was certain that the confusion had been sorted out. I did have to remind the nurses that they should not proceed with their "routine post birth protocol," i.e., silver nitrate drops in the eyes, heel stick for the PKU test, etc. until *after* receiving permission from the parents. Apparently, this had not occurred to the nurses, and my advisement aggravated them.

Max's older sister, Chelsea, did not want to be outdone by her new little brother. In her toddler and preschool years, each time someone recounted her brother's birth story to family or friends, she would add, "And I was born in the *front* seat."

Design Your Birth Plans

Optimizing the comfort and safety of your birthing experience is your prerogative. The gift of life is our most precious gift. Many resources are available to give you ideas and lists of supplies for your birthing plan. Consult several sources while preparing these plans. These preparatory steps are empowering, even if your baby changes them. The time spent thinking about, planning, and preparing for your baby's birth helps to cultivate the mother baby bond. Your plan will also instill confidence and ensure that your partner, family, and healthcare practitioner are aware of your desires. Taking ultimate care to avoid or minimize the trauma to baby, mom, and family is paramount.

My sister, Lori, had selected and packed her favorite relaxing music and fragrances for Max's birth, but she did not have a chance to use them. You may wish to create multiple plans in case your "official" birth plan doesn't go quite as you have designed. While having a plan or plans is always a good idea when preparing for the birth of your child or children, flexibility is important.

Planning for an intervention-free pregnancy and birthing experience is a wonderful goal, quite in harmony with nature. This is also an achievable and richly rewarding goal. If more moms and families opted for intervention-free pregnancy and births this would dramatically reduce unnecessary physical and emotional trauma to countless newborns and moms.

For many families, home-birthing allows for the most relaxed and natural setting. However, the setting that "feels right" in your heart is the right one for you. Think *and feel* your way through these decisions. Be sure to have a back-up plan and a "what if" plan as well. Plan, prepare, and rehearse.

Consider studying Hypno-Birthing® as a gentle, yet powerful birthing tool. Many beautiful babies have been born to relaxed moms who practiced self-hypnosis with their spouse or partner for months in advance, preparing for a more comfortable birth. Being able to adapt to unexpected circumstances is admirable, not a reason to take on guilt. If you planned for a beautiful, simple homebirth, but ended up with a caesarian-section, rejoice in the birth of your child and move forward. Your child will need all the attention and nurturance you can provide.

GENETICS AND YOUR BABY

The initial research and development of genetics is attributed to Gregor Mendel, an Austrian monk who studied the propagation of the common garden pea. Mendel noted certain traits, such as color of the blossoms, and the transmission of this and other traits to subsequent generations. After nine years of methodical research, he presented his professional paper in 1866. Mendel's viewpoint relied on the predictable mathematical behavior of genes within the chromosomes.

Mendel worked out charts for dominant and recessive traits in humans. Brown eyes are dominant, he noted, while blue eyes are recessive. He also explained many aspects of genetically inherited traits and issues, and his theory was adopted by the scientific community in approximately 1900.

Since Mendel's time, the core premise of genetic identity has been that one's identity is based solely on the order of DNA components. That is, in the moment when the human egg cell is fertilized, when mom's half-strand of DNA and dad's half-strand join together to form the human egg, or zygote, the genetic code (DNA sequence order) for baby is locked in; her or his destiny firmly and immutably cast.

Over time, however, as our powers of observation and technology have developed, baffling quirks and exceptions to the Mendelian rules kept cropping up, such as in cases of identical twins. The "genetic **NATURE** versus **NURTURE**" controversy continued, and was never resolved. The question has been: Was it the prevalent impact of nature (genetic model) or that of nurture (environment, lifestyle, life experiences, parenting, etc.) that has played the biggest part in forming the end product, your child?

Epigenetics and Your Baby

In 1939, Conrad Waddington, a prolific writer, presented an unpopular theory in his work titled, *An Introduction to Modern Genetics*. In this, he reframed the classical approach of traditional Mendelian genetics. Waddington, a British man, was a developmental biologist, a paleontologist, geneticist, embryologist and a philosopher, who had received several honors and accolades for his previous work.

Waddington introduced the "epigenetic landscape" as a more accurate and better scenario for understanding genetics, inherited traits and genetically transmitted disorders. Initially, his audience was small, and his work remained relatively unnoticed for decades. But, since the human genome study and report culminated in 2000, the scientific community has been forced to take a broader view than traditional Mendelian genetics provides.

Epigenetics is defined as, "heritable modification in gene EXPRESSION without any variation in the DNA sequence."[1] The essence of the concept is that a variety of external influences can and do influence the EXPRESSION or NON-EXPRESSION of individual genes. This directly relates to the appearance or emphasis of a trait *if expression is augmented*. Epigenetic "down-regulation" or suppression of a trait will dilute or eliminate it.

Epigenetics is a new science, and its findings are giving rise to the science of biomedicine — drugs designed to affect and alter your genetic expression are available and are now considered "hot commodities" in the financial markets.

While some of us may find ample reason to shy away from the biotech side of this new science, it bears investigation. Read more about both the traditional and designer-drug approaches to pharmacology in Chapter 14: *Drugs: Just Say NO THANKS!* Learn about drug side effects and body-friendly alternatives.

The principles of epigenetics relate dynamically to the optimizing of your baby's health. If indeed our genes can be influenced in expression by "external" or environmental factors, we have stronger scientific confirmation of some timeless and simple truths, such as:

- You are what you eat.
- Your thoughts beget your being.
- Unaware, you become your environment.
- Your happiness comes from within

Therefore, realize that your children will prosper and grow in health and wisdom by being surrounded by the richly proactive, nurturing lifestyle and home-life you build.

Another definition of epigenetics is: "Environmentally induced long-lasting [potentially intergenerational] chemical modification to the DNA affects gene expression.[3]

Changing the Future, Today

A list of traits that seem to be passed on from one generation to another, yet cannot be explained exclusively by following absolute Mendelian rules of inheritance, include:

- Health potential
- Academic performance
- Personality traits
- Artistic ability
- Criminal behavior
- Disease potential
- Athletic performance
- Lifestyle preferences
- Musical ability
- Substance abuse behavior

We know that, despite the fact that identical twins share the same DNA, they may manifest the above traits (and other traits) in quite divergent patterns. This can now be explained through epigenetics.

Epigenetics asserts that the potential activation or inactivation of specific genes (leading to traits) of a child, is courtesy of their parents, grandparents and other ancestors. An epigenetic

> **About Twins**
>
> "One strange but true fact about identical twins is that they have the same DNA, yet they always have distinctly unique finger prints."
>
> — Lecuit T, Lenne P. *Cell surface mechanics and the control of cell shape, tissue patterns and morphogenesis. Nat Rev Mol Cell Biol.* 2007; 8; 633-644.

change, either positive or negative, due to dietary and lifestyle factors in the life of a grandparent may be passed on to his or her children, grandchildren and likely beyond! And it goes on and on: Epigenetic change to your child's DNA functionality will pass on to his or her children, grandchildren, and beyond!

Epigenetic changes to the functionality of DNA (not its specific sequence) may occur due to blood-line transmission *prior to* conception, or due to *in-utero environmental* stresses and exposures. Of course, once a baby is born and is exposed to environmental toxicity or other negative factors, less desirable epigenetic changes may then be imparted. These could impact the growth and development of the child herself, and/or his or her descendents. We need to put all of this sobering information into perspective. The fact is that most babies are born with normal morphology (size and shape of torso, limbs, head, and organs) and physiology (body and organ functions).

> OPTIMIZING BABY'S ENVIRONMENT, LIFESTYLE, AND NUTRITION = OPTIMIZING BABY'S HEALTH

Never Too Late to Change

As a female baby is developing in her mother's womb, she is developing cells that will become her egg cells (gametes). The fetus is thus a potential mother! During her fetal development, this potential mother experiences "prophase I," an early step of *meioses* (a reproductive cellular and DNA division and recombination), which mixes and diversifies DNA in chromosomes from mother and father. This genetic information is actual DNA, along with **any** epigenetic modifications from mother and father. Thus, the mother and father, who are the potential grandparents of their children's children, are actually "creating" (influencing) the traits of their grandchildren.

The finalization of the egg cell development within the human female occurs *after* her birth and her eventual maturation at puberty and beyond.[4] This allows for several years of additional epigenetic modification, depending on lifestyle and emotional and environmental factors. Therefore, we can see how proactive health and lifestyle-enriching choices are worth incorporating at **any** point in one's lifetime.

A healthful, positive, supportive and nurturing environment will lead to epigenetic up-regulation, and hopefully a fuller expression of human potential for yourself *and* your child. Here is where we can actively guide our choices and our children's choices for greater health, performance and emotional fulfillment in life.

PRENATAL TESTING

As parents-to-be, especially first-time parents-to-be, you both may be anxiously anticipating the birth of your child. Many confusing thoughts may rush through your minds—about potential birth traumas or defects or inherited conditions. These questions may not be easily answered prior to birth for most parents. Yes, genetic testing is available to couples prior to conception, and it can be costly. However, if genetic testing and counseling is desired, it may prove quite helpful in particular cases; but do keep in mind that such tests have their limitations.

Screening blood tests for certain genetic abnormalities are available, but they are not infallible. All laboratory tests have the potential for inaccuracy, and may cause unnecessary worry (false positives), or fail to yield important information (false negatives). Diagnostic ultrasound has been commonly used throughout pregnancy for decades; perhaps it has been overused. Lana Asprey, M.D. and her husband David Asprey, in their highly regarded *The Better Baby Book*, have this to say about ultrasound use during pregnancy:

> The observed effects of ultrasound on a fetus have included growth restriction, delayed speech, dyslexia, damage to the myelin sheaths [protective coatings of nerves], and irreversible loss of brain cells.[5]

Balancing this information and the hope of receiving enlightening information about their developing baby, the Asprey's opted to limit, but not eliminate the use of ultrasound. They underwent one ultrasound during the first trimester, as well as one in the second trimester. The second trimester ultrasound gives a summary of the presence and configuration of organs and limbs of the tiny growing baby. You too can assert your heartfelt and educated choice concerning the use of ultrasound and its frequency.

Amniocentesis, a form of biopsy, is a more invasive diagnostic procedure. This is performed with ultrasound to visually assist the needle placement. Amniotic fluid is withdrawn and sent for analysis. Amniocentesis is considered to carry a 1 in 200 risk for causing miscarriage, and an unquantified risk for infection, hemorrhage, and fetal injury.[6] Become informed about this procedure before deciding to experience it.

What If My Baby Has a Serious Problem?

If your infant or young child was born with or develops a serious condition you will need to seek ongoing support, counsel, medical and healthcare guidance. Educate yourself about your child's issues, and available help. Scrutinize any recommended procedures and treatments and don't be afraid to look "outside the box" as well. Parents of children with serious problems need support on many levels, and these resources and support groups exist online and throughout the world. Seek out that support. In essence, special needs children have all the needs that more typical children do, and a specific set of their own as well.

Carlita's Story

Carlita's parents gave birth to a son about six years before Carlita arrived. The little boy was strong, vigorous, and abundantly healthy in all appreciable ways. When their son was approximately four, the young family moved to a newly constructed neighborhood. Sadly, little Carlita was born a few years later with serious neurological deficits. She had little voluntary motor control and never learned to crawl or walk; she was blind, almost deaf, and could not swallow or speak. Sometime later, her parents learned that their neighborhood was built on top of a toxic waste dump, full of dioxin (similar to Agent Orange). Carlita's brain scans showed massive gaps indicating missing brain tissue. Several other children born in that neighborhood were afflicted with serious neurological disorders as well. The family moved away from the toxic soil.

Carlita's special needs (constant care, monitoring, and several tube feedings daily) actually galvanized and bonded the family in new ways. They stayed home more, and devised activities and entertainment that included but did not over stimulate Carlita. She learned to hum and to cluck with her tongue, and developed her own communicative lingo, which delighted her parents. Carlita was in her wheelchair all day long and was generally quiet.

Her father became a patient of mine when Carlita was about twelve years old. After his first few treatments, he requested that Dr. Burt Espy and I come to their home to evaluate Carlita. The Rydoraku test (to check the balance of her meridians—see Chapter 2) revealed very low numbers—many at 20 out of a possible 200. We used gentle soft laser to stimulate the indicated acupuncture points and recommended several homeopathic remedies. We instructed the parents to buy a quality juicer and to make fresh veggie juice for Carlita daily. They gave Carlita fresh veggie juice several times a day, and decreased the commercial tube feeding formula to just once a day.

Within a few weeks and only a few treatments, Carlita had dramatically changed. She was more vocal, more active (still in her wheelchair), and was developing a distinct personality. She indicated her likes and dislikes, and her teacher reported that Carlita now required more attention and interaction. This also pleased Carlita's parents. Her Rydoraku readings steadily increased, edging up to 40, then 60, and stabilizing at 70-75. The family moved several states away, but let us know about her continued improvement. They religiously make her veggie juice from organic vegetables daily. Her parents felt that Carlita's quality of life improved considerably from natural healthcare and some simple lifestyle changes.

BUILDING THE FOUNDATION FOR WELLNESS

Creating the foundation for wellness for children requires the same knowledge, skills and materials

> ### My Favorite Household Cleanser
>
> My favorite household cleanser is non-toxic and inexpensive. Here's what you need: 1 12-16 oz. spray bottle (readily available from a dollar store); 1 part white distilled vinegar; 1 part water. Mix briefly, spray and wipe floors, counter tops, walls, oily skillets, windows, etc. This mixture cleans, deodorizes, and disinfects … for pennies. If your young child decides to spray some in a cup and drink it, you will hear them say "yucky," but you won't need to go to the Emergency Room! For a greater disinfectant effect, add a few drops (approximately 4) of one essential oil. Choose from lemongrass, thyme, clove or tea tree. You may wish to have both a "plain" and a "super" disinfectant spray bottle.

as building a wellness foundation for adults. In fact, if you have no children at this time, but envision having a family, to refurbish your lifestyle and home environment *now* will simplify things later. For example, if your "house rules" **disallow** spray insecticide, soda pop, smoking, Twinkies, carcinogenic food coloring, and sugary sweets by the truckload, your health as potential parents will be gaining momentum and harmful epigenetic factors will be minimized. When the pregnancy test strip shows positive, you won't need to rent a forklift to haul off the piles of toxic chemicals, junk "food," and extraneous poisons. You will be primed for a healthy pregnancy. Healthy whole food choices, non-toxic household cleaners, and fly swatters (rather than pesticides) will already be customary practice in your home.

Remember to limit exposure to electromagnetic frequencies (EMF) too. Purchase and plug in one or more EMF-squelching devices. Review Chapter 9, *Unfriendly Energy: Electromagnetic*

Pollution. Incorporate into your wellness plan regular, designated times of being "unplugged" or "un-buzzed" by your favorite electronic devices. I love to be "off the grid," out in the woods, and away from electrical power lines and cell phone towers. Try your own off the grid excursions, and enjoy the calm.

To summarize: Scour your diet, lifestyle, habits … and your mind-set . Clean, upgrade, discard and substitute. Out with dingy, toxic, or non-productive lifestyle factors, and in with fresh, health-promoting innovations. If this seems overwhelming, seek guidance from a natural health practitioner. A well-built foundation creates a beautiful and strong structure to support the wellness of your entire family, both current and future members.

Be Sure Your Baby Is a Non-Smoker

Your little one has the ability to detect noxious substances. I was amazed to read about a study that reported the distress placed upon a growing fetus when the mother actively smoked during her ultra-sound exam. According to trauma experts Levine and Kline,

> Nicotine causes the placental blood vessels to constrict. Clinical experience suggests that babies in the womb adapt by squeezing their little tummies as though to narrow or restrict the umbilical cord from ingesting this poison.[7]

Epigenetic studies are confirming the transmission of physical damage caused by smoking to children and grandchildren.

> Experts have known for some time that women who smoke during pregnancy increase their non-smoking offspring's and grandchildren's risk of developing asthma. That's because nicotine appears to make changes to DNA, creating a biological legacy, according to Virender Rehan, a neonatologist and biomedical researcher at Harbor-ULCA Medical Center in California … Now comes the latest finding by Rehan and colleagues, suggesting expectant mothers who smoke may also transmit asthma to their non-smoking great-grandchildren.[8]
>
> A child whose grandmother smoked while pregnant may have double the risk of developing childhood asthma as a child whose grandmother did not smoke, according to researchers from the Keck School of Medicine of the University of Southern California (USC) … "If a woman smokes while she is pregnant, both her children and grandchildren may be more likely to have asthma as a result," said the study's senior author, Frank D. Gilliland, M.D. Ph.D., M.P.H. The findings suggest that smoking could have a longer lasting impact on families' health than we ever realized … We suspect that when a pregnant woman smokes, the tobacco might affect her fetus's DNA in the mitochondria, and if it is a girl, her future reproductive cells as well," Gilliland says.[9]
>
> "These findings indicate that there is much more we need to know about the harmful effects of in utero exposure to tobacco products and demonstrate how important smoking cessation is for both the person smoking and their family members," said Paul A. Kvale, M.D., president of the American College of Chest Physicians…They [Keck School of preventive medicine researchers] found these results:
>
> • Children whose mothers smoked while pregnant were

one-and-a-half times more likely to develop asthma early in life than children whose mothers did not smoke while pregnant.
- Children whose grandmothers smoked were more than twice as likely (2.1 times) to develop asthma.
- Even if a child's mother did not smoke while she was pregnant—but the child's grandmother did—the child had nearly double the risk (1.8 times) of developing asthma.
- If both the mother and grandmother smoked while pregnant, a child was more than two-and-a-half times more likely (2.6 times) to develop asthma.[10]

Eat a Cleaner Diet, Grow Cleaner DNA

Our nutrition and dietary intake are of paramount importance to our health and well-being. We are now at least four generations into industrialized, processed, devitalized "foods" being accepted and routinely consumed. Currently, it is common for those who are **not** aboriginal food gathers to consume 150 pounds of sugar per year,[11] and the general population commonly eats "commercial grade foods" that are heavily processed. These foods characteristically contain white, devitalized, nutrient depleted, overly hybridized flour with sugar to sweeten and transfats to bind the glob together. Many processed foods contain chemicals of one sort or another: preservatives, flavor enhancers, colorants, texturizers, dough conditioners, genetically modified components, excessive amounts of salt and sugar, hormones, pesticides and other toxins. These are not on my list (and should not be on your list) of positive outcome epigenetic catalysts. Stop rationalizing and throw out the junk!

Establishing an eating plan comprised of natural, unadulterated whole foods—real foods—is a move in the right direction. Go there, you'll love it!

Including copious amounts of pesticide-free produce in your diet is to build sturdy walls upon your foundation for wellness. "ORGANIC" certification is great, but is federally regulated, and could be redefined to be much more lax in the future than it is now. Pay attention. Better yet, become a gardener! When you grow fruits and vegetables or herbs in your own carefully monitored and maintained garden, you can maximize nutrient value by avoiding chemicals. By composting your garden and table scraps, you are ultimately adding nutrients back into your own soil. At Farmer's Markets, you can often find pesticide-free produce that may not be organically certified. Talk to the grower to learn about the purity of their produce, as it may be equivalent to organic.

What Mama Eats, Baby Eats

Did you know that our food taste preferences begin in utero? Yes, pregnant moms who are following their cravings for sugary treats, French fries, lattés, soda pops, pork rinds, potato chips, and other unsavory choices are, in effect, programming their children to be accustomed to and prefer those unhealthy tastes. If your fetus became accustomed to broccoli, kale, chard, rutabagas, asparagus, walnuts, almonds, apples, raspberries and kumquats, your toddler will take to these health promoting choices like a minnow takes to water. Don't complain that your little one won't eat broccoli if you didn't eat it regularly during pregnancy! This in utero taste-preference mechanism probably helps perpetuate the process of wildlife making correct species-specific food selections, and reinforces the wise prohibition against giving human food (especially junk food) to wildlife. Poor food choices during pregnancy may adversely affect more than one generation.

My Daddy Eats Vegetables (And Likes Them)

Dads, you are not off the hook, either! Fathers need to practice dietary accountability too. The single sperm cell that fights its way through the wall of your mate's egg cell to begin the life of your child might be the same one you almost drowned with four or five beers at "guy's night out" a few weeks ago. Taking a healthy, homemade lunch to work or to a day of fishing goes a long way toward building the healthy environment in which your sperm cells are cultivated. On the other hand, when you opt for a quick stop at a drive-thru to pick up "lunch," you certainly are consuming poisonous junk, GMO tainted food, white devitalized flour, trans-fats, food preservatives, feminizing hormones, dough conditioners, and high-fructose corn syrup (it's even in the catsup). Let's get real, Dad, none of these aforementioned ingredients grow on trees. You are gulping down large amounts of negative epigenetic factors and tainting all of your present sperm cells. Did I get your attention? You are also potentially setting yourself up for experiencing health problems that could prevent you from running, playing, or swimming with your grandchildren or even from being around to meet them, let alone your great-grandchildren.

WHAT TO FEED YOUR NEWBORN BABY?

Breast milk! It's not a hard decision, as nature makes it, and human tampering is minimal if mom eats wisely.

Look at nature. Does any other species run down to the store and load up a shopping cart with chemically-produced formulae full of six-syllable ingredients that didn't grow on trees? No. At feeding time, moms in the wild, various undomesticated mammals, do not search for a plastic bottle (with plastic cap and rubber "nipple") filled with chemical toxicants, a "Franken Formula," to which they add municipal "water" complete with chlorine, perhaps fluoride, and who knows what else. Instead, moms in the wild get into a comfortable position and let their young one(s) suckle until content.

Alcohol and Fertility

It is commonly believed that ingesting alcohol can interfere with hormonal balance. The result in men can be a relative increase of estrogen and a decrease of testosterone. Both of these factors can inhibit sperm production, sperm mobility and therefore fertility. There is little consensus among infertility specialists and organizations concerning the dilemma of safe versus problematic quantities of alcohol. Some resources, however, admonish men wishing to father children to totally abstain from these beverages. Other authorities are more liberal in their advisements. It seems that instituting alcohol abstinence prior to conception holds advantages to a man's liver, prostate, testes, sperm production and sperm quality, and is a valuable and proactive lifestyle choice. Alcohol serves as a solvent, and actually renders numerous nutrients unusable in the human body. Of most interest in this scenario is vitamin A, which is critically important to the proper development of sperm (or any developing tissue cells). Ingesting alcohol as new cells are developing may result in decreased numbers of cells, or deformities of these cells due to vitamin A deficiency.

MOTHER'S MILK IS SPECIES SPECIFIC

I became intrigued with the variances in species-specific mother's milk while I was whale watching off the coast of Massachusetts. The milk of a momma whale has a whopping 34.8 percent protein. Her baby needs to gain thousands of pounds in the first few months in order to survive migration. A human infant, on the other hand, may only gain one-quarter to one-third of its potential adult weight prior to weaning, if nursed for approximately five years. Human mother's milk has been analyzed to contain only 4.5 percent protein content.

Nature provides the perfect formula, as mother's milk is species specific. For fast growing mammals—like cats, deer, dogs, reindeer, grey seals, and whales—the protein content is higher. Species that require the most climatic protection have the highest fat contents in their milk. Mammals in Polar Regions have some of the highest fat content milk, which rapidly increases the protective and insulative subcutaneous fat layer in their infants. Moms in equatorial and hot desert climates have higher fat content milk to conserve water for their own survival.

The mammals with more need for brain and neurological development create mother's milk with higher lactose (milk sugar) or carbohydrate content. Human breast milk weighs in at 6.8 percent lactose. Donkey and mink milk barely surpass that level at 6.9 percent.[12] Horse milk contains 6.1 percent lactose, which is a carbohydrate, and also brain fuel.

The **Milk Composition Species Table**, opposite, lists data for the composition of human mother's milk and fifteen other mammals, chosen because they are common to household and farm settings (such as cows, goats and sheep), providers of milk for human consumption in other cultures or countries (like reindeer in Lapland, horses in Mongolia), or simply interesting to compare (for donkey milk used in the Victoria era, and camel milk for Bedouins of Sahara Desert). Yak milk too is rich, and used in the form of milk, cheese, and butter by the Tibetans. The domesticated water buffalo is found in many warm climate countries: India, Pakistan, Egypt, Iran, Sri Lanka, the Philippines, Brazil, Venezuela, Argentina, and Columbia. Water buffalo milk is rich in butterfat, and has become famous in Italy for a rich and creamy mozzarella, Mozzarella di Bufala Campana™ (protein content of 19 percent, fat content 21 percent). Bulgaria is highly acclaimed for its superior quality of water buffalo meat and dairy products. Further north, moose dairies are found in Sweden and Russia. Llamas are milked by the indigenous people of the Andes.

After reviewing the Milk Composition Species Chart, it should be obvious that proportions of constituents in the various mother's milks of each species are specifically designed to meet the needs of their respective infants.

In comparison to other large mammals, human babies are born many months physiologically premature. While other mammals remain pregnant longer to ensure the healthy development and well-being of their babies, human mothers are pregnant for less time. At birth and for months after, a human infant is much more dependent on its parents than infants of other species. If you've ever observed a newborn foal, calf or fawn you have probably marveled at the fact that the newborn animal is walking around within minutes and is able to find its way to mother in order to nurse almost immediately. In contrast, the human infant is totally dependent on the love, care and nurturance of his or her parents. Breastfeeding, nurturance from the mother to child, is the most natural and

Milk Composition – Species Table*

Species	Fat %	Protein %	Lactose %	Ash %	Total Solids %	Average Birth Weight	Average Weaning Age	Average Adult Weight (Pounds)	Typical Life Span (Years)	Age when considered fully grown OR Sexual maturity
Camel (dromedary)	3.6	3.0	4.4	0.8	11.7	80 pounds	4-18 months	1,000-2,000	40-50	4-6 years
Cat	10.9	11.1	3.4	---	25.4	3.5 oz	8 weeks	8-10	12-15 (indoor)	1 year
Cow, Holstein	3.5	3.1	4.9	0.7	12.2	80-100 pounds	5-8 weeks	1500	6-15	2-3 years
Deer	19.7	10.4	2.6	1.4	34.1	4-8 pounds	2 months	88-290	10-16	1.5 years
Dog	8.3	9.5	3.7	1.2	20.7	1-23 pounds	8-20 weeks	30-45	13-20	8-30 months
Donkey	1.2	1.7	6.9	0.45	10.2	25 pounds	4-6 months	606	25	1.5-3 years
Elephant	15.1	4.9	3.4	0.76	26.9	117-330 pounds	4-5 years	10,000-13,000	70	8-13 years
Goat	3.5	3.1	4.6	0.79	12	4-11 pounds	3 months	22-380	8-12	4-7 months
Horse	1.6	2.7	6.1	0.51	11	85-100 pounds	5-7 months	840-2200	25-30	4 years
Human	**4.5**	**1.1**	**6.8**	**0.2**	**12.6**	**6.2-8.2 pounds**	**13-18 months**	**136.7**	**70-80**	**18-21 years**
Monkey	3.9	2.1	5.9	2.6	14.5	1.5 pounds	1 year	12-30	16-30	8-10
Reindeer	22.5	10.3	2.5	1.4	36.7	10 pounds	52-104 weeks	300	8-10	1-3 years
Seal, Grey	53.2	11.2	2.6	0.7	67.7	26 pounds	2-3 weeks	220-680	30-40	3-6 years
Sheep	5.3	5.5	4.6	0.9	16.3	5-8 pounds	2-3 months	120-250	6-11	4-8 months
Water Buffalo	10.4	5.9	4.3	6.8	21.5	80 pounds	1 year	1200-2200	20-30	2-4 years
Whale, Humpback	34.8	13.6	1.8	1.6	51.2	2000 pounds	26-52 weeks	80,000	50-65	10 years

* Robert D. Bremel's course notes and information from *The Handbook of Milk Composition*, edited by Robert G. Jensen, were relied upon to produce a comprehensive chart depicting numerous constituents of mammalian milks.[13]

best way to ensure a baby's well-being outside of the womb.

Each human mom and infant pair has an exquisitely synchronized system for providing individualized nutrition. Miraculously, the baby's body seems to energetically signal specific nutrient needs to mom, as if selecting from a menu. The mother's body immediately responds by providing the necessary "side orders." The mechanism of this amazing process has not yet been completely analyzed, but the rapid fluctuation in milk composition is documented. Wouldn't you lavishly tip a waitress who intuitively pinpointed your specific nutrient needs on a moment-to-moment basis? As the infant's system requires a little extra calcium for bone and tissue building, or extra zinc for a momentary immunity challenge, mom's body immediately responds by providing an increase in the required nutrients. If baby's nervous system needs calming, a little more tryptophan migrates from mom's system into her milk supply, and quickly into baby's tummy. By the way, the tryptophan creates serotonin and that physiologically strengthens the emotional bond between mothers and their nursing infants. Can you imagine a more perfect design for beginning life?

The Milk Composition Species table addresses the macro nutrients: fat, protein and carbohydrates (lactose). Many other important nutrients and biologically-active milk constituents have been analyzed and charted. Important examples include: vitamins, electrolytes, minerals, amino acids, enzymes, hormones (including insulin and thyroid hormones), anti-infection agents (including antibodies and live, active white blood cells: macrophages and T-cells), and immune system activators such as tumor necrosis factor-∂. Likely, mother's milk provides other factors that are yet to be discovered and named. Certainly some epigenetic factors are transmitted through mother's milk.

Necessary Probiotics—Another Support for Breastfeeding

A few years ago, we only had a partial answer to the question of how our intestinal tract received the good bacteria necessary for healthy digestion, healthy life.

1) That obvious answer was and is: during a normal vaginal birth, the baby gets some lactic acid bacteria exposure from traversing, and being squeezed through, mom's vaginal tract. Lesser amounts of the good bacteria are found in the intestines of Cesarean-section babies.

These Cesarean babies can be supplemented by using probiotics. Optimally the baby is breastfed and mom has taken probiotics containing the strains Bifidobacterium infantis, Bifidobacterium longum, and Lactobacillis acidophilus since or before conception. Combinations with other strains are fine. In the case that an infant is not breastfed, directly administer the above mentioned strains of friendly bacteria, and Lactobacillus helveticus. That strain is found to normalize the colonization of bottle-fed babies to an extent.[14]

2) Exposure to amniotic fluid builds the intestinal flora on a daily basis. Swallowing and ingesting this fluid brings good bacteria into the developing infant's digestive tract. If a baby goes to full term and is delivered vaginally, its exposure to **amniotic fluid (AF)** is maximized, and a greater number of beneficial bacteria are directly ingested prior to and at birth. Necrotizing enterocolitis (NEC) is a serious and often fatal intestinal infection which afflicts preterm infants. The disease is more serious, and often fatal if the baby is not breastfed. NEC affects 10 percent of all human preemies and 25 percent of those have a fatal outcome.[15]

Note the following research findings from the *American Journal of Physiology*, which studed preterm piglets that were fed amniotic fluid after birth and had a decreased rate of necrotizing entero colitis: "Like colostrum, AF may reduce NEC development in preterm neonates by suppressing the proinflammatory responses to enteral (by mouth) formula feeding and gut colonization when provided before the onset of NEC."[16]

The areola of mom's breast secretes a small amount of mucous that contains similar constituents to amniotic fluid. This secretion smells like amniotic fluid, and attracts the infant. When laid on the mother's abdomen or chest, even a human newborn **can** wiggle and follow the scent to find a breast and latch onto it unassisted.[17]

3) Evidence that friendly intestinal bacteria are sometimes transported to your skin has been examined and verified. This phenomenon is most documented in mothers-to-be late in their pregnancies. Apparently, immune cells with "arms" (dendrite immune cells) physically latch onto Lactobacillis acidophilus in the small intestine and somehow drag them to the outer skin. It is speculated that some (but not all) of the bacteria may be moved into the mom's milk. Sometimes in late pregnancy a little breast milk escapes from the breast. It seems that this is not by mistake, but indeed by design. The surface of mom's nipple and areola becomes inoculated with good bacteria from her intestines. This is a way to be sure that the baby's intestines gain plenty of these vital bacteria from yet another source.

> However, recent molecular studies have shown that milk secreted by the mammary glands during the weeks previous to labor (and thus not submitted to any kind of infant contact) contains bacterial species similar to those isolated from fresh milk obtained after labor (35). Dendritic cells have been described to penetrate the intestinal epithelium to take up commensal bacteria from the gut lumen (36), to reach the systemic circulation, and to retain even live bacteria for several days (37); recently, the transfer of intestinal bacteria to the mammary glands within dendritic cells has been proposed.[18]

4) Breastfeeding provides hundreds of different varieties of beneficial bacteria. Human colostrum has been fully analyzed to contain at least 700 different varieties.[19] Many of these varieties persist throughout breastfeeding and the proportions of various beneficial bacteria strains change as the baby grows and develops.

This vital importance of breastfeeding as immunity building in addition to providing nutrition is being emphasized and reinforced by scientific studies consistently. Breast milk provides several other factors which assist the intestinal biome, or good bacteria ecology.

- Lactoferrin is an important milk protein. Newborns cannot digest this protein, but require it to promote the growth of good bacteria, and to bind onto pathogenic bacteria, keeping them from attaching to the mucosal lining. The pathogens eventually are flushed from the body.
- Alpha-lactalbumin attacks tumor cells quite effectively.
- Lactose based complex sugars are being studied. It seems that they are indigestible by infants, but provide food for a particular bifidobacterium, a newly identified descendent of Bifidobacterium longum (a new sub species).

> Scientists have discovered that an ingredient in human breast milk protects and repairs the delicate intestines of newborn babies. The ingredient called pancreatic secretory trypsin inhibitor, or PSTI, is found at its highest levels in

colostrum—the milk produced in the first few days after birth. The new study highlights the importance of breastfeeding in the first few days after the birth.[20]

I hope you find these little known facts to be enlightening. I also hope you will incorporate this information into better lifestyle choices for yourself, and enthusiastically share with others. We can glean information relevant to adults from these studies. There is no question that having a healthy and diverse microbiome (a grouping of various beneficial bacterial colonies) in our intestinal tract is a requirement for our health.

Nature's plan provides for diversity of the microbes and multiple pathways to deliver them to the developing intestinal tract. Mother Nature considers the supply of these beneficial microbes to be of utmost importance, we all should as well. Adding probiotic mixtures to our daily regimens both from food sources and supplemental sources is a wise form of insurance. These beneficial bacteria promote intestinal and whole body health throughout your lifetime.

Commercially manufactured infant "formula" cannot begin to provide these individual and dynamic amenities, particularly the probiotic ones. "Franken formula" does provide rich sources of toxic chemicals and preservatives, synthetic vitamins, non-bio-available minerals, genetically modified organisms, and immunity suppressing milk substitutes. Comparative research studies dating back as far as 1885 and into relatively recent times indicate that infants who were bottle fed had a significantly higher relative risk (RR) of mortality than breast fed infants in numerous studies, in a variety of countries.[21]

More Than Nutrition

I absolutely believe that breastfeeding is best from numerous perspectives. Breast is the best for your baby's nourishment, growth, intestinal health, immune function, emotional health, self esteem, bonding, and countless other factors. Breastfeeding is best for mothers for bonding, relaxation time, momma brain time (time spent thinking about your baby and family instead of solving the world's problems), hormonal balance, breast cancer prevention, time efficiency, and many other factors. Breastfeeding is best for the environment—less packaging and dishwashing. Breastfeeding fosters less agricultural, commercial, landfill, and transportation waste and pollution.

> Generally, breastfed babies don't cry as much as bottle-fed babies. They don't have to wait for food, since mother's milk is always ready.
> —Ryan and Auletta, *Breastfeeding, Your Priceless Gift to Your Baby and Yourself*

Muscle Testing for Baby's Food Needs

Just ask your baby's body to tell you how much it likes breast milk or infant formula. This is best accomplished by Surrogate Muscle Testing—a simple variation of muscle testing for infants, children, or anyone who is unable to perform the muscle test themselves. The testing is performed on the surrogate (an adult) who is holding or touching the infant or child (the subject). Often, mom holds the young one while dad, grandma, doctor or a skilled friend performs the muscle tests.

In preparation, the surrogate should first be tested for muscle strength and readiness while *not touching* the child. If all systems are "GO," then proceed to test, asking questions of baby's body.

Mom, or whoever is the surrogate, should focus on the baby and look at her or him while holding out the free arm to the testing person. Small containers of pumped breast milk and infant formula can be tested by placing the testing samples one by one on baby's body, and then proceeding to do the muscle test. To more fully engage the baby's consciousness, say the baby's name and ask if they like to drink this milk or the formula you are testing.

"Baby Beth, do you like to drink this milk?"

"Baby Beth, do you like to drink this formula?"

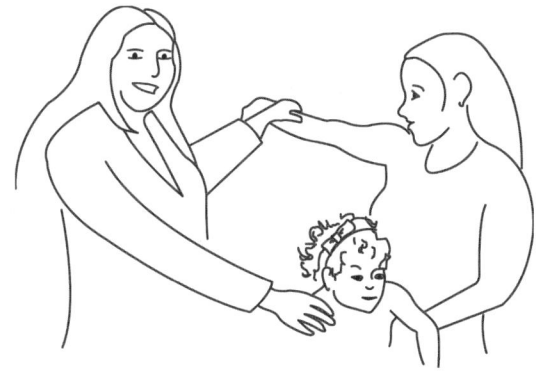

Test the various samples more than once to gain a good understanding. Then, let the baby nurse or drink the best milk or formula, since the questions primed the baby for quenching their thirst.

Lita's Story

Nancy and Rick were so pleased to have a new baby girl—their Lita was a darling. And, she simply did not want to nurse. Nancy and Rick brought Lita to my office where we did Surrogate Testing for several infant-formula recipes and found the best energetic match for Lita. Her parents truly nurtured her and were very perceptive about her needs. Lita had a few treatments and I advised she be given some additional nutrients. She thrived. I've kept in touch with the family over the years. The latest update is that Lita is in college undertaking a double major program: mechanical engineering and aeronautical engineering. Apparently, she escaped the potential maladies that commercial infant formula may trigger.

Challenged to Nurse?

What if you think you are fully unable to nurse or sufficiently nurse your infant? Take a deep breath, call a lactation specialist, your midwife, your holistic health care professional, or someone else whom you trust and feel is competent. Very few women are truly *unable* to breastfeed.

The fact that most breast feeding problems are preventable or can be treated is not widely known by mothers or health care workers.[22]

Bottles, schedules, and the separation of mothers and babies are interventions in breastfeeding in just the same way as inductions, the use of Oxytocin® in labor, and cesarean sections are interventions at birth.[23]

Also, these birthing intrusions (termed interventions) can impede or delay the milk letdown. A mother may feel that her body has failed, when it simply has not recovered from trauma. Work diligently to solve the specific problems that have been identified by your midwife, lactation consultant, or other expert. Correctly identifying the issue is required to allow for finding the appropriate remedy. Often the issue is as simple as positioning. In any case do your best to maintain a calm equanimity and be kind to yourself.

For some women, the chief obstacle to breastfeeding easily may be hypothyroidism or a predisposition to the condition. This may be elusive and difficult to document or identify with standard testing, but consulting with a holistically-oriented doctor or natural healthcare practitioner who is willing to help you unravel this issue can be helpful. A little known thyroid imbalance called hypothyroidism type 2 is often characterized by seemingly "normal" thyroid blood levels, yet the body's tissues are unable to properly utilize the thyroid hormones. Testing your basal temperature with a thermometer tightly held in your axilla (armpit) for ten minutes upon awakening, and before moving or getting out of bed, is the best test to evaluate this problem. You can gather this data at home for ten days and bring the results to your holistically-minded practitioner.

> Reproductive failure and lactation failure also preceded thyroid dysfunction and goiter. —J V Joshi, et al.[24]

Your history, family history, symptoms, and physical and kinesiological findings may help you understand if you may have a hormonal obstacle to nursing your baby. Treating mom's thyroid or hormonal balance may be a solution, or may help you set the stage for success in nursing your next baby. This condition will be expanded upon in my upcoming book about our aging bodies.

Deficiency of either mineral, iodine or manganese, may hamper thyroid function and impede breastfeeding. Further understanding about the thyroid from unconventional, but realistic and valid, viewpoints are available in: *Hypothyroidism, the Unseen Illness* by Broda O. Barnes, M.D. and *Hypothyroidism: Type 2*, by Mark Starr, M.D.

If your situation, your life, your health, or any other factor looms large enough to disrupt or disallow breastfeeding, *do not take on guilt*!

Attempt to find the best alternative(s) for your particular situation and find additional moments and methods to nurture and enjoy bonding with your beautiful baby.

Resources and Alternatives

Many helpful resources are available, including videos about breastfeeding and commonly encountered problems (see Resource and Product Guide.) If all efforts don't allow you to comfortably and efficiently breastfeed, and yet you are able to produce and pump your milk, this is your next best option.

In the absence of mother's milk from the baby's mom, providing your baby with human breast milk from a breast milk bank or willing community member is a wonderful option. The long term benefits to baby will far outweigh any perceived inconvenience involved in obtaining donor milk.

Herbalists and midwives have traditionally recommended a variety of herbs to aid the nursing mother. Fenugreek seed tea is a classic galactogogue (or lactation stimulator).

> Consider using fenugreek to stimulate greater milk production ... Blessed thistle is also helpful in stimulating milk production. Blessed thistle and fenugreek can be safely used together.[25]

These herbs may be used as tea, or taken in capsule or tincture forms. Stinging Nettle is another galactogogue. I am acquainted with Ed Smith, a medical herbologist in Oregon. "Herbal Ed" is the founder and owner of HerbPharm™, an organic herb company in Oregon. I hold Ed Smith in high esteem for his commitment to product purity and green practices at his farm and processing facility. In his book, *Therapeutic Herb Manual,* Ed suggests the use of a lactation tonic for nursing mothers to enhance the quality and quantity of breast milk.

Mother's Lactation Tonic by Herb-Pharm™ from Ed Smith, Medical

---

Say No to Guilt

If you find yourself slipping into guilt, STOP. Obtain some of the Bach Remedy pine. Take it often: 4 drops several times per day. Reread Chapter 4, *Divine Energy: The Chakras*. Find a suitable holistic practitioner who does emotion balancing and clear out the guilt and negative emotions quickly. You have important work to do.

Herbalist: chaste tree berry, fenugreek seed, caraway seed, fennel seed, anise seed

He says:

> Especially indicated in cases where the production of breast milk is lacking or scanty ... this compound can also serve to allay nausea and relieve intestinal gas in the mother, and ... her breast feeding child.[26]

In the event these options are unworkable, or provide less than a sufficient supply, then consider the Weston A. Price Foundation's infant formula recipe.[27]

You may wish to see more recipe versions and information at www.WestonAPrice.org.

Adding Ch'i to Your Child's Food

This Weston A. Price foundation recipe is tried and true. Many infants have been nourished with this original formula, or slightly modified versions. Making your own natural and real food formula will add ch'i or life force to your baby's nutrition. Remember from Chapter 2, that ch'i

---

Infant Formula Recipe[28]

2 cups whole raw cow's milk*, preferably from pasture-fed cows. 1/4 cup homemade liquid whey**
   (*See recipe for whey on following page*)
4 tablespoons lactose***
1/4 teaspoon bifidobacterium infantis
2 or more tablespoons good quality cream (preferably not ultrapasteurized), more if you are using
   milk from Holstein cows
1/2 teaspoon unflavored high-vitamin or high-vitamin fermented cod liver oil or 1 teaspoon regular
   cod liver oil
1/4 teaspoon high-vitamin butter oil (optional)***
1 teaspoon expeller-expressed sunflower oil***
1 teaspoon extra virgin olive oil***
2 teaspoons coconut oil***
2 teaspoons Frontier brand nutritional yeast flakes***
2 teaspoons gelatin***
1-7/8 cups filtered water
1/4 teaspoon acerola powder***

*In place of cow's milk, please substitute a potentially less allergenic, and more-constituent-similar milk if possible. Donkey and horse milk have similar lactose proportions to human breast milk. Water buffalo milk is considered a good hypoallergenic choice.

**Do NOT use powdered whey or whey from making cheese (which will cause the formula to curdle). Use only homemade whey made from yoghurt, kefir or separated raw milk.

 ***Available from Radiant Life 888-593-8333, www.radiantlifecatalog.com.

> ## Whey Recipe[29]
>
> Makes about 5 cups.
>
> Homemade whey is easy to make from good quality plain yoghurt, or from raw or cultured milk. You will need a large strainer that rests over a bowl.
>
> If you are using yoghurt, place 2 quarts in a strainer lined with a tea towel set over a bowl. Cover with a plate and leave at room temperature overnight. The whey will drip out into the bowl. Place whey in clean glass jars and store in the refrigerator.
>
> If you are using raw or cultured milk, place 2 quarts of the milk in a glass container and leave at room temperature for 2-4 days until the milk separates into curds and whey. Pour into the strainer lined with a tea towel set over a bowl and cover with a plate. Leave at room temperature overnight. The whey will drip out into the bowl. Store in clean glass jars in the refrigerator.
>
> Source: *Nourishing Traditions* by Sally Fallon with Mary G. Enig, Ph.D. New Trends Publishing Inc., 2000.

is the pure, harmonizing and free-flowing energy that sustains all of life.

Even if you are using commercially-produced infant formula, you can imbue it with ch'i, life force, love, and or energetic nurturance by your intention. Mindfully mixing and administering a formula preparation to your infant, blessing it or praying over it will provide an opportunity to supercharge the value and benefit of the formula or feeding. This same principle applies to feeding meals, snacks and beverages to your older children, adult family members, and of course, to yourself.

Why Prepared Formula Is the Last Alternative

The facts in the chart on page 255 have been gleaned from reliable sources. Hopefully, within the time interval of writing these words, and your reading them, one or more superior-quality all-natural, and well-balanced prepared formula(e) will be available.

However, if you must choose to use a commercially-prepared infant formula, avoid mixing the formula with tap-water. Use filtered and purified water from a Berky®, Multipure® unit, or use natural spring water. Avoid "nursery water," which is tap water fortified with excess fluoride, a known carcinogen.

Always avoid microwaving the formula since this reduces the life force or ch'i, and adds harmful radiation. Microwaving milk, formula, or any food for that matter, denatures the protein molecules, rendering them virtually impossible to digest and process. I have found that the best way to warm your baby's milk for bottle feeding is to put it in a glass or ceramic pan and gently warm on your stove top to approximately 99-101 degrees Fahrenheit (37.2-38.3 degrees Celsius). Make sure to test the temperature of the milk or formula before giving it to your baby. You can do this by putting a small drop on your forearm.

Consciously making these and other preparations with your best intentions for your child's health and wellness is a powerful tool. Ask your natural healthcare practitioner about additional nutrient supplementation, such as infant multi-vitamins, extra vitamin D_3, extra iodine (topical application is best), mild digestive aids and liquid colostrum.

REASONS TO AVOID USING COMMERCIALLY PREPARED FORMULA[30, 31]

IMMUNOLOGICAL
- Decreased Normal Flora Development
- Increased Allergies
- Increased Diabetes
- Increased Diarrhea
- Increased Ear Infections
- Increased Childhood Cancers
- Increased Illness
- Increased Hospitalization
- Increased Eczema and Skin Issues
- Increased Doctor Visits

ENVIRONMENTAL EXPOSURES
- Increased Exposure to BPA and Other Toxins from Packaging, Baby-Bottles, Etc.
- Increased Exposure to Toxins in Tap Water—Pollutants, Chlorine, Fluoride, Etc.

LEARNING
- Decreased Acceptance of Tastes of Newly Introduced Foods
- Decreased IQ
- Increased Learning Disabilities
- Increased Missed School Time

POTENTIALLY FATAL CONSEQUENCES
- Increased Risk of SIDS
- Increased Failure to Thrive
- Increased Risk of Mortality(All Causes)
- Increased Heart Disease
- Increased Childhood Cancer
- Increased Diabetes
- Increased Necrotizing Enterocolitis (Bleeding Intestines)

PSYCHOSOCIAL, EMOTIONAL, SELF ESTEEM
- Decreased Tryptophan and Serotonin
- Decreased Bonding
- Decreased Nurturance
- Decreased Sense of Self
- Decreased Independence
- Increased Irritability

GASTRO-INTESTINAL PROBLEMS
- Decreased Normal Bacterial Colonization
- Decreased Iron Levels from Intestinal Bleeding
- Increased Diarrhea
- Increased Intestinal Bleeding
- Increased Digestive Disorders of All Types, Life Long

POTENTIAL ADULT HEALTH ISSUES (ADULTS CONSUMED COMMERCIAL FORMULA AS INFANTS)
- Increased Cholesterol Levels
- Increased Coronary Artery Disease
- Increased Asthma
- Increased Cancer of Lymph Glands
- Increased Digestive Disorders
- Increased Ulcerative Colitis
- Increased Crohn's Disease
- Increased Leaky Gut Syndrome

HOW LONG SHOULD I NURSE MY BABY (OR PROVIDE THE BEST POSSIBLE SUBSTITUTE)?

There is little consensus on this issue. The American Academy of Pediatrics advocates exclusive breastfeeding for at least six months, and longer if comfortable and desired by mother and infant.

Holly Smith studied twenty-one species of various primates. Her extensive study concluded that the weaning age of apes and monkeys typically coincided with the eruption of the first set of permanent molars. Human children generally receive their first molars between 5 ½-6 years, approximately the time that the immune system reaches maturity. Often these facts and others are used to encourage breast-milk feedings for several years.

I am a proponent of extended breastfeeding. Even when suckling is no longer desired, moms can pump milk to be served to active toddlers and young school-aged children, if preferred. If you have several young children —a child who is two to six years old and a newborn, for example— breastfeed the newborn until content, then nurse the older child. Or if you prefer, pump additional milk for the older child. Continuing the use of breast milk will offer immune-system bolstering and will fend off many upper respiratory infections within the family, an ultimate benefit for the infant and all family members. And don't worry about not having enough milk, as in most cases an increased demand for breast milk automatically and naturally increases the supply.

Introducing Solid Food

Adding solid food to the nutritional regimen is an important step. Adding food too early may result in numerous food sensitivities, outright food allergies, even Leaky Gut syndrome and immunity compromise. On the other hand, withholding solid food too long in a child's development may cause some nutrient deficiencies such as iron, selenium, vitamin C, vitamin D_3, and possibly vitamin B_{12}. If a nursing mom amps up on these nutrients, baby will likely have a sufficient intake. I recommend that new moms continue their use of high-quality, non-synthetic, prenatal or comparable supplementation throughout their entire lactation period. Fortifying the supplementation program with specific nutrients can be best when taken under the guidance from your holistic, natural-approach healthcare doctor or practitioner.

Your baby will provide unmistakable clues that he or she is ready to explore solid food by grabbing interesting morsels from your plate and testing them out. Allow this process of adding foods to be a slow progression. It is recommended that no more than one new food is introduced per week in order to prevent and detect the occurrence of any food allergies or sensitivities. Interact with your baby for each experiment and speak aloud the name of the food currently under investigation.

> Learning to accept new foods, new tastes, and new textures is a progressive journey. It may take up to fifteen separate taste offerings before the item passes your toddler's taste test. Many parents give up after a few exposures, and stop offering food candidates too soon.
> —Carruth, B.R. et al, *Journal of the Academy of Nutrition and Dietetics* [32]

Neither forcing nor harshly withholding foods will allow your child to evolve a healthy approach to eating and thus encourage an overall health relationship with food. This may lessen the likelihood of emotionally-charged eating and may even deter the development of eating disorders of all kinds.

During this time, refrain from serving inappropriate foods—too hot in temperature or spiciness, those that are likely to be choking hazards, or those known to pose potential life threatening risks if consumed before a certain age. Such caution needs to be exercised with infants less than one year old ingesting honey (due to a botulism contamination), peanut butter (due to an allergy and choking hazard), or ice-cream (due to a potential of contracting the listeria bacteria). Nursing or breast milk bottle-feeding for the months during the gradual introduction of chosen foods is a good approach to transitioning to a solid food diet.

> Many sources advocate giving honey to children only after their first birthday. This is due to the junctions in the intestinal lining being "loose" and able to allow botulism spores from honey to easily migrate into the bloodstream. This is *only* known to happen in infants. The junctions typically tighten sufficiently by 10-12 months.

A BIRTHING EXPERT WEIGHS IN

Suzanne Arms, author, photojournalist, filmmaker, and founder of Birthing the Future® (a birth center) has written several books on the importance of natural birth and breastfeeding. Her website, birthingthefuture.org, is also a plentiful resource of information for all mothers and caregivers of infants and children. Suzanne Arms is an activist and has been the leader in the natural childbirthing and breastfeeding movements since the 1970s.

During the construction of this chapter I was in close communication with Suzanne Arms, exchanging multiple emails and having periodic telephone conversations. She was an invaluable resource. Her ideology and methodology are totally aligned with nature and she is an advocate to mothers and children, first and foremost. During our correspondence she stated:

> Modern life is full of pollution and a developing fetus (or "prenate") is not designed to handle the manmade chemicals and toxins that are present everywhere today. Think about it: parents, especially the woman, in and from whose body this baby develops, are truly the *architects* of their child's brain and body. When you think about it that way, you're likely to take yourself—and your lifestyle—more seriously during pregnancy. Start with the importance of getting enough clean water to drink, lots of it, getting exercise, and getting enough rest as well as sleep. These are important not only in pregnancy, but when you have a baby in your arms… You want to do everything you can to be in peak health during pregnancy. Acupuncture, homeopathic remedies, and Chiropractic care can be very helpful in preventing and reducing common problems in pregnancy and birth. This includes "morning sickness," difficulty sleeping, lower back or sciatic pain, and even high blood pressure. Chiropractic in particular can correct misalignment of your pelvic bones so your baby can move through your pelvis more easily, easing labor…
>
> Intervention-free pregnancy and birth is how babies are meant to be born; and it helps ensure the baby's full development. Natural birth means no drugs, anesthesia, or interventions in labor—like not being allowed to eat and drink in labor, or being forced to lie in bed and not being allowed to get up and move around, as well as

major interventions like cutting (an episiotomy), pulling the baby out with vacuum extraction or having cesarean surgery. It also means allowing labor to start when the baby chooses, not artificially inducing. Research shows that the two most commonly practiced interventions: artificial induction and epidural anesthesia, are also the two most likely to lead to a cesarean.

Suzanne Arms gives parents, especially mothers, the encouragement and support to honor their health and their baby's health from pregnancy and labor to birth, infancy, and childhood. She also states:

> Circumcision and vaccinations and other shots are serious decisions and you need information to make wise choices. This means doing research and discussing them well ahead of birth, just as you'll want to plan ahead for how you will be able to stay at home with your baby full-time in the beginning, and how you will breastfeed exclusively for six months or more. Breastfeeding is not a lifestyle choice for your baby; it's a matter of your baby being able to get the right nutrients and to build its immune system, jaw, gut, and teeth properly. Returning to work just weeks or months after giving birth and also not fully breastfeeding is not only very hard on your baby and deprives it of full development, but it's tremendously hard on a new mother's body and psyche as well.

Circumcision may be a matter of religious belief or even family tradition, but new research shows that this practice is becoming less common in mainstream society. It is important to research the initial surgery and procedure, as well the life long side effects that ensue from the cutting and subsequent removal of a baby boy's foreskin. There is more discussion about circumcision in Chapter 12: *The Male Energetic System*.

Vaccinations are also an important decision to consider. I have heard the horror stories from patients, friends and family members about their experiences of hospital births and the relentless pressure these recovering mothers are subjected to, even minutes after giving birth, to poke, prod, and inject their newborn babies with toxic, sometimes deadly, serums. It is of utmost importance to research vaccinations and then practice theoretical responses that can be given to nurses, doctors, family members and any others who may question a mother's right to *not* have her newborn baby vaccinated. Further commentary on vaccinations can be found in Chapter 6, *Energizing Your Immune System*. Look for more information in Chapter 14 regarding the deleterious effects of many drugs on our bodies.

WHAT TO DO WITH LEFTOVER BREAST MILK

Regard leftover breast milk as a precious, highly bio-active health remedy. The pumped or expressed milk that you may have stored in your freezer for baby's nutritional use also has powerful and numerous medicinal uses.

Colostrum is the immune-factor-rich "first milk" that each birthing mother secretes just after giving birth. Colostrum is produced for roughly forty-eight hours after birth, as the milk is "coming in." The milk continues to contain some immune factors and countless helpful nutrients, in a less concentrated amount, throughout lactation. Therefore, breast milk is beneficial to humans of all ages for assisting the body to overcome practically any immune system challenge.

Human breast milk (and essentially any raw mammalian milk) is helpful for most skin issues, even rashes, insect bites and stings. Simply apply some pumped or expressed breast milk to areas of acne, eczema or cradle cap. For instance, massage or dab it on, then allow the milk to be absorbed and to dry. Use cotton balls, a soft washcloth or your fingers for most skin issues.

If you are using breast milk as eye, ear, or nose drops, do your best not to touch the child's body with the dropper, and to wash it well after each use. If you are intrigued with the many health uses of breast milk found in the following chart, but do not have access to breast milk, you may substitute colostrum in supplemental form. Most often colostrum is in capsules, but may also be found in loose powder. For most uses listed below, dissolve some of the powder in a small amount of purified water or raw milk and proceed. DO NOT USE THIS SUBSTITUTE IN THE EYES.

USES FOR BREAST MILK

BABY'S SKIN	EVERYONE'S SKIN	BABY'S IMMUNITY BOOSTER	EVERYONE'S IMMUNITY BOOSTER
Diaper rash-prevention and for treatment			
Eczema, rashes, cradle cap	Eczema, rashes, warts	Prevention for childhood illnesses	Prevent and treat autoimmune issues
Acne	Acne	Breast feed frequently during any illness	
			Adjunctive measure for many cancers and digestive diseases: IBS, etc.
Insect bites, stings	Insect bites, stings	Cough, cold, upper respiratory infection	Cough, cold, upper respiratory infection
Abrasions, cuts	Abrasions, cuts	Nasal congestion (a few drops in nasal passages)	Nasal congestion (a few drops in nasal passages)
	Breastfeeding mom's sore or cracked nipples		
	Sunburn, localized burns		
Pink eye* (conjunctivitis), clogged tear ducts (use a few drops 4-6 times per day)	Pink eye* (conjunctivitis), clogged tear ducts (use a few drops 4-6 times per day)	Ear infection (a few drops every few hours) (also consult your child's doctor)	
Poison ivy* Poison sumac*	Poison ivy* Poison sumac*		Sore throat (gargle and swallow)
Chicken pox*	Shingles*		
	Cold sores, fever blisters*		

* Prevent cross-contamination; refer to instruction box on the following page.

> ### * OOZING TOXINS INSTRUCTION BOX
>
> For skin lesions with oozing toxins (poison ivy) or infectious agents (chicken pox), be sure to wear disposable gloves and to avoid spreading that agent around the affected area. DO NOT be conservative about using numerous cotton balls-one dab per cotton ball. Immediately discard each used cotton ball appropriately in the trash so that no one can access it. When the dabbing is finished, carefully remove your gloves, turning them inside out. Again, be sure to dispose of the contaminated cotton balls and gloves appropriately so that they're **completely inaccessible** to anyone, especially children.

> ### Help for Mom's Nipples
>
> For moms with cracked, chapped, or sore nipples, the use of expressed breast milk is very helpful. Another simple remedy is to use a good quality food grade coconut oil. This is rich in emollients, and safe for your baby. One of my patients actually had mastitis and her baby had thrush. I counseled her to use the coconut oil topically several times a day, and both problems were resolved quickly. The lauric acid in coconut oil is antibacterial, antifungal, and antiviral, but does not disturb your good intestinal bacteria.

OTHER CRITICAL FACTORS FOR OPTIMIZING YOUR CHILDREN'S HEALTH

In this section we will deal with other important health-optimizing factors. A detailed presentation on all subjects would require several books, but we can at least address them here in philosophy and principle, if not in detail. These next topics will be generalized for all ages, and you will be able to use your discretion and best judgment to individualize those that are appropriate for your own children.

Heartfelt, Truthful Communication

Communication is the bonding agent of any relationship. Maintaining that communication in a respectful and meaningful fashion is one of our greatest challenges. Stylizing communication to each family member and tuning the communication to each person's age and receptivity is well worth the effort. Listening to and acknowledging each child's discoveries, opinions, concerns, fears and joys will foster their self-esteem and feelings of security. This applies to an infant discovering her toes, a toddler mastering his tricycle, or teens telling about their athletic or academic accomplishments.

Accurately explaining actions, events and changes to your children is an important use of communication. Examples include explaining what you are doing for them and with them and why. "Sarah, now I need to change your diaper." "Johnny, it's time to take a dose of elderberry and one of colloidal silver to help your sore throat." Communicate behavior boundaries and your expectations for your children's behavior by example as well as verbally.

"Monkey see, monkey do" is a principle that begins before birth. In fact, during their time in utero, babies learn a lot about their external environment. They learn to recognize the voices of various family members. They learn about family dynamics, about respectful and disrespectful styles of communication for each dyad of family members. The baby's emotion-detecting radar is functioning on a 24-7 basis, and they easily internalize the information. A tiny person, whether in mom's warm safe uterus or out in the bright world, is constantly soaking up all manner of data and is driven to construct some type of meaningful interpretation about the new environment that surrounds them.

Grant's Story

Charlotte brought her nine-month old son, Grant to me because she was concerned about his fear of being alone for any amount of time, failure to robustly thrive, and his pattern of frequent ear infections. In fact, Grant's pediatrician repeatedly prescribed antibiotics, which Charlotte dutifully administered. The result was abatement of the infection … for ten to fourteen days … followed by a reoccurrence. After six or eight cycles of this, Charlotte knew Grant's problem would never be solved with antibiotics. Charlotte told me that Grant had four older siblings, none of whom had any of his problems and were very healthy. Charlotte was careful with the family diet and prepared most meals at home from fresh ingredients. She exercised during the pregnancy and began again fairly soon after Grant's birth. When we talked about the late pregnancy and the time of Grant's birth, important facts came to light.

Charlotte's mother, Gina, had cancer and was deemed terminal about midway through Charlotte's pregnancy with Grant. Charlotte went to see her mother often, and helped her as much as possible. The mother and daughter were very close. In the last few weeks of Gina's life, Charlotte cried often as she was truly grieving. The day Gina died, Charlotte began labor, a few weeks before her due date. She developed complications, and had an emergency cesarean section. It was obvious to me that little Grant had heard (and felt) too much crying and sadness in utero. An emotional defense system against that could be called upon, the defense of diminishing his sense of hearing. Thus began Grant's cyclical ear infections, actually a physical malady, yet also an emotional defense mechanism. I believe that Charlotte's grief and torment, her totally uncomfortable state, precipitated Grant's preterm birth. These circumstances created his fearfulness. He could not begin to comprehend the concept of death as an adult could, yet he had heard his Grandmother Gina's voice from his protective womb-cave many times. When Gina's voice disappeared, I believe Grant was instinctively fearful that his mother would disappear also.

> During development the fetus adapted to a new environmental condition as if that condition would be permanent. In modern pediatrics and developmental psychobiology, this adaptation is called "fetal programming" or "prenatal programming." It's a new concept. The general idea is that during development important physiological parameters can be reset by environmental events—and the resetting can endure into adulthood.
> —Agin, Dan. *More than Genes: What Science Can Tell Us about Toxic Chemicals, Development, and the Risk to Our Children.* New York: Oxford University Press, Inc., 2010. 6-7.

I worked with Grant to build up his immunity. During each visit, he received very gentle and specific Chiropractic adjustments. It is well documented that Chiropractic treatment strengthens the body's immune response. (Noteworthy studies were reported in 1989[32], 1991[33], and 2000[34].) We used the soft laser for his thyroid, and also for the triple warmer meridian to stop the ear infection cycle. Charlotte gave Grant immune stimulating herbs at home. We worked with Charlotte and Grant both to balance chakras and emotions, and release fear and grief. Grant never had another ear infection and soon became a confident "independent" toddler.

Skin To Skin and Other Non-Verbal Contact

"Skin to skin" contact is a vital form of non-verbal communication between parents and newborns. Begin this loving process immediately after birth. Skin to skin contact provides many well documented physiological benefits—such as regulation of your infant's body temperature and metabolism. Less often discussed are the communication and bonding benefits of skin to skin contact. What better way exists to successfully communicate to your newborn: "Yes, I love you. I'm constantly here to protect you and to care for you"? Remember, your newborn was attached to mom's body and shielded from the external world for the first nine months. Skin to skin contact and snuggling with either parent, and nursing at mom's breast are the most similar and familiar environmental conditions that parents can provide a newborn. These actions non-verbally convey a sense of security which will foster self-esteem, as well as trust, the foundation for relationship building. Also, skin to skin contact is a biological pathway to bring mom's and dad's healthy skin microbes to baby's skin, and colonize beneficial bacteria on your baby's skin.

> Love is not measured by how many times you touch each other, but by how many times you reach each other. —Author Unknown

As your child grows and matures, continue using positive reinforcing nonverbal communication. These may include various forms of appropriate and mutually comfortable touch—hugs, kisses, a pat on the shoulder—all

> **Skin to Skin**
>
> Breastfeeding helps babies to bond well because of more skin-to-skin contact and touching. This helps babies to feel secure. When premature babies are held skin-to-skin against mother's chest (this is called "kangaroo care"), they grow and gain weight more quickly. Skin-to-skin contact helps a baby to relax. It can help to regulate a baby's heart rate and breathing pattern. —Ryan and Auletta, *Breastfeeding: Your Priceless Gift To Your Baby And Yourself*

meaningful from the toddler to the adult stages. Read your child's response to your gestures and offerings of familial close connecting. At some point, when their peers are constantly present, your child may reject parental physicality, perhaps for a decade or so. Reset your non-verbal communication appropriately for the greatest comfort level of all parties.

Hopefully you have instituted using direct eye contact, and the stance of giving your full attention to your child during conversation. Now at the preteen age, these will be your mainstays of non-verbal communication. Small acts of kindness, like secretly packing your child's favorite fruit or healthy snack, or a new pen or pack of neon sticky notes in their backpack will convey your continuing love and concern without the "embarrassment factor." For teens, it may be best to leave the sweet surprises in the kitchen with a note, if they have a great propensity to be embarrassed by parental caring and concern being witnessed by their peers.

Attention, Respect and Guidance

Give your children, at all ages, the same attention and respect that you appreciate receiving. Keep the communication door open by ensuring that your children know that you value their opinions, input and observations. Patiently listen to your children and their concerns, and imagine you are conversing with one of your adult friends. In ten or twenty years, you could have a meaningful adult- to-adult conversation with an adult (perhaps who has their own child or children in tow) who just happens to be *your* offspring! Thinking of your child as a potential adult will likely yield decades of fulfilling communication.

Children do require guidance, parenting, correcting and teaching. When parents carry out these functions respectfully and lovingly, the relationship deepens and grows. Provide simple reasons for house rules and protocols. Explain that the rules provide for safety, order and family harmony. This makes the rules more understandable, if not more palatable.

Most children "push the envelope" and challenge or rebel. Hopefully your household has studied about and decided upon a parenting style and a consistent method or philosophy for correcting or redirecting the children's behavior early on. Some situations are extraordinary. Some families have more issues and difficulties than others. Seek counsel as needed. Parenting is not an exact science. Keeping the focus on love is paramount. As a parent, focusing on unconditional love, and remembering that you are your child's guarding guide and teacher, as you help them navigate life's winding path, will be a simple guideline for successful parenting.

Let's go to a *mythical land of perfection* for a moment, here we find the utopian ideal for family functioning. In this mythical realm, all family members practice continually receiving each other in a state of unconditional love. This practice of unconditional loving is second nature since each member received such selfless love from their family of origin during their entire life. Each child is confident and many parental actions have assured them that their parent's unconditional love is much stronger than any failure to perform, any misdeed, or mistake on their part.

Now we must leave utopia, and return to our real world, which is probably a few steps away from that utopian ideal. However, we can each make efforts to incorporate segments, even fractions, of such an ideal into our family life, and our daily communications. If your child openly acknowledges his or her responsibility for spilling the milk, soiling the carpet, letting the dog escape, parking the car two-inches beyond the garage wall, and can admit their error to a loving parent without terror in their eyes, your family is moving closer to utopia than average. If your child is then able to ask your forgiveness for the misdeed and you are able to genuinely grant your forgiveness, kudos to you both. Effective trauma reduction and relationship healing have been achieved! Unconditional love has been affirmed. Approaching errors, mistakes, neglect of responsibility, and *even* premeditated disobedience as opportunities to guide your child in problem solving and planning for a better outcome next time holds many merits.

Trauma Avoidance and Healing

A key role for most parents is that of averting potentially traumatic experiences for their children. Each person experiences and reacts to traumatic events in their own particular way. This is determined by many factors, including a person's age, size, sense of vulnerability, state of mind just prior to the event, and other variables.

I helped an adult patient release an entrapped traumatic experience that had been internalized since approximately age nine. Ralph displayed difficulty with attention and staying focused, was jumpy, and self medicated at night with alcohol believing he could calm himself. He had spent several years in the military, which amplified his propensity to be on edge with loud noises, especially gunfire.

Ralph's problem apparently started in grade school. One day, he was one of the last children to finish lunch, and was left alone seated at a long lunch table that could fold in the center for storage. Somehow the safety lock released, the table folded up and trapped Ralph between the two halves. He received direct head trauma, and remembered that the noise was deafening.

As time went on, Ralph seemed to recover, and the event was "forgotten." The adrenaline release, the fear of being trapped and unable to move, the pain, and the loud noise were all internalized and held in his memory and his nervous system, altering his perceptions for years to come.

Ralph actually sought treatment for his chronic headaches, which were evaluated with Clinical Kinesiology, history, and a physical exam. Beyond the typical treatment consisting of Chiropractic treatment, cranial adjustments, and acupuncture, trauma release techniques were instituted. While touching his head, I had Ralph do a memory regression to the time of the injury and work himself forward and backward in time in conjunction with visual imagery and cranial treatment. We undertook the task to "rewrite" history, and went down the path of Ralph visualizing himself sitting at the table, finishing lunch, and then walking away from the table with no trauma. This process was repeated with variations three to four times. Ralph felt significant relief of all his symptoms.

Other methods of trauma release are quite effective as well. I am very impressed with Peter A. Levine's and Maggie Kline's work, Somatic Experiencing®. This is discussed in their book *Trauma Through a Child's Eyes*. It is a wonderful tool for parents. Levine and Kline impart this wisdom:

Trauma happens when *any* experience stuns us like a bolt out of the blue; it overwhelms us, leaving us altered and disconnected from our bodies…The younger the child, the more likely she is to be overwhelmed by common occurrences that might not affect an older child or adult.[35]

Many daily events could seem traumatic to a child, and not be recognized as such by parents. This may include harsh words, some punishments, loud noises, "routine" visits to an allopathic doctor's office, falls, injections, hospitalizations, the loss of a pet, a poor score on a test, and many other common and unavoidable experiences.

Preparing your child for new experiences in advance, explaining and familiarizing your child with new people, surroundings, odors, sounds, procedures, etc. can be helpful.

If an unforeseen event or trauma does occur, be very supportive and talk through it with your child to the best of your ability. Seek counsel or treatment as needed. Sometimes a trauma occurs and is psychically linked to a seemingly unrelated factor, such as a certain piece of music playing, wearing a certain color, or the wind blowing fiercely. The seemingly unrelated factor can act as a trigger for the fear or may catalyze reliving the feelings from the initial trauma. Treatment to unlink the trauma and the trigger will render much appreciated relief.

One way to minimize trauma to children, and the family as a whole, is to appropriately minimize allopathic (or conventional medical) healthcare interventions, reserving them for true emergencies, and situations that you feel loom larger than common sense, homeopathic remedies, or your natural healthcare provider may effectively handle.

Beware of Head Injuries

Go directly to the Emergency Room for suspected concussions, as this situation requires

IMMEDIATE evaluation and the child deserves neurological screening. As soon as possible after a head trauma (or any injury) administer the homeopathic Arnica. This remedy is appropriate for injury, bruising, swelling, and trauma. Poor Ralph (whose story I relate above) should have gone to the ER and should have been evaluated for traumatic brain injury, and he should have had several doses of Arnica. Ralph should have also been taken out of sports and physical education classes for up to three weeks to eliminate that chance of a second head trauma in close succession (called "second impact syndrome"). A second head trauma seriously complicates the treatment and recovery.

Today, imaging techniques clearly depict the physical state of the brain, its coverings (meninges), and its fluid, as well as the presence or absence of intracranial hemorrhage. The C-T scan will disclose fractures, if any. By all means, use the Emergency Room for *actual* emergencies. Do not clog the emergency department with children who have simple colds, mild rashes, surface abrasions, and uncomplicated health issues that can easily be handled at home.

Grady's Story

Grady is the grandson of one of my patients. When he was approximately a year and a half, he managed to fall out of the shopping cart onto a concrete floor. Luckily, his mom was well prepared and had homeopathic Arnica in her purse. She gave him a dose immediately and repeated the treatment every ten minutes. They went to the Emergency Room, where an imaging study revealed a skull fracture.

Grady's aunt is a Naturopathic physician and met them at the ER. There the doctors explained that they expected Grady's brain to swell and for his intracranial pressure to be increased by bleeding around the brain. Typically this would happen quickly, and an emergency surgery would be performed to relieve the pressure and prevent brain damage.

The ER doctors expected to find it necessary to remove a piece of Grady's skull bone for a period of time. They expected that some time would be required for the swelling to subside. The next phase of the anticipated plan would have been to replace the removed piece of bone with a metal plate. Grady's parents and aunt continued to make sure he received a dose of Arnica every ten minutes. This averted the brain swelling and all of the worst case scenario potentials. Grady was in the ER for over three hours, receiving both homeopathic and allopathic medical treatments, while being closely observed by his family as well as the hospital staff.

This story has a happy ending as Grady suffered no neurological damage from this incident. He had the advantage of both homeopathic and conventional medical care, immediately, and ongoing treatment with homeopathic remedies during his recovery for bone healing, etc. Happily, Grady avoided surgery and its potential consequences. The key is, as shown here, to persistently repeat the homeopathic treatment.

Self Help and Skilled Guidance

Parental discernment, education, and experience will be called into play for the host of children's health concerns that are neither a dire emergency, nor a simple booboo meriting a Band-Aid®. This applies to the concerns of all family members, as well.

Continue to educate yourself about the human body, its physiology, and its cycles. Practice listening to your own body when it tells you about its needs, as this ability will be your most important tool not only for your own health, but in listening for and to the needs of your children.

Your natural healthcare provider is a valuable resource for those health concerns between the minor scrape and the emergency situation. You may prefer to consult both ends of the professional spectrum—consider a Chiropractor, Naturopath, or acupuncturist, as well as an allopathic or medical doctor. *You* should be the ultimate decision maker, however. Use the opinions of these providers, your knowledge of your child and their idiosyncrasies, your wisdom and inner knowingness (gut feelings) when making important healthcare choices.

FIRST-AID AND REMEDIES FOR COMMON CONDITIONS

The following charts are simplified and generic, but can be used as a reference or reminder for potential natural solutions for uncomplicated health concerns. These charts are NOT intended as a substitute for appropriate healthcare, guidance, diagnosis, or treatment. Consult with your trusted healthcare practitioner, or practitioners. Ask their advice concerning these or any other possible remedies for your child's health condition.

ASTHMA	
HERBAL	**HOMEOPATHIC**
• Butterbur • Ginkgo Biloba • Khella • Licorice • Mullein • Pau d'arco • Turmeric	• Aconite • Antimonium tartaricum • Arsenicum album • Pulsatilla
OTHER	
• Colostrum • Vitamin D_3 • Omega 3 fatty acids • Probiotics • Reduce omega 6 fats • Regular exercise • Avoid pasteurized milk—notorious for making asthma worse	• Have your child evaluated for food allergies and sensitivities—eliminate suspects—wheat and pasteurized dairy are typically culprits • Look for household allergens: dust, pet dander, detergents, cleansers, etc. sequester these from your child
WARNING	
Aspirin, Advil™, Chemotherapy, and antibiotics can cause asthma attacks.	

CHICKEN POX	
HERBAL	HOMEOPATHIC
• Andrographis • Burdock root • Echinacea • Ginger • Pau d'arco • St. John's Wort	• Antimonium crudum • Antimonium tartaricum • Pulsatilla • Sulphur • Rhus toxicodendron
OTHER	
• Colostrum • Probiotics • Vitamin D_3 • 2 Tbs marigold flowers; 1 tsp witch hazel leaves; 1 c. water; Soak overnight; Apply on rash* • Breast milk applied to lesions* • Drink lots of water and fruit juices • Bath of cool water and ginger	• See impetigo advice—it is applicable, read cautions for topical applications. • Replace towels and washcloths daily or more often. • Add 10 drops of tea tree oil to each load of laundry * With topical applications—do not spread toxins to other skin areas

COLD	
HERBAL	HOMEOPATHIC
• Andrographis • Black elderberry • Echinacea • Honey suckle (Lonicera) • Licorice • Marshmallow root • Mullein • Thyme • Wild cherry bark—avoid long term use • Yarrow • Yin Chiao Pills®	• Aconitium (especially in the first 24 hours) • Allium Cepa • Arsenicum album • Gelsemium • Natrum muriaticum
OTHER	
• Colostrum • Probiotics • Vitamin D_3 • ADD ESSENTIAL ONE OR MORE OILS TO A CARRIER OIL AND RUB ON FEET OR CHEST • Bergamot essential oil • Cedar wood essential oil • Clove essential oil • Eucalyptus essential oil • Frankincense essential oil • Ginger essential oil • Lemon essential oil • Melaleuca essential oil • Peppermint essential oil (do not use topically)	• Sandalwood essential oil • Tea tree essential oil • Thyme essential oil • Keep baby or child hydrated • Humidifier or pot of water on the stove—may add one or two essential oils • Steam treatment-use a towel to cover your head and baby's head as you breathe in the steam • Breastfeed so baby receives antibodies (nurse in upright position). • Sleep in upright position holding your baby so mucus can drain. • Manuka honey (IF OVER 1 YEAR OLD) 2-4 year olds: ½ t. daily; over 4: 1 t. daily

COLIC, NAUSEA, AND DIGESTIVE ISSUES	
HERBAL	HOMEOPATHIC
• Anise—digestive aid • Catnip • Chamomile • Cat's claw—digestive aid, soothing • Fennel-colic and digestive aid • Ginger • Peppermint-nausea-best choice	• Arsenicum album • Belladonna • Alba • Chamomillia—upset stomach-crankiness 6+months
OTHER	
• Colostrum • Probiotics (especially lactobacillis reuteri, lactobacillis rhamnosus, and streptococcus thermophalis) • Chamomile essential oil • Rose essential oil • Warm water bath or warm compress on abdomen • Breastfeeding moms need to investigate their diet-eliminate suspicious foods or beverages, pasteurized milk is the most common culprit, coffee, sugar, chocolate, citrus, spicy foods, and gas forming foods-beans, berries, broccoli, cauliflower, Brussels sprouts, are also suspects. Mom and baby may benefit from mom using a digestive enzyme. Note: Herb Pharm's "Mother's Lactation Tonic®" will support mom's milk supply while helping the infant's colic symptoms. It comes through the milk. A few drops can be placed on the parent's finger and into the baby's mouth as well.	

COMMON FLU	
HERBAL	HOMEOPATHIC
• Andrographis • Black Elderberry • Echinacea • Honey suckle (Lonicera) • Licorice • Yin Chiao Pills®	• Aconitum napellus (1st 24 hours) • Anas barbarie (Oscillococcinum®) • Arsenicum album • Babtisa • Bryonia alba • Eupatorium perfoliatum • Ferrum phosphoricum • Gelsemium • Influenzinum (30x once a month as a preventative; also for lingering symptoms) • Nux vomica • Rhus toxicodendron
OTHER	
• Colostrum • Probiotics • Vitamin D_3 • For congestion: Cedar wood, clove, eucalyptus, ginger, lemon, melaleuca, rosemary, sandalwood, thyme essential oils in a carrier oil and rub on feet or chest. • Keep baby or child hydrated.	• Humidifier or pot of water on the stove. • Steam treatment—use a towel to cover your head and baby's head as you breathe in the steam) • Breastfeed so baby receives antibodies • Nurse upright • Holding your baby upright to sleep so mucus can drain • See cold recommendations; they are applicable.

CONJUNCTIVITUS OR "PINK EYE"	
HERBAL	HOMEOPATHIC
• Andrographis • Eyebright drops • Fennel • Tea of golden thread	• Apis mellifica • Ferrum phosphoricum • Hepar sulphur • Pulsatilla
OTHER	
• Colostrum • Probiotics • Vitamin D_3 • Calendula—oral or tea used as eye wash; cooled to body temperature. • Snapdragon tea from flowers and leaves—Used as eye wash; cooled to body temperature • Thinly sliced potatoes on eyes • Breast milk drops in eyes • Breastfeed so baby receives antibodies. • Recipe: 2 t. chamomile flowers; 1 t. Oregon grape root; 2 c. boiling water; sit 20 min.—use as eye wash	• Colloidal silver drops in eyes • Conjunctivitis is very contagious. Use great caution not to spread it from an affected child to other family members. All should be more careful with hand washing. Replace towels and washcloths daily or more often. • Add 10 drops of tea tree oil to each load of laundry. • Read impetigo information, especially about avoiding contamination and cross contamination.

CROUP	
HERBAL	HOMEOPATHIC
• Colt's foot as a tea—short term use—consult with a holistic doctor after 5 days. • Echinacea • Lung wort • Marshmallow root • Mullein—tea or tincture • Slippery elm bark tea	• Aconite • Belladonna • Hepar Sulphur • Spongia tosta
OTHER	
• Colostrum • Probiotics • Vitamin D_3 • Use essential oils individually or in combination with a carrier oil on chest • Eucalyptus essential oil • Peppermint essential oil • Rosemary essential oil • Use a humidifier • Moist or hot air from shower	• Taking a well wrapped child out into the cold night air. • Vitamin C and Zinc Lozenges • Cloth on skin with onion plaster made of cooked minced onion over the cloth* • Humidify air—either warm or cool • See flu recommendations, they are applicable. • Warm moist pack over throat * Specific instructions at yourbodycantalk.com

DIARRHEA	
HERBAL	HOMEOPATHIC
• Blackberry tea • Ginger tea	• Aethusa • Arsenicum album • Calcarea carbonica • Chamomilla • Cuprum • Pulsatilla
OTHER	
• CONSULT A DOCTOR FOR INFANTS WITH DIARRHEA; THEY CAN BECOME DEHYDRATED QUICKLY. • Colostrum • Probiotics • Brown rice water: prepare brown rice with twice the amount of water (normally 2 cups water to 1 cup dry rice so for brown rice water, use 4 cups water to 1 cup dry rice). Cook about 45 minutes. After cooling a few minutes, strain and serve excess water, a potent mineral replacement fluid. Serve the water as a broth. Many times mild to moderate diarrhea stops after one or two cups are ingested. If no response to above treatment, consult child's doctor. • Search for cause, often it is an infection or a dietary incompatibility; address the cause appropriately.	

EAR ACHE	
HERBAL	HOMEOPATHIC
• As a prevention and treatment: 1/3 Echinacea tincture, 1/3 elderberry tincture or syrup, and 1/3 anise seed tincture blended in a mix. • Grapefruit seed extract added to vegetable glycerin • Chamomile	• Aconite • Belladonna • Chamomilla • Hepar sulphur
OTHER	
• Colostrum • Probiotics • Chamomile essential oil • St. John's wort essential oil • Collodial silver as an ear wash (warm to body temperature) • As ear drops: mullein and garlic oil blend; St. John's wort; calendula (warm to body temperature) • As a topical/external: lavender oil, tea tree oil, chamomile oil • Feed upright when bottle feeding to avoid milk in ear canals • A daily dose of fish oil for prevention • Lemon balm, Catnip, Ginger, Licorice, Spearmint, and Chamomile herbal teas to drink • Infants should get 1t. of teas 3-4 times daily; children ½ c. 3-4 times daily • Use several drops of one or more of these essential oils (lavender, roman chamomile, tea tree) added to heat pack of rice, flax or buck wheat placed in a soft sock or washcloth (secured to prevent spillage) Warm a little above body temperature and then place over the aching ear while nursing or cuddling your child.	• Prop head at 30° angle while lying down • Limit exposure to known or expected allergens • Vitamin C and Zinc • Vitamin D_3 • Massage around ear • Cranial therapy—seek a professional • Remember ear aches are most often caused by a viral infection and typically will not respond to antibiotics. Accept antibiotics ONLY if a throat culture is positive for pathogenic bacteria, and you are convinced it is necessary. Treat at home while the culture is growing for 2 days. Your child should improve immensely by the time you learn the culture results. If not, you can NOW make an informed decision.

EYE IRRITATION	
HERBAL	HOMEOPATHIC
• Snapdragon tea • Eyebright tea	• Sterile homeopathic eye drops
OTHER	
• Colostrum • Probiotics • Warm or cool compresses (use the most relieving one)	• Colloidal silver drops in eyes • Breast milk drops in eyes • See conjunctivitis—most recommendations apply

GROWING PAINS	
HERBAL	HOMEOPATHIC
• Stinging nettles as a tincture, tea, or steamed vegetable	• Calcarea phosphoric • Causticum
OTHER	
• Magnesium is the primary mineral to use; add calcium if magnesium had little or no effect, use oral or topical—See the *Product and Resource Guide* regarding topical magnesium. • Vitamin D_3 • Massage legs or painful area (be sure to preventatively use the favored remedy after sporting events and on days of great physical exertion, before pain manifests.)	• Essential fatty acids • Be sure your child is well hydrated, especially before and after physical exertion • Zinc or a multi-mineral if magnesium, then calcium did not help. • Use warm Epsom salt baths

IMPETIGO	
HERBAL	HOMEOPATHIC
• Astragalus • Echinacea	• Antimonium crudum • Arsenicum album • Graphites • Hepar sulphur • Lycopodium • Rhus toxicodendron
OTHER	
• Colostrum • Probiotics • Vitamin D_3 • Apple cider vinegar • Breast milk • Colloidal silver drops • Coconut oil • It is best to dilute one or more of these essential oils with a carrier oil, such as almond oil, jojoba oil, or olive oil. (Mix a small amount in a small cup, discard remainder after each treatment) • Eucalyptus essential oil • Helichrysum essential oil • Lavender essential oil • Tea tree essential oil • Impetigo is very contagious. It may spread to affect more areas of the affected child, or may be easily spread to infect others. Be very careful when administering topical treatments. Use disposable gloves, use cotton balls for one dab only. Discard cotton balls and gloves carefully and	securely. Do not contaminate the container of the remedy. Example: use a clean spoon to take out a small amount of coconut oil. Place the coconut oil in a small cup or saucer. Then take the cup or saucer, gloves, cotton balls to the bathroom and administer the treatment, discard all waste securely. Wash your hands well. Wash, sanitize, and scald the cup or saucer. A little carelessness could infect the entire family. Be aware that impetigo is often spread in daycare centers, schools, and swimming pools. Observe the other children for signs of impetigo; leave the area immediately if you see the classic yellow to honey colored, weepy, and crusty lesions on anyone's skin. Supply fresh towels and washcloths in your home daily. Add 10 drops of tea tree oil to each load of laundry until all evidence of impetigo is gone from your family. These are effective impetigo topical treatments if you carefully avoid recontamination.

TEETHING	
HERBAL	HOMEOPATHIC
• Catnip—soothes nervous system • Chamomile tea	• Aconite—for a distressed teething infant • Belladonna—use if Chamomilla fails • Chamomilla—institute first
OTHER	
• Breast milk has a pain reducing effect—massage onto gums • Baltic Amber teething necklace—it releases succinic acid (a natural anti-inflammatory) • Chilled hard fruit or vegetables such as a large carrot to gnaw on • A wet, cold washcloth—could even freeze it for a while to make colder. • Teething toys • Rescue Remedy—4 drops in mouth; can also massage onto gums • Plantago major (plantain) tincture—massage drops on gums • Pure vanilla extract—massage on gums; it is relaxing	

NOTE: In July 2014 the FDA issued a warning against the use of the gel form of 2 percent lidocaine for teething in infants and toddlers. During the first half of 2014, twenty-two cases of serious adverse reactions were reported, including six deaths, and three additional life-threatening events.

The uniqueness of your child and his or her specific health picture must be honored always. The "whole personness" of each child must also be considered. Dana Ullman, M.P.H., is the author of *Homeopathic Medicine for Children and Infants*, a wonderful guide for parents and healthcare practitioners alike. He makes the following comments:

> Children with fevers higher than 103.5 degrees (taken orally) that do not respond to the above remedies [in the previous charts] or general homecare within six hours should be given prompt medical care. Infants less than six months old should receive medical care for any fever higher than 100.5 degrees. Infants less than two months old should receive medical care for any fever. Also, when a child has any fever with extreme irritability, lethargy, and mental confusion along with stiffness of the neck, seizures, recurrent vomiting, or labored breathing, seek medical care immediately.[36]

I sincerely hope that you have learned a great deal about optimizing your children's health. This is a valuable topic which receives so little emphasis in our modern culture. Please pass along the concepts of pre-conception lifestyle planning and improvement, and how vital it is to make wise choices TODAY. Your lifestyle choices build your future, and that of your children. Searching for drugless solutions to everyday health problems is nature's simpler and kinder approach to nurture your child with less trauma and virtually no side effects.

Listen to your body talk and learn more about how to properly care for it. Model this ability for your children and admire them as they begin to master the art of being in tune with themselves. Always look for a Natural Solution.

As so many of us are looking for a drug-free approach to thrive in our daily lives if at all possible, I have chosen to present a chapter on this topic. Deciding whether or not to take a medication with known side effects is a serious question to ponder. Several generations of people have silently submitted to each prescription presented to them, without undertaking due diligence. Learning about any proposed drug, its actions, side effects and other consequences first, and then making a truly informed decision is the most responsible approach. It is my sincerest hope that my readers, patients, family, friends, and associates will adopt this approach and will frequently benefit from the simple, natural, and gentle alternatives described in Chapter 14, *Drugs: Just Say NO THANKS!*

CHAPTER 13 SUGGESTED READING

Aamodt, Sandra and Sam Wang, Foreword by Ellen Galinsky. *Welcome to Your Child's Brain: How the Mind Grows from Conception to College.* New York: Bloomsbury, USA, 2012.

Agin, Dan. *More than Genes: What Science Can Tell Us about Toxic Chemicals, Development, and the Risk to Our Children.* New York: Oxford University Press, 2010.

Daniel G. Amen, M.D. *10 Steps to Building Values Within Children: An Audio/Workbook Program.* Newport Beach, Calif: MindWorks Press. 2006

Arms, Suzanne, Chloe Fisher and Mary Renfrew. *Breastfeeding: How to Breastfeed Your Baby.* Berkeley, Calif.: Celestial Arts, 2004.

_____ *Immaculate Deception I: A New Look at Women and Childbirth in America.* Boston: Houghton Mifflin, 1975.

_____ *Immaculate Deception II: Myth, Magic and Birth.* Berkeley: Celestial Arts, 1996.

Asprey, Lana, M.D.; Asprey, David. *The Better Baby Book: How to Have a Healthier, Smarter, Happier Baby.* Hoboken, N.J.: John Wiley & Sons, Inc., 2013.

Ellison, Katherine. *The Mommy Brain: How Motherhood Makes Us Smarter.* New York: Basic Books, A Member of the Perseus Books Group, 2005.

Levine, Peter A., Ph.D and Maggie Kline. *Trauma Proofing Your Kids: A Parents' Guide for Instilling Confidence, Joy and Resilience.* Berkeley: North Atlantic Books; and Lyons, Colorado: ERGOS Institute Press, 2008.

Levine, Peter A., Ph.D and Maggie Kline. *Trauma Through a Child's Eyes: Awakening the Ordinary Miracle of Healing.* Berkeley: North Atlantic Books; and Lyons, Colorado: ERGOS Institute Press, 2007.

Losey, Meg Blackburn, Msc.D., Ph.D. *The Children of Now: Crystalline Children, Indigo Children, Star Kids, Angels on Earth, and the Phenomenon of Transitional Children.* Franklin Lakes, N.J.: New Page Books, A Division of The Career Press, Inc., 2006.

Martin, Chia. *We Like to Nurse.* Chino Valley, Arizona: Hohm Press, 1995.

Natterson, Cara., M.D. *Dangerous or Safe?: Which Foods, Medicines, and Chemicals Really Put Your Kids at Risk?* New York: Hudson Street Press, Published by Penguin Group, 2009.

Neustaedter, Randall, O.M.D. *Child Health Guide: Holistic Pediatrics for Parents.* Berkeley: North Atlantic Books, 2005.

Ryan, Regina Sara and Deborah Auletta. *Breastfeeding: Your Priceless Gift to Your Baby and Yourself.* Chino Valley, Arizona: Hohm Press, 2005.

Schmidt, Michael A., M.D. and Lendon H., Smith, M.D. *Childhood Ear Infections: What Every Parent and Doctor Should Know About Prevention, Home Care, and Alternative Treatment (The Family Health Series).* Berkeley: North Atlantic Books, 1990.

Sears, William, M.D., Martha, Sears, R.N., Robert Sears, M.D.; and James Sears, M.D. *The Baby Book, Revised Edition: Everything You Need to Know About Your Baby from Birth to Age Two (Sears Parenting Library)*. New York, Boston, London: Little, Brown and Company, 2013.

Siegel-Maier, Karyn. *Happy Baby, Happy You: 500 Ways to Nurture the Bond with Your Baby*. North Adams, Mass.: Storey Publishing, LLC, 2009.

Spector, Tim. *Identically Different: Why We Can Change Our Genes*. New York: Overlook Press, 2014.

Strickland, Elizabeth, MS, RD, LD. *Eating for Autism: The 10-Step Program to Help Treat Your Child's Autism, Aspergers, or ADHD*. Cambridge, Mass.: DaCapo Press, 2009.

Ullman, Dana, M.P.H.; foreword by Richard Solomon, M.D. *Homeopathic Medicine for Children and Infants*. New York: Jeremy P. Tarcher/Putnam, a member of Penguin Putnam, Inc., 1992.

Wakefield, Andrew J.; foreword by Jenny McCarthy. *Callous Disregard: Autism and Vaccines: The Truth Behind a Tragedy*. New York: Skyhorse Publishing, 2011.

Wiessinger, Diane, Diana West and Teresa Pitman. *The Womanly Art of Breastfeeding*. New York: Ballantine Books, 2010.

Young, Mary. *We Like to Nurse Too*. Chino Valley, Arizona: Hohm Press, 2009.

Zibners, Lara. *If Your Kid Eats This Book, Everything Will Still Be Okay: How to Know If Your Child's Injury or Illness Is Really an Emergency*. New York: Wellness Central, Hachette Book Group, 2009.

PART IV

THE MEDICATION DILEMMA

CHAPTER 14

Drugs: Just Say NO THANKS!

Payton brought his mom, Polly, to my office one afternoon. Polly told me that she could no longer drive—for about two weeks she felt dizzy and saw large greenish-yellow halos around all lights. She was fatigued, her appetite was diminished, and her memory had suddenly declined; her quick mind had slowed dramatically. "For one thing, I can't keep up with my bridge game; it's not fair to my partner," she said. I took notes as she continued her stories. "Why, just a month ago, I had no confusion, no headaches, plenty of energy, no halos, and no diarrhea. The amazing part is I just had my yearly physical exam about one month ago."

When I asked her about the exam findings she related mostly "good results," except that, while she still had high blood pressure, "now they've diagnosed mild heart failure."

When I asked which new drugs had been added to her program., Polly reported that she was prescribed Digoxin® and Spironolactone® for the mild heart failure, along with Lisinopril®, also for blood pressure and heart failure and Lipitor® (atorvastatin calcium) for cholesterol. This was on top of the baby aspirin and a Lopressor® (metropolol) that she had been taking for five years, Polly described.

I knew that the Digoxin® can cause the side effect of seeing halos around lights.[1] Combining Digoxin® with Spironolatone® potentiates or exaggerates that effect. All of her other new "symptoms"—aka adverse **side effects:** dizziness, fatigue, diminished appetite, declining memory, declining cognition, visual disturbances, bruising (Polly's arms and hands were covered with purple, maroon, and yellowish-green bruises), and diarrhea—could also be attributed to her list of medications.

"You know, Dr. Levy," she confided, "I feel like I'm watching my life go by and I'm not actually living it." Obviously, Polly was not able to process the quantity of medication going into her system on a daily basis. Polly discussed taking seven drugs at once, then recalled an eighth—Plavix®. She had been told it would reduce chances of forming serious blood clots. Now I knew why she has so many bruises.

The "math" was straightforward. One month ago, active, alert and busy; then, a new physical exam, five *new* prescriptions resulting in eight new problems. Polly was obviously moving in the wrong direction: greater dis-ease, less normal function, less quality of life.

After documenting the facts of this nonsensical equation, I immediately referred Polly to a

> 2 old drugs + 5 new drugs = new problems > old problems

respected osteopath who modified, and gently reduced her reliance on prescriptions. He was attentive to the overlapping of drug actions and wary of adverse drug **interactions**, and ultimately discontinued several of the offending chemicals for Polly, with excellent results! Five weeks after the first visit, Polly drove herself to her second visit at my office. She was happy and conversant; in fact, she was jubilant! Her quality of life was renewed and revitalized.

We worked together on a lifestyle plan and a treatment program to support her cardiovascular system. She streamlined her diet to a whole foods approach. Polly traded her daily donuts, French fries and pie for lush salads, broccoli, kale, quinoa other healthy seeds, limited whole grains, fresh fruits, coconut oil, turmeric, and pomegranate juice. She also joined a senior's walking club and returned to all of her previous activities.

Based on Polly's history and Clinical Kinesiology findings, we began a weekly treatment program that included gentle chiropractic, acupuncture, soft laser, vibrational energy frequencies, and guided imagery especially designed to support her cardiovascular system.

Polly's body seemed to have tolerated the daily intake of two medications, aspirin and Lopressor®, without balking. Yet, her body chemistry did not withstand the addition of five new drugs, each with its own toxicity, side effects, and interruptions to normal body rhythm and function (physiology). Her physical and mental deterioration within a short period of time was proven to be drug-induced, i.e., iatrogenic (doctor caused). She rapidly recovered lost function and viability after the offending toxins were removed from her daily regimen.

WHY INCLUDE A CHAPTER ON DRUGS?

Drugs are powerful tools for changing functions in your body. All drugs have physiological effects, which is why we use them, but some of these consequences are unwanted, producing adverse side effects. Therefore, some study, wise evaluation and intelligent pro-active conversations with your healthcare provider are called for. While it is beyond the scope of this book to impart a thorough background knowledge of chemistry, biochemistry, physiology, pharmacology, herbology, etc., it is possible to present a common-sense approach for helping you determine the appropriate questions to ask of your doctors, and resources for finding their answers.

My goal for you is that, by reading and considering this chapter, you will be able to avoid the pitfalls that Polly experienced. You will learn to use proactive approaches first to bolster your health and fine-tune your lifestyle, and ultimately learn to systematically examine and cross-examine the crucial question: *Should I actually take this proposed drug?*

For example, the questions that follow are all challenging and often difficult to ask of your doctor, **and** to answer for yourself. An important step in proactive natural self-care is to seek more information and feel informed prior to making a crucial decision (taking a new medication). You can ask your healthcare provider (and investigate for yourself):

- What are the potential adverse side effects of this proposed medication?
- Do I already have an issue with those conditions (Such as insomnia, skin rashes,

nausea, weight gain, visual disturbances, or diarrhea)?
- Are the contraindications (reasons not to take a drug) relevant in **my** case?
- Do I take other drugs that may not combine well with the proposed drug?
- Are there serious potential consequences (blindness, immune system compromise, internal bleeding, suicidality, cancer, or death [the Black Box warning])?
- Can I patiently explore the non-medication alternatives for a few months before taking the "plunge" into the prescription?

Seek counsel from your doctors—natural and allopathic—or an experienced pharmacist or pharmacy department at your local hospital, and study the Physician's Desk Reference (PDR) and other reliable resources. Check out the Institute for Safe Medication Practices (ISMP), a non-profit, independent watchdog organization that coordinates a medication-error reporting service and medication error prevention efforts. The ISMP medication-safety-alert newsletters are published quarterly and are archived. *The Quarter-Watch* reports give a quarterly summary of serious FDA-reported medication adverse events. *The Quarter-Watch* also informs professionals and patients about drug safety concerns. (See Product and Resource guide at the end of this book.)

Also in this chapter you will learn to scrutinize your lifestyle and institute positive changes that strengthen your body and total being. You will learn how foods, nutrients, herbs, homeopathics, affirmations, and other self-help measures can help move you from dis-ease to wholesome balance. You will gain a sense of empowerment to take (advised) initiative actions to gain a higher level of wellness.

HISTORY OF PHARMACOLOGY: IN A CAPSULE

Guidance from their innate human instinct and observation of nature with its rhythmic cycles began revealing self-care secrets to our distant ancestors. This, and watching animals, fish, and birds cope with their daily challenges and life cycle requirements, were the first health instructors. Historically, treatment nostrums (formulations) for human ailments were either herbal or mineral in origin. To a lesser degree, substances directly obtained from animals or fish were used.

Pharmacology's traditional roots are herbology and pharmacognosy, "Pharmacognosy" is the ancient science that studies methodology for extraction and compounding of natural medicinal substances generally obtained from plants.[2]

"Herbology" is the study of various herbs for supporting and balancing the body in a most direct and earth-resourced approach. The herb or combination of herbs may be ingested as food or tea, used as an external poultice or even dissolved in a bath. The herb may be dried and encapsulated, or tinctured in alcohol, water, vinegar, honey or glycerin. Traditionally, the herbalist's approach is to use the "whole" herb in an unadulterated form—not chemically separating and refining "active ingredients" from other important factors. This allows the natural balance of various pharmacologically active constituents—alkaloids, phytochemicals, terpines, vitamins, minerals, amino acids, and enzymes—to be preserved. Nature's balance tends to minimize unwanted (or negative) side effects. Pharmacology's traditional roots, herbology and pharmacognosy, persist today in relatively "pure" form.

BIGGER PHARMA

In contrast to the traditional approaches, the science of pharmacology and the pharmaceutical industry are forging ahead at lightning speed to produce more high-tech chemicals, biological agents, and pharmacogenetic-based treatments. Researcher Marcia Angell notes, in her book, *The Truth About the Drug Companies*, that, "It bases its reassurances on the notion that the mapping of the human genome and the accompanying burst in genetic research will yield a cornucopia of important new drugs."[3] The discovery of cellular receptor sites and the innovation of chemically based drugs that adhere to these sites have opened the door to producing a new genre of drugs.

Innovations in this field multiplied in the 1980s and 1990s, when this research was in its earlier stages, but today, the industry seems to subsidize itself by perpetuating a series of "remakes." These are often called "me too drugs," since they are structurally comparable to drugs that already exist, with only slight differences. Since a prescription pharmaceutical drug commands the highest price while it is under its original patent (typically twenty years), "…a drug company's aim is to get the drug on the shelves as early in the life of the patent as possible."[4] Therefore, speed is critical.

As the expiration date for a Block Buster drug patent looms (the industry classifies a Block Buster as one that draws over one billion dollars in a year), the NASDAQ quivers and stockholders look for the next vertical trend. As soon as the patent expires, competing producers present deeply discounted "knock-offs" to the market place. This activity has the characteristics of a feeding frenzy at a koi pond. Lately, the original patent-holder has been playing a new card, remaking the original with a combo (two-for-one) drug synthesis of two oldies but goodies.

These drugs are known as "mashups" and include drugs like Caduet®, which combines Norvasc® (blood pressure) and Lipitor® (cholesterol).

Of the seventy-eight drugs approved by the FDA in 2002, only seventeen contained new active ingredients, and only seven of these were classified by the FDA as improvements over older drugs. The other seventy-one drugs approved that year were variations of old drugs or deemed no better than drugs already on the market.[5]

Another "wild card" that pharmaceutical companies can throw down is a new method of delivery for the well paying oldie. For example, the original patent for Metformin® was in tablet form, the "new" innovation might be an extended release capsule, or a topical application or wearable patch. The goal is to obtain a new patent, with minimal research investment and ride the next wave.

The Prescription Drug Chart that follows (see next page) is a graphic description and comparison of several Block Buster pharmaceutical marvels. Star performers in eleven categories were chosen, as indicated on the left-hand heading column, such as Analgesics (pain killers), Antibiotics, Anti-Cholesterol, etc.

Understanding the Chart

The Prescription Drug Chart has several columns for each example drug. **Name and manufacturer** column are obvious. For **Rank/Sales (2011),** the first digit, i.e. 1 for Lipitor®, indicates it ranks as **the most** lucrative drug in 2011. The second number, $7,668,425,000 indicates the gross sales of Lipitor® in America in 2011. The symbol -- indicates unavailable sales figures at the time of publication.

The **Rank/Rxs for 2011** lists the number of prescriptions written for the specific drug in 2011. In the case of Lipitor®, its rank of 5 means it was the fifth most commonly prescribed drug in America in 2011. The **Rxs** portion of the column illustrates the number of American prescriptions written that year, 40,812,000.

The **Side Effects** for all eleven examples were simplified and grouped into categories tagged by

Prescription Drug Chart Based on IMS Institute for Healthcare[6]

	Prescription Drug	Manufacturer	Rank/Sales (2011)	Rank/RXs (2011)	Side effects (simplified)
Analgesics (Opioids)	OxyContin (oxycodone)	Purdue	19/$2,880,324,000	129/--	BW, CNS, CV, D, GI, M, ND, R
Antibiotics	Levaquin (levofloxacin)	Janssen	79/--	183/--	BD, CNS, CV, D, GI, HT, I, IA, M, MSk, ND, VP
Anti-Cholesterol	Lipitor (atorvastatin calcium)	Pfizer	1/$7,668,425,000	5/40,812,000	BD, BW, CNS, GI, IA, M, MSk, ND VP
Anti-Depressants	Cymbalta (duloxetine)	Lilly	9/$3,666,405,000	23/--	BD, BW, CNS, CV, GI, HT,M, MSk, ND, R, SD
Anti-Diabetes	Actos (pioglitazone hydrochloride)	Takeda	13/$3,437,722,000	59/--	BD, BW, CV, CNS, GI,HT, IA, M, MB, ND, R, VP
Anti-Inflammatory (NSAID)	Humira (adalimumab)	Abbott	10/$3,531,157,00	--/--	BD, BW, CV,CNS,D,GI, IA, I, M, MB, MSk, ND, P, R, K, SD, VP
Anti-Inflammatory (Steroidal)	Symbicort (budesonide and formoterol fumarate dehydrate)	AstraZeneca	56/--	191/--	BD, BW, CV,CNS, IA, M, MSk, ND, R, VP
Anti-Hyper-tensive	Diovan (valsartan and hydrochlorothiazide)	Novartis	27/--	34/--	BW, CNS, CV, D, GI, I, IA, K, M,MSK, ND, R, VP,
Proton Pump Inhibitors	Nexium (esomeprazole)	AstraZeneca	3/$6,155,7700,000	11/25,660,000	CNS, CV, GI, MSk, ND, R
Platelet Aggregation Inhibitors	Plavix (clopidogrel)	Bristol-Myers Squibb/sanofi-aventis	2/$6,771,208,000	7/28,139,000	BD, BW, CVS, D, GI, HT, IA, M, ND
Sleep Aids	Lunesta (eszopiclone)	Sunovion	74/--	--/--	CNS, D, GI, M, ND

Symptom Key for Prescription Drug Chart[1]

Blood Dyscrasia (BD)	Anemia (low red blood cell count or reduced hemoglobin–chronic tiredness, shortness of breath, chilled sensation, and chest pain), Neutropenia (low neutrophil count—increased susceptibility to infection), Thrombocytopenia (low platelet count–increased susceptibility to bleeding, bruising, and hemorrhaging), Splenomegaly (enlarged spleen), and Hepatomegaly (enlarged liver)
Boxed Warning (BW)	Also referred to as "black box warning" and is required by the FDA to signify that medical studies indicate that the drug carries a significant risk of serious or even life-threatening adverse effects
Cardiovascular (CV)	Arrhythmia (irregular heart rate), Hypertension (high blood pressure), and Angina (severe chest pain)
Central Nervous System (CNS)	Seizures, Headaches, Weakness, Pain, Numbness or tingling in limbs, Confusion, Slurred speech, Excessive sweating, and Tremors
Dermatological (D)	Itching, Rashes, Blisters, Welts, Hives, and Acne
Gastrointestinal (GI)	Diarrhea, Constipation, Nausea, Vomiting, and Abdominal pain
Hepatotoxicity (HT)	Nausea, Vomiting, Abdominal pain, Loss of appetite, Diarrhea, Tiredness, Weakness, Jaundice, Hepatomegaly (liver enlargement)
Hormonal (H)	Fatigue, Acne, Mood swings, Agitation, Weight problems, Diminished sex drive, Memory problems, Breast swelling or discharge
Iatrogenic (IA)	Any condition or set of symptoms that are the direct cause of a doctor's actions and would not have occurred on its own including increased risk of infection and diseases caused by prescription drugs
Immune (I)	Fatigue, Chronic illness or Infection, Diarrhea, Insomnia, Depression, Skin problems, Swollen glands, and Fever
Malaise (M)	Abdominal pain or cramping, Enlarged lymph nodes, Fever, Chills, Flu-like symptoms, Joint pain, Missed or irregular menstrual periods, Muscle aches, Severe Fatigue, and Weight loss
Metabolic (MB)	Weight gain, Weight loss, Excessive hunger or thirst, and Loss of appetite
Musculoskeletal (MSk)	Joint inflammation and swelling, Joint stiffness, Joint pain, and Muscular pain
Nutrient Deficiencies (ND)	Diminishment of vital amino acids, vitamins, and minerals
Pancreatic (P)	Clay-colored stools, Hyperglycemia (high blood sugar), and Hypoglycemia (low blood sugar)
Respiratory (R)	Difficulty breathing, Shortness of breath, Cough, and Cyanosis (purple or blue fingernails, toenails and/or lips).
Renal (Kidney) (K)	Frequent urination, Excessive thirst, Cloudy urine, and Flank pain (side pain)
Sexual Dysfunction (SD)	Impotence, Diminished sex drive, and Difficulty orgasming
Vision Problems (VP)	Halos around objects or lights, Blurred vision, and Scotomas (blind spots or dark "holes" in the vision in which nothing can be seen)

---

[1] Symptoms related to each category may include but are not limited to those listed above. An individual may experience all, some or none of the side effects listed. Complications including adverse side effects should be discussed by your prescribing doctor. You should never discontinue any medication without your doctor's advisement.

two-letter abbreviations (BD, BW, ND, etc) in the last column. Refer to the Prescription Drugs Chart on page 282 for clarification. If a drug did not rank in the top 100 for a specific category, i.e., Oxycontin® for number of prescriptions, it will be indicated by the symbol --.

HOW DID WE GET TO BE SO UNHEALTHY AND SO OVER-DRUGGED?

Our reliance on drugs and technical medicine has been the result of years in which following "fads" has become the norm. For example, in the 1950s and 1960s there was a widely used practice of removing the tonsils of children who had two or more strep throat infections. Research later showed that those children went on to suffer a higher rate of dental cavities since the reservoirs of attack-ready white blood cells in their throats had been sacrificed, and refined sugar consumption was escalating.

Today and in the recent past, research from the University of Kentucky by Boyd Haley, Ph.D., demonstrates a correlation of amalgam (mercury containing) dental fillings and the dramatic increase of many forms of dementia, including Alzheimer's disease.[7] The domino effect of a "simple" medical intervention persists for decades with devastating effects.

At the root of the cascade of many health consequences that we see today is the sharply increased dietary intake of refined, devitalized carbohydrates in the late 1940s and beyond. This list of toxic substances masquerading as "foods" includes sugar (glucose, maltose, fructose, corn syrup, corn sweeteners, high-fructose corn-syrup, dextrose, high maltose corn syrup, maltodextrin, sorbitol, glucitol, erythritol, lactitol, maltitol, xylitol), artificial sweeteners, white flour, white rice, non-whole grain pasta, most vegetable oils, including hydrogenated and trans fats, refined salt, and others.

The devitalized carbohydrates contribute to white blood cell destruction, the resultant lowering of total body immunity, depletion of minerals and vitamins, weakening of body tissues, i.e., collagen, ligament, muscle, skin, etc. A diet high in refined carbohydrates and processed foods in general contribute to obesity, diabetes, metabolic syndrome, arthritis, multiple sclerosis, high blood pressure, generalized inflammation, arthritis, osteoporosis, Alzheimer's, and many other prevalent yet bothersome conditions, even mutagenesis and cancer.

In roughly 1990, the medical fad had progressed from tonsillectomy to the use of high-powered antibiotics. Even in the 1980s, powerful antibiotics, in my opinion, were recklessly prescribed at the first whimper of a sore throat or a sniffle. As one group of researchers notes:

> ... experienced and highly trained physicians estimated that 81 percent of the patients had strep throat. In reality, only 4.9 percent were found to have positive cultures for strep after laboratory analysis. Perhaps most alarming was the fact that 104 of the 308 patients were actually started on antibiotic therapy. Only eight of the patients required antibiotics.[8]

These prescriptions were rarely predicated on the outcome of a culture and susceptibility test.[†]

[†] During this test cultures of the specific villainous bacteria are grown in Petri-dishes and tested for susceptibility to various antibiotic candidates. If the culture and susceptibility test path is taken, a two to four day delay in starting the antibiotic may occur due to the incubation period of the culture, but at least a predictable outcome can be expected from the best performing antibiotic tested.

Standard protocol was and often still is to rush in with heavy-artillery antibiotics and blast the body with the newest (this usually also equates to most costly) "big gun" available! If this fails after a five, seven or ten day assault, then a different "big gun" is used, sometimes without the simple culture and susceptibility test ever being applied. In fact, countless antibiotic prescriptions have been written and consumed purportedly to aid an obviously viral infection. **Antibiotics are not, never have been, nor ever will be indicated for viral infections**. After years of this approach, we have artificially selected the most viable (durable) bacteria to carry on their genetic lines. The newest generations are more antibiotic resistant than ever. Thus, we have seen outbreaks of MRSA—Methicillin-resistant Staphylococcus aureus. The first hospital outbreak of MRSA was in the late 1960s in Boston, Massachusetts.

Some individuals have actually died and some have lost limbs due to MRSA infections. Since the antibiotic war is waged with pharmaceuticals, each side escalates toxicity, but neither side wins. Significant collateral damage from this war is weakened immunity (see Chapter 6: *Energizing Your Immune System*) and the consequences of Candida, dysbiosis, and leaky gut syndrome (see Chapters 7 and 8).

Domestic and farm-raised animals, birds and fish that are given antibiotics, often mixed into their feed, are subject to leaky gut syndrome, dysbiosis, weakened immunity and greater susceptibility to infection. Documented cases exist wherein a person who is allergic to penicillin and actively avoids the drug succumbs to anaphylactic shock from eating meat or dairy tainted with drug residues given to the livestock. With these constant threats, it is no wonder that the public at large is unhealthy and overdrugged.

PROACTIVE CHOICES

Antibiotics can be useful when instituted as a last resort (hopefully guided by a culture and susceptibility test). Prior to choosing any drug, however, learn about possible risks and expected benefits. Prepare yourself to minimize or to rehabilitate from the risks. An example could be to take a potent probiotic in double dose during the course of antibiotic treatment (4-6 hours before or after the drug). Then continue the double dose for approximately one month after finishing the antibiotic, graduating down to a standard dose for two or more months, or even indefinitely. Probiotics are a great health-building measure.

Keeping your dietary choices, beverage consumption choices, your sleep and activity, hygiene, and thinking habits balanced and as natural as possible are foundational to good health, and minimize the need for pharmaceuticals.

SUPPORT YOUR LIVER, AVOID TOXIC LOAD

As we consider the risks of taking drugs and the benefits of more natural alternatives, it is important to understand the concept of "toxic load" as this relates to your liver's ability to process every substance it encounters in your bloodstream.

Naturally-occurring chemicals are abundant in our bodies, and therefore must be processed by the liver. These include hormones, messenger hormones, enzymes, byproducts of daily function (metabolism), and others. The naturally occurring products of metabolism are termed **endogenous** chemicals (emanating from inside the body). For example, ammonia is a byproduct of protein metabolism and must be detoxified by the liver. If the liver is functioning well, it will break down the ammonia to less toxic components that can safely travel through the blood to the kidneys. Here, these components are filtered and concentrated. The unnecessary components are passed into the urine and excreted. With toxins being removed at each pass through the liver and kidneys, the blood is incrementally detoxified. It now delivers oxygen and other vital nutrients to the body's, cells, tissues, and organs in a purified and more useful form.

Other natural items the liver and kidneys must process include the components of our food intake. With a diet of organic unprocessed foods, the body will process the broken down food components of protein, amino acids, fats, unrefined carbohydrates, vitamins, minerals, phytonutrients, plant sterols, etc. Since these are taken into the body from an external source, these items are considered **exogenous** (or external to the body in origin). Any e**xogenous** chemical or combination, however, holds the potential for triggering an allergic response. Our wonderful bodies were created with a maximum load limitation for processing a certain amount of **endogenous** chemicals and a load limit for **exogenous** chemicals.

If the diet includes pesticides, preservatives, dough stabilizers, food coloring, artificial flavorings or other chemical additives, the work load of the liver and eventually the kidneys has been unnecessarily increased. Culturally, we seem to be quite observant of load limits for aircraft and elevators that must lift against gravity. We need to become aware of the allowable toxic load limits for our body as a whole, and the detoxifying organs in particular.

Like a chemical-processing or purification plant, the liver carries out hundreds of complex operations just for the endogenous (or body created) substances alone. In the event that you are exposed to several toxic load expanders simultaneously (like extremely polluted air, pesticides and food coloring) your liver and kidney function will be taxed and even impaired, and decreased efficiency in detoxifying your blood will be the result. Your liver may feel like the elevator that unexpectedly acquired an elephant as a passenger. Gravity always wins. Add to that load excess a few margaritas followed by several Tylenol® tablets for a headache, and the party may be over.

The liver can be totally overwhelmed and will shut down. Once that occurs, the patient is rushed to a well equipped emergency room and given an I.V. of N-acetylcysteine, which will jump start the liver and may be able to nullify the deadly ethanol (alcohol) and acetaminophen (Tylenol) combination. N-acetylcysteine is a actually a naturally occurring amino acid in your liver. Wise proactive people often use this as a supplement **and** avoid the toxic overload lifestyle. This is a way to be kind to your liver, which will thank you with efficient function.

Limiting our exogenous toxic load from all sources truly benefits our health and longevity. If

---

Support for the Liver

I often take Complete Glutathione™ from Nutri-West® because of its high quality and bioavailability. This product contains some glutathione, as well as N-acetylcysteine which will convert to more glutathione. Other times, I use and recommend Oxi-Cell™ from Apex Energetics. This is a high quality, topically applied glutathione. The dosage for either formula is appropriate for those with essentially good lifestyles and perhaps a few moderate indiscretions. However, these products do not contain an elephant in the elevator type of dose; the emergency room is required for ethanol-acetaminophen toxicity, or acetaminophen overdose.

you can choose a health supportive path and avoid a perceived need for pharmaceutical medicines, so much the better!

WHEN DRUGS ARE NECESSARY

Certainly, there are circumstances that merit pharmaceutical drugs. Sometimes, in specific instances, the short term use of a drug or even an appropriate combination of drugs can save a life, a limb or halt a downward physiological spiral. Deciding when to use these pharmaceuticals is serious business. If there is no other viable alternative at the time, obviously choose the path for the best ultimate outcome. This is the point at which you must listen to your own "doctor within" and your trusted healthcare practitioner or team of practitioners. Carefully weighing the pros and cons for your treatment is critically important. Every situation is unique and must be approached as such.

If you are already in the process of taking a prescription medication or a medley of them DO NOT STOP TAKING THEM before extensive research, study, consultation with your doctor(s). Your body physiology has probably changed by taking one or more medications. Your health conditions need to be considered, understood in depth, and perhaps re-evaluated (if appropriate). The action you can undertake TODAY is a diet and lifestyle upgrade and a choice to relieve your body of unnecessary toxic loads. Such loads, as we've mentioned, include processed sugars, fried foods, sodas, artificial sweeteners, white flour, processed foods, pesticide infused foods, and genetically modified "Franken foods," chemically-laced cosmetics, etc. My hope is to reach out to those not on medications and especially to parents who can help to keep their children on an abundantly healthy and drug free path.

Should you or your loved ones be presented with a prescription for a non-life threatening situation, please study the issue, the facts of the drug(s), the possible alternatives, and give this the consideration due a most important decision. Discuss your concerns and questions with your trusted health care practitioners. If the research and study you are doing have instilled doubt or fear, study a bit more and then study about alternative treatments. Enlist the guidance of trusted health care providers—you may be best advised by a team of one allopathic provider and one natural approach provider. Like other health-conscious consumers, you may elect a three-to-four month trial of a non-drug approach; then re-evaluate, meet with both providers and decide how to direct the next three-to-four months of treatment. If you decide upon the pharmaceutical path, you will feel good about having considered the pros, cons, and alternatives. As a final caveat: Remember that wise obstetricians counsel their pregnant patients to avoid all drugs, since they are so potent and we still have much to learn about them and how they impair normal physiology. Consider your adult body to be as precious as a developing baby's. Remember that 100,000 Americans (270 per day) lose their lives to side effects and consequences of prescribed medications yearly.[9]

The Physician's Desk Reference (PDR)

The PDR (*Physicians' Desk Reference*) is the bible of prescribing physicians. The language and format are technically oriented, so don't get discouraged. All public libraries generally have a copy of the PDR in the reference area and many have one available to check out. PDR.net is the online source.

Early in the description of each listed drug is a section titled **INDICATIONS**. This section explains reasons why a doctor would consider prescribing this patented, toxic chemical to you. This is followed by the route of administrations (by mouth, injection or skin patch) and directions for use. Subsequent topics will be the most significant, for you. These may include: CONTRAINDICATIONS, WARNINGS, PRECAUTIONS, OVER-DOSAGE, ADVERSE REACTIONS, DRUG INTERACTIONS, NON-CLINICAL TOXICOLOGY, CLINICAL STUDIES, and USE IN SPECIFIC POPULATIONS. These specific populations include:

1. Pregnancy
2. Labor and delivery
3. Nursing mothers
4. Pediatric use
5. Geriatric use
6. Patients with hepatic (liver) impairment
7. Patients with renal (kidney) impairment
8. Patients with heart failure
9. Patients with diabetes mellitus

Be advised that the category for specific populations is not present for many drugs. If present, it frequently states that insufficient studies have been undertaken for the pediatric population and the producer does not advise that the drug in question be indicated for young patients. If specifications for geriatric use are indicated, these usually refer to the need *to err on the side of caution*, using the lowest possible dosage, considering potentially diminished heart, liver or kidney function. The "boxed warning" is a most important distinction to know about. It is prominently placed just under the name of the drug you are scrutinizing. It is also frequently termed a "black box warning," which means that the drug has potential for lethality. In many cases, however, a prescribing physician will not even mention the potential of a fatal outcome from the drug itself. Your pharmacy does give you a one page print out of the highlights of data about your drug in fairly plain English, so it is a good source of information. The pharmacy version is also highly edited and may not expose the boxed warning, so search this out for yourself.

Boxed Warnings

Here is one example of a boxed warning for Oxycontin (see Prescription Drug Chart on page 282). Prescribing information and black boxed warning is generally found on the manufacturer's website.

WARNING: ADDICTION, ABUSE and MISUSE; LIFE-THREATENING RESPIRATORY DEPRESSION; ACCIDENTAL INGESTION; NEONATAL OPIOID WITHDRAWAL SYNDROME; and CYTOCHROME P450 3A4 INTERACTION

See full prescribing information for complete boxed warning.

- OXYCONTIN exposes users to risks of addictions, abuse and misuse, which can lead to overdose and death. Assess each patient's risk before prescribing and monitor regularly for development of these behaviors and conditions.
- Serious, life-threatening, or fatal respiratory depression may occur. Monitor closely, especially upon initiation or following a dose increase. Instruct patients to swallow OXYCONTIN tablets whole to avoid exposure to a potentially fatal dose of oxycodone.
- Accidental ingestion of OXYCONTIN, especially in children, can result in a fatal overdose of oxycodone.
- Prolonged use of OXYCONTIN during pregnancy can result in neonatal opioid withdrawal syndrome, which may be life-threatening if not recognized and treated. If opioid use is required for a prolonged period in a pregnant woman, advise the patient of the risk of neonatal opioid withdrawal syndrome and ensure that appropriate treatment will be available.
- Initiation of CYP3A4 inhibitors (or discontinuation of CYP3A4 inducers) can result in a fatal overdose of oxycodone from OXYCONTIN.

http://app.purduepharma.com/xmlpublishing/pi.aspx?id=o

Alternatives For Healthy Living

In this next section we will look at ten of the most common health issues (pain, digestive distress, sleep disorders, etc.) that are typically "managed" with pharmaceuticals, as prescribed by allopathic doctors (M.D.s and many osteopaths). I have compiled user-friendly Alternate Remedy Charts that can be a springboard for your health journey for any of these issues. Remember that each case is different, however, and deserves personal attention to many details. Avoid the pitfall of imagining that one or two items you read about on a chart will successfully and safely address your health issues.

How to Use the Charts & Tools

Choose an area / condition to work on: Your choice of where to start will depend upon the current need in your life, an area in which you could use encouragement or help. Are you currently taking drugs for pain relief? Are you challenged by sleep issues and wondering if sleep medication might help? Begin by reviewing the charts that follow each symptom/alternative, choose one or two, and carefully read them over. The listing below will explain an ideal approach to using a chart (see pages 292–293 for sample).

1. **Start with the first and last columns: Active Lifestyle Measures** and **Mind-Body,** which will give you an essential overview of how to address your issue. If you do nothing else, study these. Consider what is possible for you, what you expect, what you are willing to do … or not.

2. **Scan the Diet Measures column.** Decide to include a few or most of the recommended foods into your constantly improving diet. Take it one step at a time. This should be your second most vital concern as you commit to work with any health issue.

3. **Next, go on to the Movement/Activity and Treatment column.** Which of these choices seem appealing and valuable to you? Which are you willing to pursue? Who can you consult for this help? What simple step can you take *today* to move in these directions?

4. **Vocalize the suggested affirmations given in column 5.** If you like them, use them. Or look for others, or compose your own. Work with your affirmations two or more times per day. Write them on 3x5 cards or sticky notes and post them around your house or in your car, where you will see them frequently and remember to repeat them.

5. **Review the Alternative Options suggested (see columns 3, 4, 6, 7):** Herbs, nutrients, aromatherapy, organ/meridian relationship, and Bach remedies are among the most effective alternatives I have found in my practice over many years. If you are attracted to try them or feel you need them, seek guidance from practitioners who specialize in these fields.

1. Pain

Natural Pain Relief

Discussion

Each person's response to a pain-inducing cause will be unique depending upon many factors including current life circumstances (like pregnancy) and general attitude (positive or fearful) toward a situation. Other factors influencing the response to pain may include: personal state of wellbeing (physical, emotional, mental); state of one's close relationships, and stresses of financial or job-related situations. Disharmony or discontent in one or more of these areas can exacerbate pain stemming from a more direct physical cause. Age, disability, existence of other health concerns or life concerns may weigh heavily in our perception of pain. We all have individual and mutable pain thresholds.

THE PHARMACEUTICAL PATH

In a culture where instant gratification is as highly valued as a gold bar, it's no wonder that over-the-counter pain relievers (OTCs) are in nearly everyone's medicine cabinet. These include such common drugs as aspirin and ibuprophen. They do indeed "work," at least temporarily, to alleviate pain, but research shows that even with short-term use they may cause serious side effects including significant damage to the gastrointestinal system, renal (kidney) impairment, liver damage, and harm to the central nervous system. Prescription pain relievers, especially opiates (like Tylenol III, or Vicodan), are highly addictive and carry an increased risk of the side effects mentioned above, as well as sedation, drowsiness, reduced respiration, and even respiratory arrest, a fatal event.

Tread lightly here, as countless cases of addiction to prescribed pain killers have occurred.

THE NATURAL APPROACH PATH

From a holistic approach, pain is often a symptom, a signal of a much larger issue. Many of our pains indicate some type of internal organ imbalance, which is perceived on the surface as a headache, back pain, wrist pain, etc. While health restoration is the best ultimate goal, most people are focused on relief. Treating the underlying cause is the best treatment for long-term effects. You can aim to find the root cause, likely with the help of a trained and experienced Clinical or Applied Kinesiologist or other trusted healthcare practitioner. Undertaking a supportive lifestyle, making nutritional changes and including specific nutrients and treatments to correct the underlying issue(s) causing the pain will offer the greatest long-term benefit.

Do everything possible to avoid and minimize the use of analgesics, "pain relievers" or "pain killers." I suggest deep breathing, relaxation techniques, meditation, acupuncture, chiropractic and any number of natural pain relief tools.

Many of my patients have found pain reduction possible with Xango® juice. Additional tools I use in my practice include Traumeel® by Heel Inc.—a homeopathic that contains arnica and other synergistic homeopathics. In my office, I commonly recommend that patients take homeopathic Surgery/Trauma drops by Nutri-West® two weeks prior to a surgery (if it's pre-planned) and continue until at least one bottle is consumed, often three weeks. One patient, who had one-third of her colon removed due to cancer, used Surgery/Trauma drops pre- and post-op and did not need to take a single dose of pain medication after leaving the recovery room. She was offered an I.V. with a metered pump of Demerol® to be used for several days but felt no need for it.

HOW TO IMPLEMENT NATURAL PAIN RELIEF TOOLS

As the accompanying chart (on pages 292-293) indicates, numerous lifestyle measures, foods nutrients, and herbs are available to help you. Consult your holistic practitioner for guidance with details. I encourage chiropractic and acupuncture treatment as well. You may also want to seek out massage therapy, acupressure, Feldenkreis Therapy®, Alexander Technique® or trigger point therapy.

Never abruptly stop medications your body is accustomed to taking; instead, work with your team of doctors to transition off medication if that is your goal. Simply adding several proactive, natural pain relief tools may begin to diminish your body's perceived need for medication. Work to find the cause of your pain and effectively address the cause. Your commitment to a regimen of diet and lifestyle improvement is crucial, as is allowing emotional processing and release on an ongoing basis. You will need to study, explore and be in frequent contact with your team of doctors if you endeavor to change your medication program.

George's Story, Revisited

Pain is an early warning system, acting as a proactive and protective sensory function. Pain warns you of malfunctions, developing disorders, and injury. Whenever you experience pain, you should look for the actual cause and work to correct or eliminate that cause. George's story, told in Chapter 1 (pages 8-9), is a case in point.

Prior to his fatal (and unanticipated) heart attack, George had experienced a series of pain signals indicating a state of moderate heart distress. His body was *talking loudly* for at least fifteen years, yet no one truly listened and interpreted the messages. All of the warning messages were clearly related to the heart meridian:
- 15 years prior to heart attack, George experienced elbow pain—Golfer's elbow.
- 10 years prior to heart attack he sustained whiplash injury—prolonged pain and poor healing; and a burning sensation.
- 7-0 years prior to heart attack he had four or five episodes of severe chest pain—never evaluated.

Please listen to your body much more closely than George did.

NATURAL PAIN RELIEF

Active Lifestyle Measures	Diet Measures (Foods to include in diet)	Alternative options: Herbs and Nutrients	Aroma Therapy
AVOID: • Blindly drowning out pain without understanding its cause • Holding harsh thoughts and emotions **INCLUDE:** • If the pain is due to a musculo-skeletal injury, Ice intermittently and gently stretch or mobilize as tolerated • Large amounts of pure water • Practice compassion and forgiveness • Research cause of dysfunction, seek treatment with a natural health care practitioner. • Therapeutic touch gently over area of concern by self or other	• Chia seeds • Chili Peppers* • Cherries • Cherry juice • Flax seed • Ginger tea (both ingested and topical) • Green Tea • Herring • Mackerel • Pineapple • Sardines • Walnut oil • Walnuts • Wild salmon	Herbs: • Devil's Claw • Hops • Kava kava • Meadow sweet • Pau d'arco • Turmeric • Zostrix (topical capsaicin)* Vitamins: • Multivitamin Others: • Alpha lipoic acid • Arnica (homeopathic) • Arnica salve (topical) • Bromelain • L-Phenyl-alanine • Melatonin • Omega 3 oils • Probiotics	• Douglas fir • Helichrysum • Many others for specific pain issues • Peppermint* • White fir • Wintergreen • Valerian
	For Headaches:	**For Headaches:**	**For Headaches:**
	• Amaranth • Almonds • Avocado • Barley • Buckwheat • Dark leafy greens • Pumpkin seeds • Quinoa • Walnuts	Herbs: • Butterbur • Feverfew • Garlic • Peppermint* • Turmeric • Willow bark Vitamins: • Vitamin C Mineral: • Magnesium	• Basil • Bergamot • Eucalyptus • Idaho tansy • Spearmint* * Blocks substance P, a naturally occurring neurotransmitter which facilitates pain perception.

(tools to avoid analgesics or pain killers)

Affirmations	Organ and Meridian Relationship	Bach Remedies	Movement/Activity and Treatments	Mind-Body
• I now release all turmoil and discomfort • I am becoming more comfortable and relaxed • I effortlessly move through life • I enjoy improved body function	• Brain Receptors (pericardium meridian) • Refer to Chapter 2 (*Acupuncture: The Healing Energy*)	• Agrimony • Aspen • Beech • Gorse • Impatiens • Rescue Remedy • Willow	• Any enjoyable, well tolerated exercise • Appropriate health promoting recreation • Appropriate therapeutic music, rhythm or sound • Consider: acupuncture, acupressure, chiropractic, Jin-Shin, massage, polarity therapy and/or reflexology • Ice to acute injury • Qi Gong • Swimming • Tai Chi • Warm bath (best with Epsom Salt) • Water therapy • Yoga	• Acknowledge, observe, experience your emotions • Allow time to process emotions, then seek support or guidance as needed • Center yourself • Cherish and enhance relationships • Creative visualization • Gratitude expression • Journaling • Learn more about your health concerns and treatment options • Meditation • Relaxation techniques • Spiritual practice • Unwind, review the day, organize concerns and release the burden before sleep

2. Infections and Other Immunity Challenges

Immunity Builders

Discussion

Our immune system was intelligently designed to protect our body and to maintain its delicate equilibrium. Antigens (markers) on the surface of foreign substances (splinters, bacteria, and viruses) are read and interpreted. If they are recognized as friendly, no immune response ensues. If the antigens are not on the "authorized guest list," then the foreign antigens stimulate an antibody response. Our immune system, through a process termed "chemotaxis," uses chemicals in the body to communicate and direct the appropriate white blood cells, i.e. macrophages, B cells, etc., to the specific location of the intruders. Refer to Chapter 6, *Energizing Your Immune System*.

THE PHARMACEUTICAL PATH

The allopathic approach, since the availability of antibiotics, has been to "shoot first and ask questions later." The shooting has been with penicillin, sulfa drugs, tetracycline® and their derivatives, and on to Levaquin® and the like. Each "generation" of new antibiotics is more powerful due to the genetic selection of killing off weaker bacteria and thereby allowing the more deadly (virulent) strains to survive and propagate. Unless life or limb is threatened, take the time to determine the exact organism in question by using a culture and susceptibility test (c&s). By waiting for the test results, you have "bought" a two-to-four day window to actively try natural measures to support your own immune system, hopefully enough to do its own job. When the results of your c&s test are available, you may then be given a prescription; taking responsibility for being an educated consumer you can research and then decide about using the prescribed drug or not. Refer to Chapter 8, *Leaky Gut and Your Digestion* and to Chapter 6, *Candida, Causes and Treatments*.

THE NATURAL PATH

When an infection seems eminent or has already occurred, adhere to anti-infection lifestyle measures, more stringently; and begin using herbs, vitamins, minerals, etc., to augment your immune system. I recommend Kinesiology self testing to make some of the choices; or you may consult with a knowledgeable and well-trained natural health practitioner/Kinesiologist. It is generally safe to use several natural immunity builders concurrently for an active (and short term) condition. It is more effective to take multiple doses daily (five to eight) for an acute infection, such as a cold or flu, than to take a larger dose only two or three times a day.

How To Implement Immunity Builder Tools

Consult your holistic practitioner for guidance with the details. I encourage chiropractic and acupuncture treatment as well. Never abruptly stop medications your body is accustomed to taking; instead, work with your team of doctors to transition off medication if that is your goal.

If you have an auto-immune disorder, realize that you do not have a drug deficiency, you have an excess of inflammation and toxicity. Your body may need to be re-trained to work harmoniously again. If you are warding off or have succumbed to an acute infection, work diligently to avert the infection, then diligently rebuild your immune system. If you feel you are losing the battle, however, you may need to consult your allopathic doctor and consider the antibiotic choice as a last resort.

Adding several proactive immunity-building tools may begin the process to diminish your body's perceived need for medication or amount of medication. Your commitment to a regimen of diet and lifestyle improvement is crucial, as is allowing emotional processing and release on an ongoing basis.

Colds and Sore Throats

Treatment for Two

Pauline brought her two daughters, Kayla (6 years) and Rae Lynn (4 years) to my office with sore throats and colds. This was the third round of illness for the girls over a three-month span of time. As soon as Kayla and Rae Lynn complained of colds and sore throats the first time, Pauline took them to an emergency care center and they were both given antibiotics. No testing was done to detect strep or to determine sensitivity toward a particular antibiotic. The girls seemed to improve, but within a month, both had reoccurrences. After the same treatment yielded the same results, Pauline was ready for a new path and a new outcome.

After taking their health histories and doing some basic examination, I gave both girls a rapid strep test. This test gives an immediate reading for the presence or absence of streptococcus bacteria with a great degree of accuracy. It was negative for both girls. We proceeded with herbal and homeopathic remedies, and a few treatments including laser and ultrasound over their throats and lymph gland areas, and Chiropractic treatments. At home, Pauline improved their diets and kept the girls on probiotics for six months, and called to say the girls were thriving.

IMMUNITY BUILDERS

Active Lifestyle Measures	Diet Measures (Foods to include in diet)	Alternative options: Herbs and Nutrients	Aroma Therapy
AVOID: • Antibacterial soap • High fat diet • Holding harsh thoughts and emotions • Minimize natural sweeteners • Over exertion • Poly-unsaturated oils • Refined sugars • Sleep deprivation **INCLUDE:** • Exercise 3 times per week • Exposure to sunlight for 30 minutes daily • Good hygiene measures • Positive outlook on life • Practice compassion and forgiveness • Regular hand washing • Sufficient sleep	• Apple • Bananas • Beets • Blueberries • Cabbage • Celery • Celery seed • Coconut • Chicken soup • Citrus fruits • Cranberries • Garlic • Jerusalem artichokes • Lemon water • Lime • Manuka honey • Mushrooms (especially shitake and maitake) • Olives • Onions • Papaya • Plum • Seaweed • Sauerkraut (homemade) • Watermelon • Yogurt	**HERBS:** • Astragalus • Basil • Bearberry • Black elderberry • Cardamom • Cinnamon • Cumin • Echinacea • Garlic • Goldenseal • Horseradish • Nutmeg • Osha • Red root **VITAMINS:** • Multivitamin • Vitamin A • Vitamin C • Vitamin D_3 • Vitamin E **MINERALS:** • Colloidal Silver • Selenium • Zinc **OTHERS:** • Colostrum • Grapefruit seed extract • Probiotics • Propolis honey • Tea tree oil (topical)	• Basil • Clary sage • Cypress • Eucalyptus • Frankincense • Lavender • Lemongrass • Marjoram • Melaleuca (tea tree) • Mountain savory • Myrrh • Neroli • Nutmeg • Oregano • Peppermint • Roman chamomile • Rosemary • Spike lavender • Thyme

(tools to avoid antibiotics)

Affirmations	Organ and Meridian Relationship	Bach Remedies	Movement/Activity and Treatments	Mind-Body
• I now focus my inner strength on an upsurge of wellness • I release disharmony, discord and weakness • I see my body functioning at peak performance	• Lymphatic (heart and pericardium meridians) • Thymus gland (triple warmer meridian) • Thyroid (triple warmer meridian) • Refer to Chapter 2 (*Acupuncture: The Healing Energy*)	• Elm • Gorse • Olive	• Any enjoyable, well tolerated exercise • Appropriate health promoting recreation • Appropriate therapeutic music, rhythm or sound • Consider: acupuncture, acupressure, chiropractic, Jin-Shin, massage, polarity therapy and/or reflexology • Qi Gong • Tapping over the thymus gland (under the breast bone)* • Therapeutic touch • Water therapy • Yoga * This activates the immune system.	• Acknowledge, observe, experience your emotions • Allow time to process emotions, then seek support or guidance as needed • Center yourself • Cherish and enhance relationships • Creative visualization • Gratitude expression • Journaling • Learn more about your health concerns and treatment options • Meditation • Relaxation techniques • Spiritual practice • Unwind, review the day, organize concerns and release the burden before sleep

3. Heart Disease, Atherosclerosis

Blood Vessel Protection

DISCUSSION

Cholesterol is a prominent building block in the human body. It is vital to our daily health and is moved through the bloodstream to repair damaged cells and to be a substrate for the construction of hormones, bile acids and body-friendly vitamin D. In fact, our bodies produce about 800 milligrams of cholesterol a day, "about half of which is oxidized to form bile acids, which are important in the digestion of fats and in removing cholesterol from the body."[10]

If you've held the misconception that cholesterol is your enemy, pay attention! Every cell in the human body has a cellular membrane. This intelligent membrane works like a guard at a gated community. All body fluids and chemicals must have appropriate identification and pass codes to enter or leave the cell. This process is called "osmosis through a semi-permeable membrane." Your cell membrane is the guard.

Your cell membranes are essentially 50 percent saturated fat, **primarily cholesterol** with its lipoprotein coating. This can allow for osmosis of qualified water-soluble and fat-soluble substances at a regulated pace. We all need to have well constructed and well functioning cell membranes whose guardian function is keenly tuned in.

Statin drugs (like Lipitor® or Crestor®) were formulated to inhibit critical enzymatic processes in your liver that are necessary for cholesterol biosynthesis. **This limits your body's production of cholesterol for all purposes.** This imposed biochemical change also blocks the ability of your body to make a necessary endogenous nutrient, Co-enzyme Q_{10}.

Cholesterol serves another vital function, that of cushioning and protecting your nervous system. Nerves are delicate and may be easily traumatized. After an accident, the most persistent, lingering pain is typically pain of nerve trauma. Some nerve injuries do not resolve for 6-18 months since repair and regeneration of nerves requires more time than regeneration of skin, muscle, ligaments or bone. It behooves all of us to retain every molecule of nerve protection we have. Specifically, the sheath of protection over your nerves is the myelin sheath. **Your myelin nerve sheaths are comprised largely of cholesterol.** With an intact sheath, the nerve impulses are smoothly transmitted. Erratic and subnormal nerve conduction is caused by various "demyelinating" diseases, like multiple sclerosis and Gullian-Barre syndrome.

Many people have been diagnosed with what is called "atherosclerosis" sometimes referred to as "hardening of the arteries or blood vessels." Why atherosclerosis forms in our blood vessels has no simple, definitive answer. But one predisposing factor is whole body inflammation. Ingesting exogenous toxins and chemically-altered substances trigger the immune response and typically lead to inflammation. These non foods include trans-fats, which are generally chemically-altered, un-natural, and poorly digested. Sugar (in all its various forms from fructose to xylitol) is devoid of important minerals to help your body properly process the refined carbohydrates that are inflammatory agents.

Other sources of inflammation are chlorinated water, smoking and tobacco use and even pasteurized dairy products, which can and do cause damaging reactions in the lining of your blood vessels, the *intimae*.[11]

Foreign chemicals travelling in the blood stream may nick or scratch the delicate intimae. Your body is programmed to patch up these divots—using free cholesterol to patch the artery wall. This is for your greater good, attempting to keep the blood vessels intact. The continued intake of chlorine attracts calcium to the patched area at a greater than normal rate—the patch grows and hardens, and atherosclerosis is the result.

Vitamin K_2, a fat soluble vitamin, helps your body direct calcium to its appropriate locations. With sufficient vitamin K_2, you receive protection against atherosclerosis, as well as protection against osteoporosis and tooth decay. When deficient in vitamin K_2, an accelerated buildup of plaque may occur in the arteries—the absence of K_2 did not direct the free calcium in the blood to bony tissue, rather, it took the easier path of going to soft tissues. In this case, the arteries are "hardened," and the teeth and bones "soften."

With a consistently poor diet, full of unnatural inflammatory agents, the patchwork to mend your blood vessels continues to progress. As the patchwork infrastructure grows, it may also become brittle. Ultimately, chunks may break off. If an atherosclerotic particle flows to the heart and blocks an artery, heart attack or myocardial infarction may result. If a particle flows onward to the brain and lodges in an artery, it may cause a stroke or cardiovascular accident! Eating organic eggs, butter and raw dairy (from pasture-fed cows) does not increase these occurrences.[12]

THE PHARMACEUTICAL PATH

The widely held misconception that higher blood cholesterol equates to higher heart disease and higher rates of cardiac death was mistakenly propagated by a flawed research study begun in 1954, and published in 1970. This study wrongly implicated a direct connection between natural, unadulterated dietary fat and heart disease. The false premise—known as the "lipid hypothesis" was formally adopted by the American Heart Association and the United States government. "Big Pharma" jumped on the bandwagon.

Most of your body's cholesterol is enmeshed in your cell membranes, brain tissues, myelin sheaths, hormones and bile salts. Soon after the lipid hypothesis was popularized, drugs were developed to either bind or incapacitate the cholesterol on its way to work or to block synthesis (production) of this vital endogenous chemical at the factory (the liver).

Subsequent studies overturned the lipid hypothesis and demonstrated much of the opposite. Review the prescription drug chart (see page 282), notice that Lipitor®, Pfizer's darling and $7.6 billion a year Block Buster drug carries a **Black Box Warning** and threatens multiple side effects, including various nervous system issues, muscle weakness, and degradation of muscle tissue (Rhabdomyolsis). This rapid muscle tissue breakdown can clog the kidneys and cause kidney failure and death.

Statin drugs—which **limit your body's production of cholesterol for all purposes**—were formulated to inhibit critical enzymatic processes in your liver that are necessary for cholesterol biosynthesis. Statin users statistically have a greater incidence of new diabetes diagnoses, higher cancer rates, lowered immunity and higher rates of infection. Female statin users are more prone to breast cancer than non-statin using females. All statin users become deficient in Co Enzyme Q_{40}, an endogenous nutrient that is **mandatory for life**, integrity of all muscles, including cardiac muscles, all cells, and DNA strands. Statin use correlates to an "increase in all-cause-deaths in those who use statins."[13]

THE NATURAL PATH

Prevention is always the best intervention. Reduce inflammation in your body by feeding it with

BLOOD VESSEL PROTECTION

Active Lifestyle Measures	Diet Measures (Foods to include in diet)	Alternative options: Herbs and Nutrients	Aroma Therapy
AVOID: • Chlorinated (tap) water to include water-based commercial and restaurant food and beverages • Holding harsh thoughts and emotions • Saturated fats • Trans-fatty acids • Tobacco **INCLUDE:** • 5-7 servings of fruits and vegetables daily • 30 minutes of exercise 3-5 times per week • Almonds • Flaxseed • Large amounts of well filtered or spring water and use this source for water-based foods and beverages • Organic soy protein • Practice compassion and forgiveness	• Almonds • Almond oil • Apples • Avocados • Avocado oil • Barley • Beans • Bee pollen • Blueberries • Broccoli • Carrots • Cashews • Chia seeds • Cinnamon • Coconut oil • Cranberries • Eggplant • Flax seeds • Garlic • Grapefruit pulp • Green tea • Herring • Lentils • Mackerel • Oatmeal • Oats • Olive oil • Onion • Oranges • Peanuts • Pine nuts • Pomegranate • Rice bran • Sardines • Seaweed • Sesame seeds • Shitake mushrooms • Spinach • Tahini • Walnut oil • Walnuts • Wild Salmon	**HERBS:** • Aloe Vera • Andrographis • Astragalus • Bilberry • Cinnamon • Garlic • German chamomile • Ginger • Guggul • Hawthorn • Hyssop • Milk thistle • Scutellaria (skullcap) • Snow fungus (moon fungus) • Turmeric **VITAMINS:** • Coenzyme Q10 • Beta Carotene (Vitamin A) • Multivitamin • Niacin (B_3) • Vitamin D_3 **MINERALS:** • Selenium **OTHERS:** • Beta sitosterol • Melatonin • Omega 3 • Probiotics • Quercetin • Red yeast rice extract • Resveratol • Rutin • Serrapeptase	• Cypress • Frankincense • Helichrysum • Lemon grass* * Strengthens blood vessel walls

(tools to avoid atherosclerosis and statins)

Affirmations	Organ and Meridian Relationship	Bach Remedies	Movement/Activity and Treatments	Mind-Body
• I embrace total love, and invite it into my life. • I feel my body cleansing and releasing all unnecessary debris • I love opening my heart and sharing it with others	• Liver • Thyroid • Thymus gland (triple warmer meridian) • Refer to Chapter 2 (*Acupuncture the Healing Energy*)	• Chestnut bud • Crab apple • Gentian • Holly • Impatiens • Rock rose • Vine • Willow	• Any enjoyable, well tolerated exercise • Appropriate health promoting recreation • Appropriate therapeutic music, rhythm or sound • Consider: acupuncture, acupressure, chiropractic, Jin-Shin, massage, polarity therapy and/or reflexology • Swimming • Walking • Yoga	• Acknowledge, observe, experience your emotions • Allow time to process emotions, then seek support or guidance as needed • Center yourself • Cherish and enhance relationships • Creative visualization • Gratitude expression • Journaling • Learn more about your health concerns and treatment options • Meditation • Relaxation techniques • Spiritual practice • Unwind, review the day, organize concerns and release the burden before sleep

wholesome, unadulterated foods, drinking pure water, avoiding smoking and tobacco products.[14] Fresh vegetables and fruits from your organic garden get the most points. Search out organic and non-GMO (genetically modified organisms) food. Look for wholesome, organic eggs, dairy, meats, when possible cage-free, range-fed or pasture-fed, and wild caught fish, if these are in your diet. Spring water is potentially the purest source, artesian is next. You may choose to have the water tested or ask for test data of commercially sold water. Distilling and purifying water are options. I prefer the Berky® water purification system and use it daily. I am also comfortable with the Multipure® filtration system. Avoid ingesting chlorine. All processed foods and beverages that contain water (unless labeled "filtered water") will contain chlorine and other toxins as well. These simple guidelines are health promoting and help avoid many disease states, especially keeping your arteries open and flexible.

How to Implement Blood Vessel Protection Tools

Carefully assess the measures described under the Lifestyle and Mind-Body columns in the chart on pages 300–301, and begin using diet enhancements. Use affirmations and actively visualize clear, open blood vessels with smooth linings. (Refer to visually explicit diagrams before you do your visualizations.) Incorporate movement and activity and treatments. Consult your natural healthcare provider for the alternative options: herbs and nutrients, aromatherapy, and Bach remedies which seem most appropriate for you. I encourage chiropractic and acupuncture treatment.

Never abruptly stop medications your body is accustomed to taking; instead, work with your team of doctors to minimize or transition off medication, if that is your goal. Simply adding several proactive tools may begin the process to diminish your body's perceived need for medication or amount of medication. Your commitment to a regimen of diet and lifestyle improvement is crucial, as is allowing emotional processing and release on an ongoing basis.

Carl's Story

Carl was a hardworking wheat farmer and cattle rancher, working long days for decades. He also enjoyed the wonderful desserts his wife made daily, and smoked about a pack of cigarettes each day. When he first came to my office, Carl was 72. He had experienced several episodes of chest pain and had been through the tests his medical doctor had recommended. His medical doctor convinced Carl to stop smoking, which he did over a two month period prior to coming to my office. He wanted to walk "the natural path" to improved blood vessels.

Carl and his wife made great strides at improving their diet—adding whole foods and discarding processed foods. He also remained a non-smoker and convinced his sons to quit as well. I recommended an oral chelation regimen that Carl faithfully followed for nine months. He also took supplements designed to lessen inflammation and to support his heart and cardiovascular system. Carl received treatments frequently for three months, then at progressively wider intervals for about two years.

Ultimately, Carl had no further chest pain and gained more energy and endurance. He told me he felt we had added several years to his productive life.

4. Depression

Feel Good, Be Happy

DISCUSSION

Our lives are an unpredictable series of events and actions, but with experience we may learn methods to safely moderate our reactions to such circumstance, and to control our actions wisely. Human emotions come and go as both external conditions and our inner awareness or focus changes. Emotional and whole-self wellness is enjoyed when we allow ourselves to *experience* and *release* our emotions. Generally, the best pattern for that process is: FEEL the current emotion, examine it a bit, respectfully express it as appropriate, then RELEASE the emotion, letting it float away as a puff of grey smoke dissipates, with no trace. Refer to Chapter 3, *Energy and Emotions*, and particularly note the Balloon Meditation on page 58. "Stuffing and holding emotions inside, encourages energy to stagnate and often emerges as second-hand anger, fear or depression, which is the most self-denying of the three.

If you experience depression (or what you believe to be depression) you are not cursed with a disease. You may be reacting to events, actions, situations, disappointments, self reprisals, losses or the like, and/or suffering from a biochemical imbalance caused by dietary or other factors. If you cannot work through these "lows," on your own, get guidance and help. Often depression is a symptom of one sort of life dysfunction or another. Solving this deeper problem—whether it entails emotional stuffing or hoarding, persisting in a destructive or demeaning job or relationship, etc.—will mitigate the depression in most cases. Peter Breggin, author of the *Antidepressant Fact Book* writes:

> Depression is, above all else, a signal that our lives are not going well. Emotional pain should direct our attention to the source of the suffering and motivate us to face the conflicts and stresses in our lives, including the ones that have seemed too painful to think about. Remember that the depth of our despair often reflects the contrasting desire that we have to live a more joyful, creative, and meaningful life. I often explain to my patients that they should be encouraged by the intensity of their psychological suffering because it confirms the depth of their feeling about life and their potential to bring enormous energy to a more constructive approach to living. If they did not strongly desire a much more fulfilling life, they wouldn't be so despairing over one that they have.[15]

Kelly Lambert, Ph.D., describes the concept of an effort-driven rewards circuit in her book, *Lifting Depression*. She explains that our historical and ancestral patterns of creatively working, especially with our hands and producing a tangible result, is immediately rewarding. Crafting a new or improved physical item enriches and strengthens the actual neural circuitry of our brains and forestalls depression. This type of creative activity builds our self esteem and self-perceived social value.

> Keeping the effort-driven rewards circuit well engaged helps you interact effectively and efficiently with challenges in the environment around you or in your emotional life…doing certain types of physical activities, especially ones that involve your hands. It's important that these actions produce a result you can see, feel, and touch, such as knitting a sweater or tending a garden. Such actions and their associated thoughts, plans and ultimate

results change the physiology and chemical makeup of the effort-driven rewards circuit, activating it in an energized way. I call the emotional sense of well-being that results effort-driven rewards.[16]

The modernization, industrialization and technological advancement of our societies have deprived us of many forms of physical activity, artistic expression and prowess. We are less in touch with our creativity, our skills, our neighbors and our communities. All of these deficiencies may contribute to depression.

The diet of most Americans today (I refer to it as the S-A-D, Standard American Diet) was birthed by agrifarming and commercialized food processing. Sadly, it yields a frighteningly nutrient deficient diet. The plethora of sugar (in all its many forms), refined carbohydrates, pesticides, stabilizers, dough conditioners, preservatives, food colorings, artificial flavorings, artificial sweeteners, synthetic hormones, genetically modified organisms and other chemicals contained in this diet creates a tragedy with dire consequences. The brain requires a consistent supply of glucose, a variety of amino acids (building blocks of neurotransmitters), essential fatty acids (including Omega 3s) and many vitamins and minerals for normal function. **The SAD diet does not supply the necessary nutrients for either brain or body function.** Continuing the SAD diet continues to diminish brain and body dysfunction. Vast research confirms that the prevalence of sugar creates dramatic swings in the blood sugar and promotes depression.

> SAD DIET = SAD PERSON

Various symptoms of hypothalamic imbalance can accompany depression. These can different sleep or appetite disorders, along with a tendency to become less active, more irritable, more reclusive and less communicative. Some people react to chronic pain, chronic or long term illness and many physical disorders with depression. For some, the manifestation of depression is symbolic of giving up or not feeling up to the challenge. Sometimes those struggling with depression are plagued by feelings of worthlessness; they question the value of their life. They may feel ineffective, unsuccessful or inadequate.

Obtaining proper guidance and becoming **proactive** can move the person in a positive direction. If you or someone you know is despondent or potentially suicidal, seek help NOW, not tomorrow. Crisis help lines are available nationwide through the National Suicide Prevention Lifeline. They can be reached by phone at 1-800-273-8255 or on the web at www.suicidepreventionlifeline.org. No one needs to be alone during the darkest hour. Emergency care or hospitalization may be needed. A short term regimen of medication may be useful, but generally a lifelong reliance on medication will not be needed if the true cause of the depression is discovered and addressed.

As recommended with all conditions, anyone taking antidepressant or other psychotropic drugs should not stop or diminish the dose without medical supervision and a clear plan. Stopping the use of psychotropic drugs abruptly is dangerous, fraught with many side effects and may precipitate suicidality.

THE PHARMACEUTICAL PATH

This path looks like a train wreck, too much collateral damage. In fact, a great deal of documentation exists to prove that actual brain damage on a

> ### Drug Withdrawal Help
>
> When you plan to wean off your psychotropic drug, you and your prescribing doctor should reference a valuable resource, such as *Psychiatric Drug Withdrawal*, a guide for prescribers, therapists, patients, and their families. This in depth, well referenced guide was written by Peter Breggin, M.D. in 2013. I consider Dr. Breggin to be the leading authority on both psychiatric drugs and their morbid problems. *Ethical Psychology and Psychiatry* is the title of a cutting edge scientific journal he founded. "The Dr. Peter Breggin Hour" is available on the Progressive Radio Network, both live and in archived form. Another helpful resource is *Point of Return™: A Safe and Sensible Withdrawal Method for Benzodiazepines & Antidepressant Drugs* by Dr. Bill Code, M.D. with Alesandra Rain, Andrea Crocker.
>
> Help is available, but you must search it out.

cellular level is caused by anti-depressants and other psychotropic drugs.

The pharmaceutical approach negates the whole person ideal. It is based simply on the model of altering brain chemistry with toxic chemicals. Prozac® was the first SSRI, selective serotonin reuptake inhibitor, to be marketed in America. Serious consequences have followed.

> In 1956 Eli Lilly patented LSD and in 1987 they gave us Prozac…LSD, the most notorious of the psychedelic drugs, was first marketed by Sandoz in Europe with the suggestion that it be used to chemically induce insanity in "normal subjects" with the hope of discovering how mental illness is produced. Yet in December 1955, two months before Lilly obtained their patent on LSD here in America, *TIME* magazine featured the drug, declaring that LSD *"may actually help psychiatrists clear up mental illness."* It was also promoted as a *cure for alcoholism* and as an *"aid in facilitating psychoanalysis"*. Now, a generation later, many of these same marketing claims are being made for Prozac that were once made for LSD…As our latest panacea, it is being prescribed for everything from headaches and flue to acne and home sickness. Yet, *according to FDA spokespersons, there have been more adverse reaction reports on Prozac than any other medical product.* We are being media blitzed to believe these new mind-altering chemicals have a large margin of safety, but will time prove otherwise or has it already? Considering the wide spread use of these products, we have no time to lose in learning the answer.[17]

And more:

> The influence of the drug companies on federal agencies cannot be exaggerated. In the midst of the controversy over Prozac causing suicide and violence, Steven Paul, director of research at NIMH, was hired away to become vice president of Eli Lilly and Co. During the transition, he defended Prozac at a critical time of controversy about the drug's capacity to cause suicide and violence.
>
> The Food and Drug Administration (FDA) has forsaken its watchdog role. Instead, FDA officials climb like puppies into the laps of drug company executives who might someday hire them at enormous salaries. Paul Leber was for many years the director of the FDA's psychiatric

drug section; now he makes a living as a consultant to drug companies.[18]

The potential risks for all psychotropic drugs are broad, far-reaching and often devastating. I recommend that you explore many other harmless remedies prior to desperately plunging into the pharmaceutical path. The use of psychotropic drugs sometimes spawns aggression, suicidality, violent and homicidal behavior. These morbid effects are not predictable for any given case. These extreme results are not present in the majority of cases, yet extraordinary caution is warranted.

THE NATURAL PATH

Watching comedy movies seems like a fantastic alterative. Actually, Norman Cousins, the respected editor of the *Saturday Review*, rented Charlie Chaplin movies and spent several days in a hotel room totally absorbed in watching and laughing at slap-stick comedy. He effected great relief for his severe arthritis pain in this fun, drug-free fashion. Patch Adams, M.D., has generated great joy from making people laugh. Making time to engage in life enriching activities which truly bring enjoyment is helpful.

Looking for the cause of your sadness or discontent is a constructive step. This is to understand your reactions, not to validate blaming people or circumstances for your misery.

Misery, sadness, depression and similar states of mind are changeable and mutable. We can work with emotions such as pain, grief, sadness, etc., to keep them from freezing (like water) into a rigid state within us. By adding an appropriate therapeutic input, we can process and eliminate the stagnant emotion and transmute it to a less dense state. In essence, this will remove the old emotion from your being, current experience, and consciousness. A variety of treatment approaches and self help tools are available to aid individuals in achieving "the happy place," such as meditation, visualization, EFT™ (the Emotional Freedom Technique), the Sedona method™, NLP™ (Neuro-Linguistic programming), Psych-K™ (Psychological Kinesiology), the Emotion Code™, various emotional clearing techniques, mind-body techniques and neuro-emotional remedies (review Chapter 3, *Energy and Emotions*). Some of these techniques are simple enough to be a self help modality. Many of these techniques work best when administered by a trained therapist or practitioner. I evaluate the patient and their situation and often integrate more than one technique. I often incorporate color and sound therapy with one or two other methods. Frequently, I suggest affirmations for the patient to repeat during the treatment session and continue at home.

Aromatherapy with pure essential oils of medicinal and seemingly common place flowers and herbs are very effective. Ann Blake Tracy, a psychologist, recounts case histories of several patients who used the tool of aromatherapy to bolster their mood and feeling status enough to both terminate taking Prozac® and feel that their depression had totally resolved. Again, I will caution you to never stop taking any prescribed drug, especially psychotropic drugs, without diligent study and professional guidance.

Nutrition has everything to do with how your brain functions and how your thoughts are generated and processed. Refined sugar in all its forms causes erratic changes in blood sugar levels and alters the consistent supply of glucose to the brain. The use of these refined carbohydrates, white sugar, white flour, white rice, etc., depletes and causes a relative deficiency of many components of the B vitamin complex. These fast-burning carbohydrates also deplete many, if not most, minerals, especially chromium, vanadium, and trace minerals. Those minerals are necessary to maintain blood sugar stability and tissue integrity and to help process the next bites of carbohydrates ingested. Simply stated, your mood and outlook on life will be much better two hours after snacking on slices of an organic apple and a few raw almonds, than it will be two hours after a candy bar or a sugary soda.

Eating a wholesome diet should be the goal of every health-minded person. The three macronutrients we need are protein, carbohydrates and fats; and eating a balance of each type in their natural unadulterated state is key. Vitamin D_3, B vitamins, Omega 3 oils, other essential fatty acids, and many amino acids are super-brain, mind, and mood nutrients.

A lack of sunlight (and therefore, vitamin D) may contribute to feeling down. Using full spectrum fluorescent lights in the home for lighting and using them therapeutically can be helpful. I only use full-spectrum fluorescents. In winter or lessened sunlight conditions, sun exposure for 30 to an aggregate of 120 minutes daily can be very helpful. If you use a longer sunlight exposure time, consider increments of 30 to 45 minutes.

> Vitamin D deficiency may play a role in depression and possibly other mental disorders…It could play a role in supplementary treatment of depression… Vitamin D may be an important nutrient for women's physical and mental well being.[19]

Proactively addressing your issues and challenges will help your emotional health. Feeling, processing and releasing your emotions will help you with your emotional dexterity. Embracing life with all its unexpected twists and turns give you emotional flexibility. Practicing compassion and forgiveness will provide you with a calm satisfaction. Counting your blessings daily will let you more easily experience your humble and your gracious facets. Loving unconditionally will invite love from many directions.

How to Implement the Feel Good, Be Happy Tools

Refer to the following chart for encouragement and guidance. Rejoice! You will find numerous lifestyle measures, foods, nutrients, and herbs are available to help you. Consult your holistic practitioner for guidance with the details. I encourage you to find an empathic, psychiatrist or psychologist if you are now on medication or believe that this type of support will be beneficial. I advocate chiropractic and acupuncture treatment as well. Never abruptly stop medications your body is accustomed to taking; instead, work with your team of doctors to minimize or transition off medication, if that is your goal. Simply adding several proactive Feel Good, Be Happy mind-body tools may begin the process to diminish your body's perceived need for medication or amount of medication. This is a personal journey. Your commitment to a regimen of diet and lifestyle improvement is crucial, as is allowing emotional processing and release on an ongoing basis. You will need to study, explore and be in frequent contact with your team of doctors if you endeavor to change your medication program. Remember to stop and smell the roses, and make a little time to be playful!

FEEL GOOD, BE HAPPY

Active Lifestyle Measures	Diet Measures (Foods to include in diet)	Alternative options: Herbs and Nutrients	Aroma Therapy
AVOID: • Alcohol • Any drugs which may worsen depression • B vitamin deficiency • Caffeine • Holding harsh thoughts and emotions • Refined carbohydrates • Sugar **INCLUDE:** • Exposure to sunlight for 30 minutes daily • Appropriate emotional guidance or therapy • Constructive goals • Creative activities or projects • Exercise (At least 3 times per week) • Group activities • Laughter • Learn coping skills • Practice compassion and forgiveness • Volunteering	• Chia seeds • Chiso (Japanese beefsteak leaf) • Flax seed • Flax seed oil • Garlic • Green leafy vegetables • Green tea • Herring • Lentils • Mackerel • Oat straw tea • Oats • Peas • Rice • Sardines • Walnuts • Walnut oil • Wild salmon	**HERBS:** • Chamomile tea • Melissa • Licorice root • Oregano • Saffron • St. John's Wort • Rhodiola rosea • Turmeric **VITAMINS:** • B vitamin complex • Cobalamin (B_{12}) • Folic acid (B_9) • Multivitamin • Vitamin D_3 **OTHERS:** • L-Theanine • L-Tryptophan • Melatonin • Omega 3 oils • Oxitriptan (5-HTP) • Probiotics • S-Adenosyl-methionine (SAM-e)	• Basil • Bergamot • Chamomile • Cypress • Frankincense • Grapefruit • Jasmine • Lavender • Lemon • Lime • Mandarin • Neroli • Orange • Peppermint • Roman chamomile • Rose • Sandalwood • Sweet orange • Tangerine • Verbena

(tools to prevent depression)

Affirmations	Organ and Meridian Relationship	Bach Remedies	Movement/Activity and Treatments	Mind-Body
• I am ready to move forward and experience the beauty and grace of my life • I am now joyful and happy • I gratefully accept and remember my blessings • I love myself • I am loveable	• Adrenal • Brain (pericardium meridian) • Liver • Thyroid (triple warmer meridian) • Refer to Chapter 2 (*Acupuncture the Healing Energy*)	• Gentian • Gorse • Hornbeam • Mustard • Oak • Sweet chestnut	• Aerobic exercise • Any enjoyable, well tolerated exercise • Appropriate health promoting recreation • Appropriate therapeutic music, rhythm or sound • Creative activities or projects • Consider: acupuncture, acupressure, chiropractic, Jin-Shin, massage, polarity therapy and/or reflexology • Dancing • Swimming • Tai chi • Team sports • Walking	• Acknowledge, observe, experience your emotions • Allow time to process emotions, then seek support or guidance as needed • Center yourself • Cherish and enhance relationships • Creative visualization • Gratitude expression • Journaling • Learn more about your health concerns and treatment options • Meditation • Relaxation techniques • Spiritual practice • Unwind, review the day, organize concerns and release the burden before sleep

5. Diabetes and the Problem of Refined Dietary Sugars

Balanced Blood Sugar

Discussion

Unbalanced blood sugar is a sign that your body's fuel is not being processed correctly. Imagine being behind a car whose combustion mixture is too "rich." You will see black smoke coming out of the tailpipe, and even smell raw, uncombusted gasoline vapors. The pancreas is analogous to the carburetor and is responsible for the oxygen/fuel mixture. If the mixture is off and the combustion is not properly catalyzed (facilitated by insulin), then "black smoke" (or out of bounds glucose) runs wild throughout your body. The excess underutilized fuel causes strain and overwork for the heart, blood vessels, liver, kidneys, nervous system and eyes.

Glucose is the most basic fuel for your body. Carbohydrates are broken down in your stomach to yield glucose and other by-products. If your fuel processing system is working well, insulin from your pancreas quickly comes on site to bind with the glucose and assist it (or actively transports it) into muscle tissue. Within the muscle tissues, the glucose either is called to use immediately or waits to be called into action at a later time. If it waits, it converts to glycogen and fat for storage.

Your pancreas secretes insulin and glucagon, the two hormones involved in processing, storing, and releasing glucose. These processes rely on good functioning of both the pancreas and the liver. Cell receptor sites accept glucose that is bound to insulin. When your "fuel processing" and insulin-glucose delivery functions are in a state of malfunction, glucose is not expediently nor securely delivered inside the cells. Two results of this include: Type II diabetes mellitus, a form of insulin resistance, and Type I diabetes, formerly termed juvenile onset diabetes. Other blood sugar imbalances and pancreatic dysfunctions also exist, but will not be considered here.

THE PHARMACEUTICAL PATH

There is no "magic pill" to cure diabetes. Diabetes is an adaptation of the body to an incompatible environment, lifestyle, and food supply. In fact, using numerous pharmaceuticals in an attempt to

---

Diabetes Facts

- There are 24 million U.S. diabetes sufferers.
- There are 221 million people with diabetes worldwide.
- Every 3 minutes an additional person is diagnosed with diabetes (from 2009 study).
- A British study in 2007 revealed that children living now might be expected to die one decade earlier than their parents, primarily due to obesity and diabetes.
- When excess glucose is in the blood (unable to enter cells and be metabolized as fuel), it becomes an inflammatory agent. If this persists, the inflammation damages the intimae of blood vessels triggering atherosclerosis and heart disease. This may lead to kidney disease, peripheral neuropathy (impaired sensation), and foot, leg or bed sores or diabetic retinopathy.
- Every 30 seconds a diabetes-triggered amputation occurs worldwide.
- The leading cause of blindness in adults is diabetic retinopathy.

relieve the symptoms of diabetes can be extremely dangerous.

> The results of the ACCORD trial (Action to Control Cardiovascular Risk in Diabetes) in 2008 found a 22 percent increased rate of death in diabetic patients who were treated aggressively versus those who were given fewer drugs and combinations of drugs. In fact, the study was halted early in February 2008 for ethical reasons.[20]

Many class action suits and recalls for diabetic drugs such as Avendia® or Actos® are on record. On June 14, 2007, an article in the *New England Journal of Medicine* reviewed forty-two trials completed with rosiglitazone maleate (Avandia®). Researchers tracked heart attacks and death from cardiovascular causes. The average age of death in these trials was fifty-six years. The researchers concluded that rosiglitazone maleate (Avandia) "was associated with a significant increase in the risk of myocardial infarction (heart attack) and with an increase in the risk of death from cardiovascular causes that has borderline significance."[21] Suzy Cohen, in her book, *Diabetes Without Drugs*, discusses another article on the subject, from the *New England Journal of Medicine* (December 2008):

> In a nutshell, the study proved that aggressive use of blood sugar-lowering medications to prevent heart disease was a complete and utter failure…Recent evidence has found that intensive treatment with medications does not improve cardiovascular function. It may cause a *higher* mortality (death rate) in people with type 2 diabetes.[22]

THE NATURAL PATH

Since diabetes is sometimes mis-diagnosed, it is important to stay current with healthcare providers concerning any recommended drug usage. Statin drugs (such as Lipitor® and Crestor®), for instance, may induce hyperglycemia (high blood sugar). Therefore, if you take statin drugs and there is any suggestion that diabetes may be the diagnosis in your case, talk to your doctor(s) about first curtailing the statin use and then re-evaluating your blood sugar status. This process may take several months. Many cases of apparent "diabetes" triggered by the statin use have resolved after dropping the statin. The high glucose that results from statin use may bring about the same physiological damage as that of an actual diabetic who is not on a statin.

If you are a diabetic who is prescribed a statin drug, reread the previous section on Blood Vessel Protection and evaluate the potential risks. Search (long and hard) to discover any potential benefits to using the proposed statin.

Most people with unbalanced blood sugar can help resolve the problem by avoiding refined carbohydrates. The first category includes all sugars (sucrose, glucose, maltose, etc.) Balancing blood sugar means avoiding soda of all descriptions, white potatoes and their many carbohydrate-rich derivatives (fries, chips, potato starch, etc.) Also avoid white rice and white flour. "Wheat flour" too presents a challenge. On a food label it implies that the product is predominantly *white processed* flour to which a little whole wheat flour has been added.

Although chlorine gas was outlawed as an agent of chemical warfare after World War I, the U.S. F.D.A. has never banned the use of this toxic agent from our food or water supply.

Realize that a **whole grain**, such as the most pure, unadulterated wheat you can find,

BALANCED BLOOD SUGAR

Active Lifestyle Measures	Diet Measures (Foods to include in diet)	Alternative options: Herbs and Nutrients	Aroma Therapy
AVOID: • Alcohol • Fast food • Gluten and flour based foods • Holding harsh thoughts and emotions • Potato Flour • Processed foods • Refined carbohydrates • Sugar • Tobacco • White potatoes **INCLUDE:** • Always consume breakfast • Consistency of meal times • Healthy protein snacks • Moderate amount of fresh fruit • Moderate exercise 3 to 5 times per week • Nuts • Plant based diet • Practice compassion and forgiveness • Seeds	• Almonds • Apple cider vinegar • Avocados • Avocado oil • Barley grass • Bitter melon tea • Blueberries • Cashews • Chamomile tea • Chicken • Cinnamon • Coconut • Coconut oil • Eggs • Fiber rich foods • Ginger • Hempseed meal • Hemp seed oil • Herring • Jerusalem artichoke • Mackerel • Marshmallow tea • Oatmeal • Oat bran • Olive oil • Onion • Papaya • Peanut butter • Pears • Pea pod tea • Rooibus tea • Sardines • Stevia • Turkey • Walnut oil • Walnuts • Wild salmon	**HERBS:** • Aloe Vera • Astragalus • Chamomile • Cinnamon • Fenugreek • Ginseng • Guggul • Gymnea sylvestre • Jerusalem artichoke • Pau d' arco • Stinging nettle • Turmeric **VITAMINS:** • Multivitamin • Vitamin A • Vitamin B complex • Vitamin C • Vitamin D_3 **MINERALS:** • Chromium • Magnesium • Vanadium • Zinc **OTHERS:** • Acetyl-L-carnitine • Alpha Lipoic acid • Astaxanthin • Digestive enzymes • L-glutamine • L-taurine • Pycnogenol • Resveratrol • Omega 3 oils • Probiotics	• Cinnamon • Coriander • Cypress • Dill • Fennel • Juniper • Myrrh • Pine • Ylang ylang

(tools to prevent diabetes)

Affirmations	Organ and Meridian Relationship	Bach Remedies	Movement/Activity and Treatments	Mind-Body
• I accept myself completely • I am full of radiant light and energy • My personal power is growing stronger every day • I can accomplish any and every goal • I savor sweetness in my life • I love myself	• Pancreas (spleen meridian) • Heart • Liver • Kidney • Refer to Chapter 2 (*Acupuncture the Healing Energy*)	• Beech • Chestnut bud • Crab apple • Gentian • Gorse • Impatiens • Willow	• Any enjoyable, well tolerated exercise • Appropriate health promoting recreation • Appropriate therapeutic music, rhythm or sound • Consider: acupuncture, acupressure, chiropractic, Jin-Shin, massage, polarity therapy and/or reflexology • Swimming • Walking • Yoga	• Acknowledge, observe, experience your emotions • Allow time to process emotions, then seek support or guidance as needed • Center yourself • Cherish and enhance relationships • Creative visualization • Gratitude expression • Journaling • Learn more about your health concerns and treatment options • Meditation • Relaxation techniques • Spiritual practice • Unwind, review the day, organize concerns and release the burden before sleep

> **When Bad Things Happen to Good Flour**
>
> To make all purpose flour, wheat kernels must be stripped of their bran and germ layers. This stripping process removes the most nutritious parts of the grain, such as the fiber, minerals, and vitamins…The flour—which is naturally brown—still needs to be whitened using a chemical that is standard in the flour industry, chlorine gas. The Environmental Protection Agency categorizes chlorine gas as a pesticide and defines it as a flour-bleaching, aging and oxidizing agent that is a powerful irritant, dangerous to inhale and lethal. Chlorine gas, when it comes in contact with wheat, also forms another substance called alloxan, which is known to destroy pancreatic function… Scientists routinely use alloxan to destroy the pancreas of lab animals, usually rodents. Alloxan looks similar to glucose, so it's readily taken up by beta cells, where it sparks tremendous free-radical damage, and kills the cells so they no longer produce insulin. When enough beta cells die, insulin production stops.[23]

contains all of the necessary ingredients to form new life. The grain is a seed. The complete vitamin E complex is contained in the whole wheat kernel. This vitamin E complex preserves the other nutrients and life giving factors in the grain. the moment the grain is milled, the vitamin E complex is destroyed and the entire grain begins to oxidize, to degrade, and lose its nutritional value. Rarely do you find organic, non-hybridized, totally non-GMO tainted wheat in today's world. Avoiding or at least drastically minimalizing the use of flour based products is a wise guideline.

How to Implement Balanced Blood Sugar Tools

Refer to the following chart for encouragement and guidance. Rejoice! Numerous lifestyle measures, foods, nutrients, and herbs are available to help you. Consult your holistic practitioner for guidance with the details. I encourage chiropractic and acupuncture treatment as well. Never abruptly stop medications your body is accustomed to taking; instead, work with your team of doctors to minimize or transition off medication if that is your goal. Simply adding several proactive blood sugar balancing tools may begin the process to diminish your body's perceived need for medication or amount of medication. This is a very personal journey. Your commitment to a regimen of diet and lifestyle improvement is crucial, as is allowing emotional processing and release on an ongoing basis. You will need to study, explore and be in frequent contact with your team of doctors if you endeavor to change your medication program.

6. High/Low Blood Pressure/Hypertension

Balanced Blood Pressure

DISCUSSION

Your cardiovascular system is a closed system of pressurized fluid, your blood. Blood pressure is a measurement of the pressure exerted by your blood against the walls of your arteries (arterial blood pressure). This pressure fluctuates in response to many factors. These include stress, both physical and emotional, age, diet, activity level, body position, time of day, and area of body used for the blood pressure reading. Obviously the inclusion or exclusion of nicotine, caffeine, alcohol, and certain medications can have a direct influence on your blood pressure.

When your heart muscle is contracting, more pressure is created in the closed system. The heart contraction phase of the cardiac cycle is called **systole.** The pressure reading obtained during systole is the systolic blood pressure. It is the higher number, the first number recorded in a blood pressure reading. The second number is the **diastolic blood pressure**, or the pressure occurring during diastole, the heart's relaxation phase. Below is a representation of the "ideal" highest limit for adult arterial blood pressure and facts about the cardiac cycle.

Blood pressure readings are measured in units called millimeters of mercury (mmHg). A greater arterial pressure moves the column of the mercury up in its glass tube more millimeters than a lesser arterial pressure will. It is necessary to have a balanced level of blood pressure for proper function of your heart, vascular system, brain, kidneys, and to a degree, lungs and liver. If the pressure is problematically too low (**hypotension**), certain organ functions will suffer, and delivery of the oxygenated blood to your vital organs (including your brain) will be compromised. This is called "impaired blood perfusion." If your blood pressure progressively lowers, and proper perfusion of blood to your brain and other vital organs is not achieved, as may happen with an injury causing drastic blood loss, death may be imminent.

On the other hand, if your blood pressure is dangerously high (**hypertension**), it can cause the rupture an important artery, resulting in a stroke. Long term continued high blood pressure may cause damage to your blood vessels, organs, and/or eyes. Sometimes people are born with a weaknesses or bulging in one or more artery (aneurysm), or later develop an area of weakness. Excess pressure may cause a "blowout," or a rupture, generally with devastating internal bleeding. This too can be fatal. Balanced blood pressure is your friend and helps keep your body working at optimum function.

The classification of blood pressure as to being "normal" or normotensive, high or hypertensive, or low—also termed "hypotensive," does not seem to be an exact science. The parameters for these categories are redefined as the decades change. Many people feel that the categories should change with a person's age and certain conditions. Years of drinking chlorinated water can make the blood vessels stiff and less flexible, and prone to forming atherosclerosis, which narrows

Name	mmHG*	Cardiac Action	Pressure	Sound (or beating noise)
Systolic	120	Heart contracting	Greatest	First of the series
Diastolic	80	Heart relaxing	Least	Fifth or last of the series

*Millimeters of mercury—described above

the arterial diameters. At this point, a higher blood pressure is required to balance the increased arterial resistance. Perhaps this person's blood perfusion to all tissues will be more complete if their blood pressure is 130/90, rather than 120/80. This "high" reading could be their best functional blood pressure state, relevant to their age and condition.

Each individual is unique and has diverse factors to consider. **Never** accept a new diagnosis of hypertension based on only **one** reading. This is particularly true if it is your first visit to a new facility or office. Be sure that your health history, blood pressure history, family history regarding blood pressure and heart disease are all available to your health care practitioner, and are considered. Be sure that your lifestyle factors: diet, basic activity level, stress level, sleep patterns, nicotine and caffeine use, and medication use are presented to your practitioner. If one blood pressure reading is high, then collect a series of readings at different times of the day, under a variety of conditions—moods, activity levels, etc, and study the facts. You must be openly communicating with your trusted healthcare practitioner(s) and evaluating the readings and treatment options. If you are experiencing a distressing life situation and do not tell your health practitioner(s), you are impeding the accurate evaluation of your case. In essence, understanding whether you truly have an issue with hypertension may follow a convoluted trail fraught with obstacles.

This book does **not** address hypertension of such a magnitude as the quote above (top right) reflects, but rather suggests ways and means of prevention to avoid a stroke, heart attack, kidney damage, retinal damage, etc.

The state of balance or imbalance for your heart, kidneys, adrenals, and thyroid may greatly influence your blood pressure. If you have low blood pressure, most likely you can help yourself

> If you have a blood pressure reading which alarms you or your healthcare practitioner(s), listen closely to their advice. This will likely be to "**report to the emergency room.**" While there is not a total consensus, generally consider that 180/120 *begins* the range for alarm, and indicates an emergent situation.

with proper hydration or rehydration, and a natural approach treatment for adrenal or thyroid imbalances, if present. The treatment paths in the chart that follows are not directly intended for helping either **severe** hypertension, or hypotension. Individuals with either of these will surely benefit from the active lifestyle measures, mind/body tools, and movement/activity and treatment suggestions on the Balanced Blood Pressure chart on page 320–321 in this section, along with more specific treatment for their condition.

THE PHARMACEUTICAL PATH

Along with antihypertensive medication, most allopathic doctors and nurse practitioners recommend some lifestyle changes. These are generally the obvious ones, smoking and nicotine use cessation, weight loss if applicable, increased exercise if appropriate and the restriction of salt (later I will note why it is controversial to restrict salt).

Several categories of medications are commonly used for hypertension. Often, two or three drugs are chosen for the anti-hypertensive cocktail, which increases chances of adverse drug interactions. Side effects may occur. In some cases, after years or months on one combination, the blood pressure may begin to elevate. Then a new mix of medications may be instituted.

Commonly the body will have a rebound reaction to the removal or rapid cessation of an anti-hypertensive drug, making the blood pressure erratic or labile. Never abruptly stop taking blood pressure medication without your doctor's advisement, as your blood pressure may shoot up **dangerously**.

Read *What Your Doctor May Not Tell You about Hypertension,* by Dr. Mark Houston, which provides a wealth of information. Encourage your prescribing doctor to reference the *Hypertension Handbook for Students and Clinicians.* These books condense Dr. Houston's years of study, research, and clinical experience with hypertension. Dr. Houston considers hypertension to be a disease of the blood vessels and their delicate lining, the endothelium.

If you take antihypertensive medication, and you may need to for some period of time, do not consider this to be a complete treatment. You **must** embrace some lifestyle improvements and inflammation-reducing methodology.

THE NATURAL PATH

Avoid hypertension in the first place! If *you* missed that boat, prepare and educate your children, grandchildren, and other loved ones so that they can optimize their potential for avoiding hypertension. Using many of the recommendations on the Balanced Blood Pressure chart one may be able to avoid developing hypertension before it is ever an issue.

If you have high blood pressure, study, and assemble a team of knowledgeable and trustworthy healthcare practitioners, both allopathic and naturally oriented. **Next, firmly resolve to improve your lifestyle as if your life depended on it, because it does.**

If you smoke, critically examine the WHY behind that behavior and find your most comfortable path to becoming a non-smoker. Seek support and help for accomplishing that goal. As you improve your entire lifestyle, it will become natural to improve individual facets of your daily life choices. If you enjoy coffee with a pastry for breakfast followed by a cigarette, change that entire regimen. Take a brief walk or do other activities to increase your heart rate, then prepare a healthy smoothie from organic nutrient-dense ingredients. Self love and self discipline will help you throughout your lifestyle evolution. Post pictures of yourself with your loved ones truly having fun alongside a list of your affirmations, goals, and/or reminders. Your improved lifestyle will benefit your loved ones as well. Your unconscious mind will associate your goals and future good times with your loved ones.

Eliminating inflammation-causing factors in your diet and lifestyle is crucial. Smoking is extremely inflammatory in nature—you are inhaling smoke and hundreds of chemical toxins into your system and putting those chemicals into your bloodstream. Alcohol is also generally inflammatory by nature. Occasional moderate use of alcohol may be acceptable, but daily use is **NOT**. Be sure to eliminate refined sugar in all its many forms. Read more about this subject in the next section on inflammation.

Eliminating processed, devitalized foods by definition eliminates excess **refined** salt. Once you eliminate canned, boxed, prepared foods, you will likely tolerate moderate amounts of added high quality **unrefined** salt.

> ### The Right Salt
>
> For many years, my favorite has been Celtic Salt®. Its 92 minerals provide a grey color. Redmond Real Salt®, mined from the Great Salt Lake basin, contains 60 minerals and appears mildly pink with rust colored mineral flecks. Another wholesome salt is Himalayan Salt®. It is pink and has 84 minerals.
>
> Any of these **unrefined** salts can be safely used by most people, even those with hypertension. The magnesium and trace minerals in these natural salts provide a balanced mineral source. In fact, Dr. Fergdoon Batmanghelidj (fondly called Dr. B.) has found that few people drink sufficient water. He suggests drinking half as many ounces of water as your weight in pounds (100 ounces of water for someone weighing 200 pounds). For proper use of the water in your cells, he recommends dissolving a small amount (1/4 tsp.) of one of these salts in your mouth just prior to drinking sixteen ounces of water, and repeating though the day. Only use this approach after reading and fully understanding his treatment. Refer to the website: watercures.org, and his books, *Your Body's Many Cries for Water* and *Water for Health, for Healing, for Life: You're Not Sick, You're Thirsty!*

Classic white table salt does not have a full complement of minerals (only Sodium and Chloride), and typically has additives for anti-caking and pourablity enhancement. Avoid it.

Municipal tap water is another inflammatory agent, as it contains chlorine. Studies since at least 1985 have correlated chlorinated drinking water with increased risk of atherosclerosis (calcium and fat residues collecting in the arteries), spawning hypertension and heart disease.

Meditation, biofeedback sessions, guided imagery, and emotional release techniques are all effective in health expansion **and** blood pressure reduction.

In my office, I look closely at the organ relationships, especially heart and kidney, as they relate to fluid balance and fluid movement in the body. Investigating any potential relationship between your adrenal glands and thyroid and hypertension is also an important step.

How to Implement Balanced Blood Pressure Tools

Refer to the following chart (see pages 320–321) for encouragement and guidance. Rejoice! You will find numerous lifestyle measures, foods, nutrients, and herbs are available to help you. Consult your

> ### Eggplant Recipe to Lower High Blood Pressure
>
> Ingredients:
> 1 eggplant cut into 1 inch pieces
> 1 gallon of spring water
>
> Instructions:
> Place eggplant pieces into bottle of spring water. Let mixture sit in refrigerator for 4 days.
>
> Remove eggplant pieces from spring water and discard (saving the spring water only). The spring water will now be light brown in color.
>
> Drink 1 ounce of the eggplant infused spring water for 14 days. After 14 days, drink 1 ounce of the infused spring water every other day until it is gone. Continue with another batch, drinking only every other day.
>
> Check your blood pressure regularly. You do not want it to drop too low.

holistic practitioner for guidance with the details. I encourage chiropractic and acupuncture treatment, massage, tai chi, yoga, and meditation. Body-mind therapy and attitudinal shifts may be life changing as well. Never abruptly stop medications your body is accustomed to taking; instead, work with your team of doctors to minimize or transition off medication if that is your goal. Simply adding several proactive blood pressure balancing tools may begin the process to diminish your body's perceived need for medication or amount of medication. This is a very personal journey. The journey may be long and feel like you are travelling a bumpy road, as hypertension is a result of a faulty diet and lifestyle. Your commitment to a regimen of diet and lifestyle improvement is crucial, as is allowing emotional processing and release on an ongoing basis. You will need to study, explore, and be in frequent contact with your team of doctors if you endeavor to change your medication program.

Ernesto's Stress

Ernesto was in his mid forties. He worked hard at his managerial position with a convenience store chain and took his responsibilities seriously. But he also internalized the stress, causing his body distress. He often worked the night shift; hired, trained, and fired the staff members; and had to cope with employee theft frequently. Ernesto developed hypertension and started medication. He then came to me asking for alternatives. His heart and kidneys required balancing.

We worked to improve heart and kidneys through Chiropractic, acupuncture, specific nutrients, detoxification, and body-mind therapy. We also worked to improve his quality of sleep and his diet. We talked about learning to not take the work stresses home and to incorporate stress reduction measures, yet he could not accomplish these. Ultimately, I suggested that Ernesto look for a less stressful job, but he felt unable to make a change at that time.

Through this entire process he attempted to wean off his medication several times. Typically he succeeded for a few weeks at a time until more stress arose. At this point, his blood pressure would climb and he would feel obliged to reinstitute the medication. Ernesto found out about the eggplant recipe to lower his high blood pressure (see page 318) and faithfully followed the regimen. That was the final puzzle piece for Ernesto. His blood pressure lowered, he successfully weaned off his medication, and his blood pressure remained in an acceptable range.

Along with the eggplant drink, Ernesto decided to relax his grip on the stresses of his job. He did balance his blood pressure while at the same job, but a few months later a new opportunity knocked on his door and he changed to a much less stressful and more rewarding job. Yay, Ernesto!

BALANCED BLOOD PRESSURE

Active Lifestyle Measures	Diet Measures (Foods to include in diet)	Alternative options: Herbs and Nutrients	Aroma Therapy
AVOID: • Alcohol • Caffeine • Cocaine • Cold remedies • Coltsfoot • Decongestants • Diet pills • Ephedra • Goldenseal • Ginseng • Holding harsh thoughts and emotions • Licorice • Oral contraceptives • Processed foods • Smoking and all tobacco products • Stress • White table salt • Yerba Maté **INCLUDE:** • DASH diet • Exercise • Laughter • Learn coping skills • Plant based diet • Practice compassion and forgiveness • Seeds • Stress reduction • Weight loss	• Amaranth • Apricots • Avocado • Avocado oil • Bananas • Black strap molasses • Brown rice • Cashews • Celery • Eggplant • Fava beans • Figs • Garlic • Lamb's quarters greens • Mackeral • Olive oil • Olives • Onions • Pomegranate • Reishi mushrooms • Sardines • Sea vegetables • Sesame seeds • Shitake mushrooms • Sorrel • Spirulina • Swiss chard • Tahini • Tomatoes • Unprocessed grey or pink sea salt • Walnut oil • Walnuts • Winter squash • Yams	**HERBS:** • Bilberry • Bitter orange • Black cohosh • Chanca piedra • Chicory • Coleus • Corn silk • Dandelion • Dong quai • Hawthorn • Horseradish • Fenugreek • Garlic • Stinging nettles • Valerian **VITAMINS:** • B vitamin complex • Choline • Coenzyme Q10 • Multivitamin • Vitamin C • Vitamin E **MINERALS:** • Calcium • Magnesium • Melatonin • Potassium **OTHERS:** • Omega 3 oils • Probiotics	• Goldenrod • Helichrysum • Lavender • Lemon balm (Melisa) • Marjoram • Nutmeg • Rosemary • Ylang ylang

(tools to prevent hypertension)

Affirmations	Organ and Meridian Relationship	Bach Remedies	Movement/Activity and Treatments	Mind-Body
• I am able to let go and enjoy moving forward • I am more and more in touch with my inner peace each day • I am calm • I love opening my heart and sharing it with others • I love myself	• Heart • Kidney • Liver • Refer to Chapter 2 (*Acupuncture the Healing Energy*)	• Agrimony • Elm • Holly • Impatiens • Rock rose • Vine	• Any enjoyable, well tolerated exercise • Appropriate health promoting recreation • Appropriate therapeutic music, rhythm or sound • Consider: acupuncture, acupressure, chiropractic, Jin-Shin, massage, polarity therapy and/or reflexology • Dancing • Qi Gong • Tai Chi • Walking • Yoga	• Acknowledge, observe, experience your emotions • Allow time to process emotions, then seek support or guidance as needed • Center yourself • Cherish and enhance relationships • Creative visualization • Gratitude expression • Journaling • Learn more about your health concerns and treatment options • Meditation • Relaxation techniques • Spiritual practice • Unwind, review the day, organize concerns and release the burden before sleep

7. Arthritis and Other Inflammatory Conditions

Cool Your Inflammation

Discussion

The classic signs of inflammation have been documented since approximately 30 BCE, described by Aulus Cornelius Celsus who noted them as:

- Redness
- Heat
- Swelling
- Pain

These four signs have been taught to doctors since that ancient era. An increased blood flow to the area of concern brings nutrients, oxygen, white blood cells, and necessary body chemicals to begin the work of protecting the affected area from its invaders (bacteria, viruses, toxins, or foreign bodies). This results in **redness** and **heat**. The local blood vessels become more permeable and fluid seeps into the area. Irritated cells release **inflammatory mediators** to guide the process. The mediators attract white blood cells to the area so they can actively engulf the offending bacteria or debris. These preliminary processes open spaces between cells in the blood vessel lining (epithelium) to allow the white blood cells and other needed components to easily pass from the bloodstream into the "target" tissue.

The fluid and cells that have moved from the bloodstream to the affected tissue account for the localized **swelling**. Your body produces several types of inflammatory mediators to perform specific tasks; one of these is to make the local nerves more sensitive to the **pain**. This fact, along with the trauma or issue at hand, accounts for the pain you feel. This description is quite simplified, but serves to give you an overview of your body's self protective process, inflammation.

When you get a large splinter, for example, your body wants to clean up this source of inflammation as soon as possible. Numerous chemical processes using many natural biochemicals, infection fighting cells and mechanisms become involved. Coordinating chemicals are also working hard to normalize the area. You can best help your body's internal process by cleaning, observing, and protecting the wound, as well as by immersing yourself in the best lifestyle patterns possible. These include proper hydration, nutrition, and rest. On the other hand, taking a dose of anti-inflammatory medication could slow the normal adaptive body process, **and** your healing.

An example of chronic or systemic inflammation could be either asthma or rheumatoid arthritis. In either case, the issue is more complicated and more pervasive than a splinter in the hand.

Enid's Case

Enid had rheumatoid arthritis, with occasional episodes of mild stiffness over a period of years. When her husband's job changed and they moved to a much smaller town in a remote area, she did not adjust well. In addition to taking on several administrative and social roles at her church and organizing their new home, she was concerned about her third-grade daughter's adjustment to a new school and classmates. Enid let her diet slide to include much more processed and pre-prepared food, even frequently picking up fast food for her family's dinner. Within a few months of the move, she had markedly increased stiffness and joint swelling. Her ability to walk was greatly impaired.

Enid came to my office saying that she felt she had suddenly aged forty years, but was strongly invested in regaining lost function, vitality, and enjoyment of life. We determined that she would undergo a fast of freshly made vegetable juices.

She received a Clinical Kinesiology evaluation to guide her treatment with chiropractic, acupuncture, and emotional balancing. She elected to maintain the juice fast for two weeks. For greater detoxification, Enid received colonic therapy, twice a week for six weeks. After her fast, other nutrients were added to her program. She was tested for food sensitivities and modified her diet accordingly. Since Enid proactively jumped into a natural care program so early in the process of developing rheumatoid arthritis, she did not suffer much actual joint damage. She did not use any anti-inflammatory medication and felt that all of her symptoms resolved. While Enid was feeding her body pro-inflammatory "foods," her body worked hard to detoxify itself, but could not keep up with the rate of **retoxification** foisted upon it by the toxins in her diet. When she detoxified her body and changed her diet, she removed the triggers for a dramatic immune response.

Enid chose to incorporate Xango® juice with its soothing xanthones into her long-term regimen. Xanthones' robust anti-inflammatory phytonutrients have helped many of my patients (and myself) for many years (see Appendix, Product and Resource Guide).

THE PHARMACEUTICAL PATH

If Enid had chosen the pharmaceutical path, she likely would have been prescribed one or two anti-inflammatory drugs at a time. She would have gone back every four to six weeks for blood tests and a brief question and answer session. The primary purpose of the blood tests would be to monitor her blood-forming cells' ability to produce adequate amounts of blood cells, both red and white. Anti-inflammatory drugs categorically damage this function. The result is termed "blood dyscrasia." If white blood cells are decreased, immune system function diminishes. Often we hear or read the term in its plural form, *dyscrasisas*, since it is typical for anti-inflammatories to block the production of **more** than one type of blood cell. For the purposes of this book, I have instituted the abbreviation of BD for blood dyscrasia. Refer back to pages 282 and 283 to review the Prescription Drug Chart and its symptom key.

If Enid did not feel some relief of symptoms, or if her blood forming tissues had suffered extensively, then her roster of medications would be changed. Some patients endure many cycles of medication changes. Enid had been trained as a registered nurse and had worked in hospitals before her daughter's birth. She had witnessed countless patients experiencing side effects of drugs. She adamantly wanted to choose a pharmaceutical-free path.

THE NATURAL PATH

Learning to pay attention to your body's signals will help minimize your inflammation. Many anti-aging specialists feel that prolonged inflammatory processes precipitate numerous older age diseases and hasten the aging process. The key is **not** to search for ways to combat your body's normal self protection mechanisms such as inflammation, but to learn how to avoid **provoking** them through clean diet and supportive lifestyle tools.

How to Implement Cool Your Inflammation Tools

Refer to the following chart for encouragement and guidance. You will find numerous lifestyle measures, foods, nutrients, and herbs are available to help you. Pour water on your fire. Drink large amounts of the most pure drinking water you can find. This will dilute the inflammatory toxins and help flush them away. When your urine is

COOL YOUR INFLAMMATION

Active Lifestyle Measures	Diet Measures (Foods to include in diet)	Alternative options: Herbs and Nutrients	Aroma Therapy
AVOID: • Artificial sweeteners • Caffeine • Chemical additives • Coffee • Corn • Corn Products • Dairy • Food preservatives and dyes • GMO foods • Holding harsh thoughts and emotions • Margarine • Red meat • Safflower oil • Shortening • Spicy foods • Tobacco • Wheat • White potatoes **INCLUDE:** • Large amounts of pure water • Plant based diet • Practice compassion and forgiveness • Seeds • Therapeutic touch gently over areas of concern by self or another person • Xango® juice	• Almonds • Apples • Avocado oil • Avocados • Blueberries • Broccoli • Brussels sprouts • Butternut squash • Cayenne* • Celery • Cherries • Chilies* • Coconut oil • Cucumbers • Currants • Dates • Flax seed oil • Garlic • Ginger • Green beans • Green grapes • Green tea • Kale • Leafy greens • Lettuce • Herring • Mackeral • Mangosteen • Olive oil • Oranges • Persimmons • Pickles • Pomegranate • Prunes • Quinoa • Raspberries • Sardines • Scallions • Seaweed • Tangerines • Walnut oil • Walnuts • Wild salmon	**HERBS:** • Aloe Vera • Andiroba oil (topical) • Arnica (homeopathic) • Arnica salve • Ashwagandha • Birch leaf • Boswellia • Bupleurum • Burdock root • Cat's Claw • Devil's claw • Feverfew • Hawthorn • Licorice root • Stinging nettles • Turmeric • Willow bark • Yucca **VITAMINS:** • Cobalamin (B_{12}) • Vitamin C • Vitamin K **MINERALS:** • Zinc **OTHERS:** • Bromelain • Chondroitin sulfate • Colostrum • Glucosamine • Omega 3 oils • Proteolytic enzymes • Sam-e • Zostrix (topical capsaicin)*	• Birch • Black pepper • Cinnamon • Clove bud • Eucalyptus • Frankincense • German chamomile • Ginger • Helichrysum • Hyssop • Juniper • Lavender • Lemongrass • Marjoram • Myrrh • Nutmeg • Oregano • Peppermint* • Pine • Spearmint* • Spruce • Tea tree • Wintergreen

* Blocks substance P, a naturally occurring neurotransmitter which facilitates pain perception.

(tools to prevent and slow down inflammatory conditions)

Affirmations	Organ and Meridian Relationship	Bach Remedies	Movement/Activity and Treatments	Mind-Body
• I am ready to release past hurt, anger and frustrations • I love myself • I am comfortable and flexible	• Liver • Thymus (triple warmer meridian) • Refer to Chapter 2 (*Acupuncture the Healing Energy*)	• Beech • Cherry plum • Honeysuckle • Rock rose • Vine • Willow	• Any enjoyable, well tolerated exercise • Appropriate health promoting recreation • Appropriate therapeutic music, rhythm or sound • Consider: acupuncture, acupressure, chiropractic, Jin-Shin, massage, polarity therapy and/or reflexology • Range of motion exercises • Qi Gong • Swimming • Tai chi • Warm bath with essential oils followed with ice pack if needed • Water therapy	• Acknowledge, observe, experience your emotions • Allow time to process emotions, then seek support or guidance as needed • Center yourself • Cherish and enhance relationships • Creative visualization • Gratitude expression • Journaling • Learn more about your health concerns and treatment options • Meditation • Relaxation techniques • Spiritual practice • Unwind, review the day, organize concerns and release the burden before sleep

practically colorless, you will know that you have diluted the inflammatory toxins and have begun to flush them out. Consult your holistic practitioner for guidance with the details. I encourage chiropractic and acupuncture treatment as well as lymphatic massage, reiki, meditation, and visualization. Serrapeptase enzymes in tablet form taken between meals can help your body to be cleansed of inflammation byproducts and offer great relief.

Never abruptly stop medications your body is accustomed to taking; instead, work with your team of doctors to minimize or transition off medication if that is your goal. Simply adding several proactive inflammation cooling tools may begin the process to diminish your body's perceived need for medication or amount of medication.

Remember that when you experience inflammation, your body senses a state of emergency, feeling that the fire alarm has been sounded. Removing inflammatory factors is necessary. Inflammatory agents may include: GMO foods, chemical additives, pesticides, processed foods, artificial sweeteners, flour based foods, refined carbohydrates, "energy" drinks, soda, tobacco products and so on. Your commitment to a regimen of diet and lifestyle improvement is crucial, as is allowing emotional processing and release on an ongoing basis. You will need to study, explore, and be in frequent contact with your team of doctors if you endeavor to change your medication program.

Avoiding the Wheelchair

A Success Story

Carla's story (page 3) at the beginning of this book tells the saga of a woman with high level inflammation and little tolerance for the myriad of strong medications she had been trying to endure. She experienced compromised function of both her kidneys and her liver. Carla suffered progressive damage to her knee and hip joints in spite of the anti-inflammatory medications **and** because she did not remove the inflammatory triggers in her lifestyle. Once Carla came to my office and was guided to better health, via a Clinical Kinesiology evaluation, she achieved her goal—avoiding the wheelchair. She was able to stop all anti-inflammatory medication, and resume many enjoyable activities. Carla and I both moved to different towns and lost contact, but unexpectedly encountered each other in a restaurant twenty-eight years later. She still did not have a wheelchair.

8. Heart Attack, Myocardial Infarction, Coronary Artery Syndrome, Stroke...

Keep the Blood Flowing

Discussion

Blood clot formation is one of your body's crucial life preserving processes. Immediately after being cut or physically traumatized, your body activates complex chemical and biological processes to minimize your blood loss. A scab over a recent cut or scratch is the most familiar form of blood clot. Biochemicals that form blood clots or scabs are stored in your skin, so the normal clotting process begins right away. If the cut is deeper or wider than your own blood clotting mechanisms can handle, it is time to go to an emergency care facility for sutures (stitches). Between the stitches, your body will form scabs to close the wound, stop the bleeding, block bacteria and debris, and thus allow for the tissues to heal. The protective blood clotting function is important and can be a life saver.

The biochemicals that form blood clots are called "thrombogenic (clot producing) factors." These are also stored in the linings of your blood vessels, primed for rapid release if the "home" blood vessel is damaged. When the blood vessel is severed, you are glad that repair materials are on site.

Platelets are fragments of a certain type of large white blood cells called "megakaryocytes." These grow and virtually explode when mature. The fragments become your platelets, providers of many required materials for the first step of blood clot formation. When your body feels that the clot is structurally sound and complete, it recruits anti-clotting enzymes to counteract further growth of the scab or blood clot around its perimeter. If your body is well balanced, your blood clotting and anti-blood clotting messengers are in a healthy equilibrium. This balance maybe disturbed by certain medications, sometimes with drastic results. Lifestyle and dietary indiscretions may also upset the balance.

As the tissue beneath the blood clot or scab heals, your wise body knows that it is time to begin disassembling the protective clot. Specific enzymes break down the clot incrementally, slowly reabsorbing the blood clot or scab. The residual scab may easily fall off, revealing newly healed tissue. This is a truly remarkable self-defense process.

Sometimes, however, this process gears up to your detriment. Blood clots may form in veins, most often the deep veins of the calf, with no apparent cut or trauma. This is called "deep vein thrombosis" (DVT), or a blood clot within an intact vein. This can be triggered by sluggish circulation, lack of activity, inflammation, and certain medications. Estrogen and testosterone are the most notorious medications known to cause blood clots. Pregnant women are more prone to DVT than non-pregnant women of similar ages because of increased weight and intra-abdominal pressure that can impede blood flow in the iliac veins (they are near the uterus). Pregnant women also have higher blood levels of hormones and clotting factors than other people. Dehydration, HIV, chlorinated water, elevated homocysteine and smoking all cause inflammation of the blood vessel linings. This inflammation causes nicks in the endothelium of the vascular system. This triggers the blood clotting mechanism and begins atherosclerotic buildup. These are lifestyle precipitators of cardiovascular disease and blood clots. Work to minimize your risk.

A deep vein blood clot puts the body in a precarious situation. If the clot should break loose, it will travel with the blood flow toward the heart. (The venous blood always moves to the heart to be reoxygenated before it moves to the arteries for delivery to the tissues.) If blood clot material has travelled from a vein in one of the limbs and moved through the heart valves, it may enter a coronary artery. Since coronary arteries are much smaller in diameter than the veins or valves, the clot will lodge, typically, in one of these narrow areas. This stops the flow of blood to the most distant muscle tissue served by that artery. If the blockage remains, the under-oxygenated muscle tissue will die. This is called a heart attack, a myocardial infarction, or coronary artery syndrome.

If a floating blood clot makes its way into one of the carotid arteries, it will travel toward the brain until it lodges in a narrow part of an artery and stops blood flow to a segment of the brain. This is called a stroke or cerebral vascular accident (CVA). If a floating blood clot goes into a vessel in the lung, it will likely cause a pulmonary embolism (PE).

THE PHARMACEUTICAL PATH

After a stroke, pulmonary embolism, heart attack, or placement of a stent (small metal tube to attempt re-opening a blocked artery), doctors will generally prescribe a platelet aggregation inhibitor (Plavix®, Xarelto®, or others) or an anticoagulant such as Warfarin (Coumadin®). One or more of these powerful medications are typically recommended for arterial fibrillations (irregular heart fluttering). These health conditions are frightening and can be life-threatening. Most people will likely feel obliged to take the suggested medication; which probably is the best decision *initially*. How long to continue is the question with no consistent answer.

To err on the safe side, doctors may counsel continuing these medications indefinitely—even for a lifetime.

If you or someone you know is in this situation look forward to the appropriate "Keep the Blood Flowing" tools in this section, if these are not contraindicated in your case.

The worst problem with these platelet-inhibiting medications is the effects that they have on your entire cardiovascular system: **all** of your blood, **all** of your veins, **all** of your arteries, **all** of your platelets. Since only a small percentage of the body can possibly benefit from the effects of these medications (the damaged or clot-prone areas), unwanted side effects are common.

On their website, Xarelto® gives this disclaimer:

> **Call your doctor or get medical help right away if you develop any of these signs or symptoms of bleeding:**
> - Unexpected bleeding or bleeding that lasts a long time, such as:
>   - Nosebleeds that happen often
>   - Unusual bleeding from the gums
>   - Menstrual bleeding that is heavier than normal, or vaginal bleeding
> - Bleeding that is severe or that you cannot control
> - Bright red or black stools (looks like tar)
> - Cough up blood or blood clots
> - Vomit blood or your vomit looks like "coffee grounds"
> - Headaches, feeling dizzy or weak
> - Pain, swelling, or new drainage at wound sites

These health conditions are serious; the medications have the potential to save your life **and** to negatively impact you as well. Educate yourself, consult your doctors, and make your best decision.

THE NATURAL PATH

Everything that you put into your body will eventually affect your blood and blood vessels. Therefore, determine to avoid the lifestyle triggers for excess blood clot formation. Proactively prevent the problem. Avoid irritants such as chlorinated water, excess alcohol, tobacco, e-cigarette vapor, processed sugar, processed foods and beverages, chronic inflammation, chronic infection, being sedentary, and taking synthetic hormones.

Choose a lifestyle that is kind to your body. Eat a nutrient-dense and varied diet of natural, unadulterated food. Drink large amounts of the most pure drinking water possible. Serrapeptase is a natural enzyme that can help deter blood clotting. Garlic and flaxseed oil on salads or steamed vegetables are gentle dietary measures for "lubricating" your endothelium, your platelets, and red blood cells.

Choose appropriate tools from the "Keep Your Blood Flowing" chart.

How to Implement Keep the Blood Flowing Tools

The following chart lists numerous lifestyle measures, foods, nutrients, and herbs that are available to help you. Consult your holistic practitioner for guidance with the details. I encourage chiropractic and acupuncture treatment as well. Never abruptly stop medications your body is accustomed to taking; instead, work with your team of doctors to minimize or transition off medication if that is your goal. Simply adding several proactive tools to keep the blood flowing may begin the process to diminish your body's perceived need for medication or amount of medication. Your commitment to a regimen of diet and lifestyle improvement is crucial, as is allowing emotional processing and release on an ongoing basis. You will need to study, explore, and be in frequent contact with your team of doctors if you endeavor to change your medication program. If you have been prescribed a platelet inhibitor after a stroke, heart valve replacement or heart stent placement, you have some serious considerations to weigh. Openly communicate with your doctors. Ask questions persistently.

Angie's Plan for Success

Angie developed blood clots after taking birth control pills for four years, and was briefly hospitalized. Her medical doctor advised stopping the pills and taking Coumadin for a while. After discontinuing that, she wanted advice on avoiding future episodes, and to keep her blood flowing naturally.

After her preliminary exam, we planned a program to keep the blood flowing without medication, thus allowing her protective blood clotting mechanisms to be available for injuries. We also considered how to balance her hormonal system with only natural remedies, since estrogen in all forms may precipitate blood clots.

Angie had been a "social smoker," and she struggled with that habit for several months, but finally succeeded in quitting. She opted for vegetable sources of omega 3s, and selected chia seed oil capsules, which tested "yes" (using muscle testing)! She added chia seeds to her diet, and planned to eat salad daily, including arugula, another omega 3 source.

Angie enjoyed walking and hiking, and she re-dedicated herself to walk or hike three times a week. This exercise of the calf muscles stimulated her blood vessels and kept her blood flowing. Altogether, it was an admirable proactive plan to protect from future blood clot episodes.

KEEP THE BLOOD FLOWING

Active Lifestyle Measures	Diet Measures (Foods to include in diet)	Alternative options: Herbs and Nutrients	Aroma Therapy
AVOID: • Animal fats • Crossing legs at the knee • Excessive alcohol consumption • Fast food • Get adequate rest • High fat diet • Holding harsh thoughts and emotions • Oral contraceptives • Processed foods • Sedentary lifestyle • Skipping breakfast • Stress **INCLUDE:** • 5-7 servings of fruits and vegetables daily • 30 minutes of exercise 3-5 times per week • Adequate rest • Coping skills • Fiber rich breakfast • Flaxseed • Onions with evening meals • Organic soy protein • Plant based diet • Stress reduction	• Almonds • Apples • Blackberries • Buckwheat • Cantaloupe • Cashews • Chia seeds • Coconut oil • Flax seeds • Flax seed oil • Grapes • Green tea • Garlic • Herring • Honeydew • Hot chili • Hot peppers • Lemon • Mackerel • Mushrooms • Oat bran • Oat meal • Olive oil • Onions • Oranges • Papaya • Pineapple • Pomegranate • Potatoes • Red wine (moderate amount) • Sardines • Seaweed • Sesame seeds • Tahini • Walnuts • Walnut oil • Watermelon • Wild salmon	**HERBS:** • Cloves • Garlic • Ginger • Turmeric **VITAMINS:** • Multivitamin • Vitamin E • Vitamin K **MINERALS:** • Calcium **OTHERS:** • Bromelain • Omega 3 oils • Probiotics • Serrapeptase	• Clove • Grapefruit • Helichrysum • Lavender • Lemon • Orange • Tangerine

(tools to prevent excess blood clotting)

Affirmations	Organ and Meridian Relationship	Bach Remedies	Movement/Activity and Treatments	Mind-Body
• I see and feel life's energy flowing smoothly through my blood vessels • I trust my body's ability to balance and heal • Unconditional love flows through my entire being	• Heart • Pericardium • Refer to Chapter 2 (*Acupuncture the Healing Energy*)	• Aspen • Crabapple • Gentian • Impatiens • Sweet chestnut	• Any enjoyable, well tolerated exercise • Appropriate health promoting recreation • Appropriate therapeutic music, rhythm or sound • Consider: acupuncture, acupressure, chiropractic, Jin-Shin, massage, polarity therapy and/or reflexology • Dancing • Walking • Yoga	• Acknowledge, observe, experience your emotions • Allow time to process emotions, then seek support or guidance as needed • Center yourself • Cherish and enhance relationships • Creative visualization • Gratitude expression • Journaling • Learn more about your health concerns and treatment options • Meditation • Relaxation techniques • Spiritual practice • Unwind, review the day, organize concerns and release the burden before sleep

9. Heartburn, Acid Reflux, Indigestion, GERD

Digestive Comfort

Discussion

Hydrochloric acid is the key to proper digestion. Your stomach produces it to break down proteins and to signal the rest of your digestive tract to gear up other functions. Your stomach lining is designed to tolerate and thrive with this acid exposure. Your gastric (stomach) acids are required to stimulate the release of bile and pancreatic enzymes, other critical players in completing your digestive process.

People who have a lack of hydrochloric acid generally develop one or more symptoms of digestive acid deficiency, including:
- Anemia (especially B_{12} related)
- Arrhythmia (irregular heart beat)
- Depression
- Elimination disturbances
- Fatigue
- Fingernail cracking and ridging
- Food sensitivities and intolerances
- Gas
- Hair loss
- Hyperemesis in pregnancy and otherwise
- Hypertension
- Impaired hearing
- Indigestion
- Muscle cramps
- Muscle weakness
- Nutrient deficiencies
- Osteoporosis
- Sexual dysfunction
- Weakened immunity
- Weakness of connective tissue, hair, nails, etc.

THE PHARMACEUTICAL PATH

This approach uses over-the-counter antacids or stronger proton-pump inhibitors (PPIs), such as such as Nexium® and Prilosec®. Both antacids and PPIs are designed to interfere with your normal gastric acid function and production. With less of the necessary acid, digestion is less efficient, and consequences begin to develop.

To complicate matters, if you have taken a proton-pump inhibitor long term, your body accommodates to it. In this case, stopping the medication may create rebound acid hypersecretion, a trained response to your stomach attempting to maintain normal function. The use of proton-pump inhibitors may induce any of the symptoms listed above, as well as increased stomach discomfort, insomnia, disturbance of the normal intestinal flora, and actually statistically doubling the risk of accident or injury due to neurological impairment.

THE NATURAL PATH

Work *with* your digestive system, **NOT AGAINST** it! Eat the right foods, i.e., unprocessed, natural, non-GMO foods. Between meals, drink pure spring or purified water in copious amounts. This will appropriately dilute and flush away the stomach acids after they have performed their job. If you are properly nourished and hydrated, your stomach will dutifully produce the next batch of necessary acid on demand. If you are experiencing reflux, scrutinize your diet and lifestyle. Your habit of eating very hot, spicy food just before bed may be the key to your reflux. Eat several hours (begin with three) before lying down. You may wish to experiment with timing variations. If you continue to have reflux, elevate the head of your bed a few inches. Some resources suggest a 7-degree elevation. Avoid tight belts and waist lines. Search out experienced Clinical Kinesiology or Applied Kinesiology practitioners who can evaluate and reposition your stomach if necessary. If you have actual pain or inflammation, soothe it with aloe vera, Xango® juice, papaya juice, or other options listed below in the tools for Digestive Comfort. Once you have improved and have no discomfort, ask to be tested for hydrochloric acid deficiency (See page 233 in Chapter 12).

How to Implement Digestive Comfort Tools

Refer to the following chart for encouragement and guidance. You will find numerous lifestyle measures, foods, nutrients, and herbs are available to help you. Consult your holistic practitioner for guidance with the details. I encourage chiropractic and acupuncture treatment as well. Never abruptly stop medications your body is accustomed to taking; instead, work with your team of doctors to minimize or transition off medication if that is your goal. Simply adding several proactive digestive comfort tools may begin the process to diminish your body's perceived need for medication or amount of medication. Your commitment to a regimen of diet and lifestyle improvement is crucial, as is allowing emotional processing and release on an ongoing basis. You will need to study, explore, and be in frequent contact with your team of doctors if you endeavor to change your medication program.

Renelda's Story

Renelda consulted me for help concerning her digestive system. She experienced acid reflux, poor digestion, and alternating diarrhea and constipation.

In years past, Renelda had a serious eating disorder and was considered bulimic. The periodic induced vomiting had eroded her tender esophageal tissues (not designed to withstand much exposure to stomach acids) and even damaged the enamel of her teeth. Renelda had been through a residential program for eating disorders in the past with good success. For many people like Renelda, reflux is a long lasting consequence of an eating disorder with forced vomiting.

After Renelda's history taking and exam, we started on a program of weekly treatments and utilized numerous healing and soothing agents for her traumatized digestive tract. On a daily basis, she consumed a smoothie including fresh papaya, papaya juice, or Xango® juice. She added an excellent quality protein powder with dehydrated organic vegetables and sprouts (Total Green® by Nutri-West™), and various pulverized supplements. This provided high density nutrients in an easily digestible form, along with soothing and tissue healing factors. Renelda was encouraged to use okra often in her simple homemade vegetable soups.

We also used the soft laser with a setting to cool her internal inflammation. I selected a mild digestive enzyme formula containing marshmallow root to further soothe while improving digestion.

Other compatible lifestyle measures and nutrients were added. We explored and released "stuffed" emotions and Renelda improved. At the end of nine months, she truly experienced digestive comfort on a daily basis.

DIGESTIVE COMFORT

Active Lifestyle Measures	Diet Measures (Foods to include in diet)	Alternative options: Herbs and Nutrients	Aroma Therapy
AVOID: • Alcohol • Antacids • Carbonated beverages • Certain antibiotics • Coffee • Chocolate • Eating while stressed • Fast food • Holding harsh thoughts and emotions • Laying down within 3 hours after eating • NSAIDS • Overeating • Processed foods • Spicy foods • Tobacco • Tomatoes **INCLUDE:** • Eating in a relaxed state • Eating in pleasant surroundings • Herbal bitters before meals • Marshmallow root tea • Peppermint tea • Practice compassion and forgiveness • Slippery elm tea • Small frequent meals • Stress management • Weight loss	• Almonds • Apple cider vinegar • Bananas • Cabbage • Cabbage juice • Carrots • Carrot juice • Garlic • Lettuce • Okra (not fried) • Olives • Olive oil • Peppermint tea • Plantain (cooked) • Seaweed • Slippery elm tea • Watercress	**HERBS:** • Aloe Vera • Calendula • Chamomile • Chicory • Cinnamon • Dandelion • Dill • Fennel • Garlic • Ginger • Licorice (DGL) • Marshmallow root • Peppermint • Slippery elm • Turmeric **VITAMINS:** • B vitamin complex • Vitamin A • Vitamin C • Vitamin E **OTHERS:** • Digestive enzymes • Melatonin • Nux vomica (homeopathic) • Probiotics • Xango® juice	• Anise • Black pepper • Cardamom • Chamomile (German and Roman) • Cinnamon • Ginger • Neroli • Nutmeg • Sweet orange • Spearmint • Turmeric

(tools to avoid heartburn, reflux and G.E.R.D.)

Affirmations	Organ and Meridian Relationship	Bach Remedies	Movement/Activity and Treatments	Mind-Body
• I peacefully digest my foods and events daily • I am nurtured by simple things • I slowly taste and savor life's joys	• Esophagus (kidney or small intestine meridians) • Kidney • Stomach • Refer to Chapter 2 (*Acupuncture the Healing Energy*)	• Cerato • Crabapple • Pine	• Any enjoyable, well tolerated exercise • Appropriate health promoting recreation • Appropriate therapeutic music, rhythm or sound • Consider: acupuncture, acupressure, chiropractic, Jin-Shin, massage, polarity therapy and/or reflexology • Swimming • Tai chi • Yoga	• Acknowledge, observe, experience your emotions • Allow time to process emotions, then seek support or guidance as needed • Center yourself • Cherish and enhance relationships • Creative visualization • Gratitude expression • Learn more about your health concerns and treatment options • Journaling • Meditation • Relaxation techniques • Spiritual practice • Unwind, review the day, organize concerns and release the burden before sleep

10. Insomnia, Sleep Disturbance

Sleep Well For Health

Discussion

Sleep is a required restorative process that should occupy approximately one-third of your day/night cycle. Sufficient sleep provides you with cellular repair and rejuvenation, mental and emotional regrouping, and prepares you for peak cognitive function. If you sleep well consistently, you will have more balanced energy levels throughout the day, increased wellness in all regards, and improved performance of all your tasks.

If you are lacking sufficient sleep consistently, you will lose your "edge" in many areas. Sleep deprivation impacts people in the mental-emotional department with impaired memory, concentration, stress handling, critical thinking, decision making, problem solving, and creativity. All of these factors increase the risk of accidents and injuries due to diminished cognitive and motor skills functions, impaired coordination and slower reaction times. Sleep deprived individuals have increased irritability, moodiness, fatigue, and often lack motivation in all areas of their lives. If you suffer from a chronic lack of sleep, you have a statistical propensity for lowered immunity, and an increased risk of infection, hypertension, heart disease, diabetes, and

Four Stages of Non-REM Sleep

Non-REM 1 stage is typically completed in 5-10 minutes. This stage is comparable to "drifting" off. You transition from beta to alpha to theta brain waves, which have a frequency between 4 and 8 Hertz. By comparison, in the fully awake state of consciousness, your brain is producing beta waves at 13-30 cycles per second or Hertz (Hz). The typical adult with no sleep disorder is in the non-REM 1 stage about 4-5 percent of their night.

Non-REM 2, you are truly asleep, though not yet in "deep" sleep. Your brain slows down and produces theta waves (4-8 Hz). In this state memory and emotions are easily processed. This stage often lasts 30 to 60 minutes and accounts for one-half of your sleep time. Heart rate and metabolism slow down. Body temperature may decrease and muscles relax. The first time you achieve non-REM 2 sleep in a night, it may only be for a span of 10 to 20 minutes.

Non-REM 3 stage is considered true deep sleep. Now your brain is producing delta waves, the slowest of all (0.5-3 Hz), as well as other faster waves. Now your body has the right conditions to synthesize proteins. They will be used for growth and for tissue repair. At this point it will be difficult for someone to awaken you. You may be in non-REM 3 stage for 10 minutes or so. Generally, most adults are in this phase of sleep for 7 percent of their night.

Non-REM 4 is the deepest level of sleep. Delta waves are predominant. These are slow waves. Generally no eye movement occurs during this phase. However, this is the phase of sleep when unusual behaviors (parasomnia) may occur, such as sleep walking, sleep talking, and sleep terrors, which are generally not remembered. It is difficult to arouse or awaken someone who is in the non-REM 4 stage of sleep. Here the body works to repair wounds, mineral loss from bones and tissues, and repair or rebuild components of the immune system. Studies indicate that older individuals, especially those over 70, spend less time in the non-REM 4 stage. Whether or not this is normal and intended remains a mystery.

obesity. Thirty percent of adult Americans are said to get insufficient sleep.

Sleep moves through five stages of approximately 90–110 minutes each. **You will be more refreshed upon awakening if you have completed several full sleep cycles.**

Two distinct types of sleep occur during each sleep cycle: REM or rapid eye movement sleep, which is the last phase of each sleep cycle and allows dreaming, and non-REM (NREM) sleep, which precedes REM sleep and is especially restorative to the physical body. Non-REM sleep occurs in four distinct stages (although some researchers now combine stages 3 and 4).

The REM sleep phase is also termed **sleep stage 5 or the R stage**. During this phase, brain activity is similar to the waking state with brain activity waves being prominent. Eye movements are common, rapid, and probably associated with dreaming, which is very much a visual experience.

REM sleep offers many benefits: increased brain development, and remembering recently acquired skills. Memory and emotions are stimulated and processed, and your visual system is stimulated. Many of your diverse immune factors are more active during REM sleep. It is quite interesting that infants born pre-term by ten weeks spend 80 percent of their sleep time in the REM state, while full-term neonates spend 50 percent of their sleep time in REM sleep. The preterm babies require more brain development, and nature provides for it. By age 2, most toddlers devote 30-35 percent of their time to REM sleep, graduating to 25 percent by age 10 and beyond. The REM phase may diminish to 15 percent in the elder population.

During REM sleep, your body's muscular functions begin to reawaken. You may experience twitching or slight movements of your limbs and face. Your metabolism, respiratory rate, and heart rate begin to increase. As the brain waves speed up, the blood pressure rises slightly. The REM sleep stage is the "theater" for most your dreams. Sometimes infants slide directly into REM sleep and demonstrate muscular twitches soon after beginning sleep. REM sleep is credited with fostering creativity and locking new information into your long-term memory.

It is clear that humans are programmed with specific, purposeful stages within their sleep cycles. Many other mammals have been studied in order to find similar, yet distinct, components of their sleep cycles.

THE PHARMACEUTICAL PATH

Many pharmaceutical agents alter or interfere with your sleep cycles. Perhaps you believe that you suffer from insomnia, but discover that your lack of sleep is truly a side effect of your antidepressant. Finding a new solution for the depression may eliminate your insomnia. Several categories of medications may disturb your sleep due to their interference with your nervous system, hormonal system, level of consciousness, or other factors. Here is a partial list of some of the more common sleep disturbing drug categories:

- ADHD medications
- Alzheimer's medication
- Analgesics (over the counter—contains caffeine)
- Antidepressants (especially SSRIs)
- Antihistamines
- Anti-hypertensives
- Anti-smoking medications
- Asthma medication
- Heart failure medications
- Statins
- Steroids
- Thyroid (synthetic—only take in the early morning)

If you take any medications, study their side effects before you decide that you have insomnia, as it may be a side effect of a medication.

A sleep aid prescription may alter the time, quality, and/or sequencing of your sleep cycle stages. The most commonly altered sleep stages are non-REM 4 and REM sleep. This means that you will miss out on the physical body repair and rejuvenation of the non-REM 4 sleep, as well as the brain restorative and memory and emotional processing benefits of undisturbed REM sleep.

….. Many sleep aid drugs are also addictive both behaviorally and physiologically. Moving out of the addictions may be quite challenging for some. Rebound insomnia after stopping these medications is often problematic. Daytime drowsiness and a propensity for auto accidents, depression, and risk of suicidality have been associated with sleep aid medications. It is wise to consider these medications **only** as a last resort.

THE NATURAL PATH

Good sleep hygiene starts with a sensible and consistent bedtime and waking time. Avoid sugar, caffeine, nicotine, and other stimulants—particularly in the afternoon and evening. Insulate your bedroom or sleep area from the maddening world—eliminate televisions, phones, computers, and other electronics. Consider using an EMF clearing device in or just outside of your bedroom. Some people actually turn off the electrical circuits to their bedroom before bed. Limit sensory stimulation—certain movies, dramatic computer games, vigorous exercise, and loud music for two or more hours before bedtime. Keep your room dark and be sure the temperature is comfortable—cool is best. Allowing for fresh air circulation is helpful.

If you have a flood of thoughts running through your mind when you go to bed, you can train your mind to do a "data dump" before going to the bedroom. With this method you begin at a desk or sitting area *in another room*. As an aid to "emptying" your mind, write your to-do list for tomorrow, or write down your creative ideas for business, projects or fun. Then, leave all of that in this other room and tell yourself to put all such thoughts away until tomorrow. Once in bed, if your mind fills with thoughts or wants to revise tomorrow's list, physically get up and go to the other room to give 5–10 minutes to your mind's whims. Then, firmly decree that all such cognitive activity must stop for the night, as you go back to bed. Eventually, you will train yourself and your unruly mind to go with the new sleep regimen. Another method is to play relaxing music *before* bedtime or even *at* bedtime to provide a restful ambiance.

Beyond these lifestyle enhancements, I check patients in my office for issues or toxins that can impair sleep. I routinely check all new patients for parasites with Clinical Kinesiology testing using the parasite handmode. Parasites can be an elusive cause of insomnia. Often I use black walnut tincture, garlic, Citricidal® grapefruit seed extract, or numerous other appropriate remedies which give a strong response to the patient's muscle test. Some people respond well to food grade diatomaceous earth mixed in water twice a day.

Another health condition that contributes to sleep problems is heavy metal toxicity. Many people harbor problematic quantities of heavy metals and suffer with digestive, neurological, and skin issues. Clinical Kinesiology testing allows for specific testing of metals. When these offending metals are known, they can be addressed individually if desired. Essential fatty acids, detoxification formulae, oral chelators, etc., may be used. Cilantro helps remove heavy metals. I find that the Aqua-Chi® footbath treatment also assists the detoxification process, as do sauna sessions. Various homeopathic remedies can also help.

I also evaluate the state of balance of the hypothalamus, an important segment of the brain. It has numerous regulatory functions. The sleep/wakefulness aspect of the hypothalamus is the critical part to examine for those with sleep difficulties. In-office treatment and nutritional support may be most helpful.

Another logical consideration is to search for a mind-body issue, a trapped emotion, or an unexpressed need. This type of issue may be difficult to identify. Once it is identified and addressed, stress and sleep difficulties may improve or abate.

How to Implement Sleep Well for Health Tools

Refer to the following chart for encouragement and guidance. You will find numerous lifestyle measures, foods, nutrients, and herbs are available to help you. Consult your holistic practitioner for guidance with the details. Research to discover the cause of your sleep dysfunction. It could be caused by a medication (even a prescribed sleep aid drug). Worry, discontent or depression could be the causative factor. Directly confronting and genuinely treating the root cause will be of great benefit. I encourage chiropractic and acupuncture treatment as well. Never abruptly stop medications your body is accustomed to taking; instead, work with your team of doctors to minimize or transition off medication if that is your goal. Simply adding several proactive sleeping better for health tools may begin the process to diminish your body's perceived need for medication or amount of medication. This is a very personal journey. Your commitment to a regimen of diet and lifestyle improvement is crucial, as is allowing emotional processing and release on an ongoing basis. You will need to study, explore, and be in frequent contact with your team of doctors if you endeavor to change your medication program. **Sweet dreams.**

I wholeheartedly encourage you to search for drugless solutions to your ailments, whenever possible. Yes, drug interventions save peoples' lives every day, most often in the Emergency Room for short term application.

But this potential benefit is overshadowed daily by the potential for damage from many medications and their often drastic side effects. Synthetically produced pharmaceutical agents are specifically designed to alter your body's normal physiology (and often conflict with this). In fact, most drugs are considered to be in a combative relationship with your body and its exquisitely designed systems (nervous system, gastrointestinal system, and immune system to name a few). If you have diarrhea after eating a contaminated food, your body institutes the best method known to evacuate the harmful bacteria and toxins from itself. Taking an anti-diarrheal drug would force your body to harbor those harmful agents, and attempts to circumvent your protective mechanism. I suggest looking for new ways to cooperate with your body. The "disease care" system itself becomes more dysfunctional as more patients obediently take a handful of new prescriptions without even researching the downside. Be a part of the solution by being proactive, becoming informed, and being assertive enough to ask the difficult questions posed on page 279–280 BEFORE agreeing to a new prescription drug.

Review Polly's story at the beginning of this chapter. She was an actual patient who did **not** research or question the addition of five new drugs to her regimen, and suffered unbearable consequences. Is there someone like Polly in your circle of friends and family or does her story remind you of

SLEEP WELL FOR HEALTH

Active Lifestyle Measures	Diet Measures (Foods to include in diet)	Alternative options: Herbs and Nutrients	Aroma Therapy
AVOID: • Caffeine • Holding harsh thoughts and emotions • Light in sleeping area • Long daytime naps • Most medications interfere with melatonin and therefore your sleep, even sleep aids • Stress • Sugar • Tobacco **INCLUDE:** • Eliminate light from bed room or sleeping area • Meditation before bed • Peaceful, low key activities before bedtime • Practice compassion and forgiveness • Soft music • Use lavender dream pillow or eye pillow at bedtime • Warm baths before bedtime	• Almonds • Baked potato • Barley • Cherries • Chia seeds • Chicken • Chicken liver • Dairy products • Dill • Flax seed • Flax seed oil • Halibut • Oatmeal • Oat straw tea • Peanuts • Pumpkin • Pumpkin seeds • Seaweed • Soybeans (organic) • Spirulina • Spinach (cooked) • Squash • Turkey • Whole grains	**HERBS:** • California poppies • Catnip • Dill • Hops • Kava kava • Lavender • Lemon balm (Melisa) • Oat seed • Oat straw • Passion flower • Rooibos • Schisandra • Skullcap • Valerian • Yerba maté **VITAMINS:** • Cobalamin (B_{12}) • Inositol • Niacin (B_3) • Pantothenic Acid (B_5) • Pyridoxine (B_6) • Riboflavin (B_2) • Thiamin (B_1) • Vitamin C • Vitamin D_3 • Vitamin E **MINERALS:** • Calcium • Magnesium **OTHERS:** • GABA • Melatonin • Omega 3 oils • Probiotics	• Bergamot • Cedar wood • Chamomile (German & Roman) • Lavender • Lemon • Neroli • Orange • Sandalwood • St. John's Wort • Sweet marjoram • Valerian • Ylang ylang

(tools to allow restful sleep without drugs)

Affirmations	Organ and Meridian Relationship	Bach Remedies	Movement/Activity and Treatments	Mind-Body
Daytime: • In this day, I will address necessary thoughts and tasks and lay them to rest before bedtime • I deserve a good night's sleep TONIGHT Bedtime: • I am prepared for luscious restful sleep • I am now ready to receive peaceful rejuvenating slumber • My mind and body are relaxed and at ease, gently drifting into sleep	• Pericardium • Liver • Large Intestine • Thyroid (triple warmer meridian) • Refer to Chapter 2 (*Acupuncture the Healing Energy*)	• Agrimony • Aspen • Honeysuckle • Vervain • Water violet • White chestnut	• Any enjoyable, well tolerated exercise • Appropriate health promoting recreation • Appropriate therapeutic music, rhythm or sound • Consider: acupuncture, acupressure, chiropractic, Jin-Shin, massage, polarity therapy and/or reflexology • Tai chi • Warm bath with lavender and or other essential oils before bed • Yoga	• Acknowledge, observe, experience your emotions • Allow time to process emotions, then seek support or guidance as needed • Center yourself • Cherish and enhance relationships • Creative visualization • Gratitude expression • Journaling • Learn more about your health concerns and treatment options • Meditation • Relaxation techniques • Spiritual practice • Unwind, review the day, organize concerns and release the burden before sleep

yourself? I hope you want to avoid the destructive waves that almost engulfed Polly. You **can** assertively and responsibly learn about keeping your body, mind, self, and entire being well. Choose a lifestyle that enriches your health. If you encounter health problems, health conditions or discomforts in life study them and natural methods to resolve them. If you are considering adding a medication to your life, **first** read as much as you can about it **and** its consequences. Can you and your doctor(s) find a way to minimize the dosage or duration of the medication? Start by delving into the healthy tools charts contained in this chapter.

SUGGESTED READING

Abraham, John. *Science, Politics and the Pharmaceutical Industry: Controversy and Bias in Drug Regulation.* New York: St. Martin's Press, 1995.

Abramson, John, M.D. *Overdosed America: The Broken Promise of American Medicine.* New York: Harper Collins, 2013.

Angell, Marcia. *The Truth About the Drug Companies: How They Deceive Us and What To Do About It.* New York: Random House, 2004.

Breggin, Peter R. *Toxic Psychiatry: Why Therapy, Empathy and Love Must Replace the Drugs, Electroshock, and Biochemical Theories of the "New Psychiatry."* New York: St. Martin's Griffin, 1994.

_____. *Psychiatric Drug Withdrawal: A Guide for Prescribers, Therapists, Patients and their Families.* New York, New York, Springer Publishing Company, LLC., 2013.

_____ and David Cohen, Ph.D. *Your Drug May Be Your Problem: How and Why to Stop Taking Psychiatric Medicines.* Jackson, Tenn.: Da Capo Press, 2007.

Code, Bill, M.D., with Alesandra Rain and Andrea Crocker. *Point of Return: A Safe and Sensible Withdrawal Method for Benzodiazepines, Antidepressants and Sleeping Pills, 2nd edition.* Oxnard, Calif.: Point of Return, Inc., 2008.

Cohen, Jay S., M.D. *Over Dose: The Case Against the Drug Companies.* New York, New York: Jeremy P. Tarcher/Putnam, 2001.

_____. *What You Must Know About Statin Drugs and Their Natural Alternatives.* Garden City Park, New York: Square One Publishers, 2005.

Cohen, Suzy, R.Ph. and Samuel M. Cohen, M.D. *Drug Muggers: How to Keep Your Medicine from Stealing the Life Out of You.* New York: DPI: Dear Pharmacist, Inc., Rodale Books, 2008.

Elliott, Carl. *White Coat, Black Hat: Adventures on the Dark Side of Medicine.* Boston: Beacon Press, 2010.

Fried, Stephen. Bitter *Pills: Inside the Hazardous World of Legal Drugs.* New York: Bantam Books, 1998.

Gold, Robert Steven, R.Ph., MBA. *Are Your Meds Making You Sick?: A Pharmacist's Guide to Avoiding Dangerous Drug Interactions, Reactions, and Side Effects.* Alameda, Calif.: Hunter House, 2011.

Graveline, Duane, M.D., M.P.H. *Lipitor: Thief of Memory.* Self published, 2006.

_____. *The Statin Damage Crisis.* Self published, 2009.

_____. *Statin Drugs Side Effects and the Misguided War on Cholesterol.* Self published, 2004.

Greenberg, Gary. *Manufacturing Depression: The Secret History of a Modern Disease.* New York: Simon & Schuster, 2010.

Houston, Mark C., M.D., M.S. *What Your Doctor May Not Tell You About Heart Disease: The Revolutionary Book That Reveals the Truth Behind Coronary Illnesses—and How You Can Fight Them.* Boston: Grand Central Life & Style, 2012.

_____. *Vascular Biology in Clinical Practice.* Philadelphia: Hanley & Belfus, Inc., 2002.

_____. Meador, Beth Pulliam, M.S.N., R.N., C.S. and Linda Moore Schipani, M.S.N., R.N. *Handbook of Antihypertensive Therapy.* Philadelphia: Hanley & Blefus, Inc., 2000

Moynihan, Roy and Alan Cassels. *Selling Sickness: How the World's Biggest Pharmaceutical Companies Are Turning Us All Into Patients.* Madeira Park, Canada: Douglas & Mcintyre Ltd., 2005.

Roberts, Barbara H., M.D. *The Truth About Statins: Risks and Alternatives to Cholesterol-Lowering Drugs.* New York: Gallery Books, 2012.

Welch, H. Gilbert, Lisa Schwartz and Steve Woloshin. *Overdiagnosed: Making People Sick in the Pursuit of Health.* Boston: Beacon Press, 2011.

Whitaker, Robert. *Anatomy of an Epidemic: Magic Bullets, Psychiatric Drugs, and the Astonishing Rise of Mental Illness in America.* New York: Crown Publishers, 2010.

CONCLUSION

Health Is Your Birthright

I have certainly enjoyed sharing the journey with you of understanding how *your body can talk*. My sincere hope is that you feel empowered to navigate your own lifestyle and health care decisions. Teach your children and other important people in your life these same commonsense, natural health principles.

I hope that the allopathic, conventional medical method of chasing symptoms with toxic drugs is not the first path you will tread on your healing journey. Please use *Your Body Can Talk* as a reference guide for your daily health decisions, and be encouraged when you review the hundreds of natural options available to you as user-friendly first alternatives.

Vibrant health stems from a harmonious balance among structural, chemical and energetic components of your whole being. Your own body remains the ultimate source of information about your health. Clinical Kinesiology energetic testing has given you but a glimpse of how your body can talk. Your healing biocomputer constantly relays new information about your body's current state of function. **Are you listening?**

Remember, a natural solution exists for almost every health condition. Your lifestyle determines your quality of life. The robust state of health that you will enjoy for years to come depends upon your choices today.

As you learn to more completely accept full responsibility for your health, include into your lifestyle those healthy measures that strengthen and heal your organs. Keep your energetic system moving forward and fully realize the radiant and miraculous health that is your birthright.

> The next major advances in health of the American people will come from the assumption of individual responsibility for one's own health and a necessary change in lifestyle for the majority of Americans.
>
> —John H. Knowles, M.D.

PART V

ADDITIONAL RESOURCES

Afterword

ORGAN MEDITATION

It's wise to do something healthy for all of our organs every day. You may want to seek the assistance of a holistic practitioner for guidance. However, in addition, an effective daily practice may involve spending a few moments meditating and visualizing each of your organs or organ systems surrounded by strong energy, in perfect balance and happy.

You may choose to work on specific organs at specific times, especially if symptoms have manifested and you want to focus on an individual organ. Or, you may use the meditation to relax, rejuvenate and renew the energy of all your organs together.

Simply have a friend read these instructions while you lie quietly and relax. Or, use your own voice to record the instructions, preferably with some soft, soothing music playing nearby.

Preparation

Prepare yourself for the meditation by doing a few moments of soft, deep breathing. Breathe in through your nose, fill your lungs completely and breathe out through your mouth. As you breathe, gently stretch the muscles of your whole body, relax and be at peace.

You may also want to picture yourself in your favorite place. For example, see yourself in a green mountain meadow surrounded by wildflowers, the dramatic blue sky and puffy white clouds above. Or, imagine yourself on a sandy beach with the ocean waves lapping just inches away, a bit of sea spray sprinkling your body.

As you address each organ individually, visualize one harmonious symphony of organs and body parts interacting, being energized and helping you to be a more functional, healthy, happy, and whole human being. As you proceed, you may also want to characterize each organ with a particular color, or specific facial characteristics, smiles, or features of your favorite animal. Take as much or as little time as you need to fully recognize each organ during your meditation.

I offer this Organ Meditation as a lasting gift to help you become healthier in body, mind and spirit. I hope you will call on this Organ Meditation at any time or in any place to help yourself along your healing journey.

The Meditation

In the event that you are missing one or more of your body parts, acknowledge the loss calmly and quietly. However, do something extraordinary!

Visualize the organ or body part as being intact, healthy, and revived. Know that in your energy body, the energetic aspect of that organ is still alive!

Allow that missing organ to express itself through all your thoughts and meditations. Encourage the energy essence of that missing part to continue to play a role in the symphony of organs.

Begin your organ meditation with the pituitary gland, a small gland in the upper forehead. In your mind's eye, see it being enveloped in white light, radiating peace and well-balanced energy. Envision your pituitary as stable, strong, and functioning perfectly. Take several deep breaths as you focus on your pituitary and its role as a master gland in your healthy body.

After a minute or two, move your focus down midway between the eyebrows to the hypothalamus. Watch the hypothalamus, your wonderful air traffic controller, directing and regulating traffic, and helping your whole energetic system to function effortlessly. Allow all thoughts to surround your hypothalamus as you relax and release your healing energy upon it.

With a calm spirit, enter inside your mouth. Notice and acknowledge your tongue and vocal chords. Know that these organs are a part of your body's deepest expression. See them well balanced, fully functioning and connecting to the thyroid as you experience complete access to all your emotions. Relax and breathe deeply.

Using imagery to designate something gentle yet strong, explore the beautiful butterfly-shaped thyroid at your throat. This powerful gland rules over your metabolism and many other important functions. See it smiling and fluttering, working well, producing its hormones, connecting to the other glands and helping them to maintain correct balance. Notice your body giving complete trust to your organs as they heal and energize one another.

Slowly, move down and discover the trachea, bronchial tubes, and lungs. Notice this entire airway filled with light. Feel it breathing the essence of life in and out of your body. Quietly experience this entire area with no restriction—freely breathing and moving air and energy into your body. Float and relax.

Lovingly touch your heart with your thought and spirit. Picture it as a beautiful valentine full of love. See your heart energetically strong, complete and full. Envision all four chambers healthy and functioning correctly. Notice all the blood vessels clear and having sufficient room for the blood flow. Recognize and trust your heart as the seat of all your emotions, full of clarity and expression, whole and unbroken. Imagine that with your attention you can gently heal any tiny cracks, bruises, or hurts from past brokenness. With loving thoughts, polish your heart to a smooth, shiny new surface. Know that your heart is smiling and happy with expression and a renewed abundance of joy.

Slowly, let your awareness travel down and acknowledge your entire esophagus from your throat to your stomach. See its pathway as clear, open and functioning well. Notice your stomach being pleased with the healthy food it is given, enabling it to function and digest and work with that food to bring nutrients and energy to your entire body. Breathe deeply and give thanks.

Meditate quietly on your pancreas, hidden under the V of the ribcage. Allow that pancreas to be confident and full of self-esteem. See it faithfully working daily to keep your digestion functioning and blood sugar in balance. Envision it being vibrant, healthy and active throughout your entire lifetime. Crossover to the right of your body's midline and acknowledge your liver and gallbladder. See the red color of the liver and the green of the gallbladder. Notice them happy and smiling, unbound by anger and resentment.

Thank your liver and gallbladder for doing their hard, hard job of cleansing the blood, making and storing bile, helping with digestion and other functions. Recognize them working like clockwork together as you pamper your liver and gallbladder through healthy lifestyle choices.

Look to the left side of the lower ribcage and visualize your spleen pleasantly participating with all of the organs to keep your blood system pure and vibrant. See the spleen keeping quality control of the blood, keeping it circulating and healthy. Infuse your spleen with confidence, character and love as you continue to energize your body.

Let your imagination acknowledge the continuous flow from mouth to esophagus to the small intestine through the ileocecal valve to the large intestine. See this continuous digestive flow of energy and the breaking down of healthy, vibrant food into the building blocks of life. Envision that energizing vital force growing from the nutrients being absorbed from your system.

Say "yes" to your kidneys happy and smiling, gleefully filtering your blood, saving the good and reusable factors and pushing out the toxins, poisons and excess fluid. At rest, see your kidneys serene and calm in response to healthy liquids and nutrients, pleased to do their work and no longer holding onto fear. Envision your kidneys full of energy and light, moving your body forward.

All women affectionately perceive your uterus and ovaries. See these inner parts as the deepest essence of the woman. Marvel at the growth potential and nurturing aspect of these loving organs. See them contentedly participating in the whole body throughout all stages of your life. Notice the uterus in synchrony with all body rhythms. Listen and see the thyroid, uterus and ovaries communicating correctly with each other and maintaining every function in proper flow. Continue to breathe life-giving energy into your body.

All men, visualize your prostate and testicles. Contemplate your prostate being of correct size and texture. Mentally remove any aspect of inflammation or overgrowth. Envision your testicles as healthy and functioning optimally with proper hormone secretion. Know that this deepest reflection of your manhood is balanced, healthy, and whole.

Through your own meditation and visualization, create the completeness that allows all your body parts to work together. Once you've acknowledged all the organs and body parts, see your total self and acknowledge your entire being: body, mind, and spirit.

Relax, rejuvenate, energize. Most of all, enjoy being in the beautiful healthy body that you have helped create for yourself, now and for the rest of your life.

Appendix

ASSOCIATIONS and PROFESSIONALS

Susan L. Levy, D.C.
Advanced Health Systems / Natural Solutions
800-770-6704
YourBodyCanTalk@gmail.com
www.yourbodycantalk.com

Dr. Susan Levy is in private practice. Available for seminars, lectures, and consultation, she also provides information, health status evaluation, saliva hormone testing, referrals, and a mail order supplement service for patient needs and requests.

Refer to Dr. Levy's website, ***www.YourBodyCanTalk.com*** *for more information concerning how your body talks to you.*

• • •

Acufinder.com
909 North Sepulveda Boulevard, 11th Floor
El Segundo, CA 90245
760-630-3600
www.Acufinder.com

Nationwide acupuncturist referrals

• • •

The Alan G. Beardall Foundation
Christopher G. Beardall DC L.Ac.
1551 North Pacific Highway
Woodburn, OR 97071
503-982-6925
www.ClinicalKinesiology.com
beardall@hotmail.com

A research and scholarship organization designed to further the work of the late Alan G. Beardall, D.C. Provides information, web classes, teaching manuals, and books for professionals who wish to learn the Clinical Kinesiology technique.

• • •

American Association of Naturopathic Physicians
818 18th Street, NW, Suite 250
Washington, DC 20006
866-538-2267 (toll-free)
202-237-8150
www.naturopathic.org

Listing of nationwide naturopathic professionals, and newsletter

• • •

American Botanical Council
P.O. Box 144345
Austin, TX 78714
512-926-4900
512-926-2345 (fax)
www.herbalgram.org

Reliable herbal medicine information and ongoing journal publication

• • •

American Chiropractic Association
1701 Clarendon Boulevard, Suite 200
Arlington, VA 22209
703-276-8800
703-243-2593 (fax)
www.ACAtoday.org

Largest professional association in the United States representing Doctors of Chiropractic. National database of Chiropractors, seminars, training and information.

• • •

American Herbalists Guild
125 South Lexington Avenue
Suite 101
Asheville, NC 28801
617-520-4372
www.AmericanHerbalistsGuild.com

Reliable herbal medicine information and ongoing journal publication

• • •

Fereydoon Batmanghelidj, M.D.
P.O. Box 3189
Falls Church, VA 22043
703-848-2333
703-848-0028 (fax)
information@watercure.com
www.watercure.com

Dedicated to the mission of educating the public about the truth of dehydration so that we will not become unnecessarily over-drugged; promoting the public awareness of the healing powers of water so that we can become healers of our own bodies; transforming the expensive sick-care system so that we can have a more nature-friendly, people-friendly health care system.

• • •

Birthing The Future®, a 501c3 non-profit
Founder-Director, Suzanne Arms
P.O. Box 1040
Bayfield, CO 81122
970-884-4005
http://BirthingTheFuture.org

Offers a wide array of educational and inspirational media to transform how we bring humans into the world, support women, and prevent trauma in the "primal period." Films, books, brochures, pamphlets, bookmarks, cards and resources on pregnancy, support in labor, natural birthing (and vbac), breastfeeding, the mother-baby bond, and fathering. "Where the heart's knowing meets the edge of science and ancient wisdom guides us home. – Suzanne Arms

• • •

California College of Natural Medicine (CCONM)
Theresa Dale, Ph.D., C.C.N., N.D., N.P.
1237 S. Victoria Av. #169
Oxnard, CA 93035
800-421-5027
928-496-2050 (fax)
www.cconm.com

Developer of Neuro Emotional Remedies Training classes; information and clinic

• • •

The Gerson Institute
P.O. Box 161358
San Diego, CA 92176
888-443-7766
www.gerson.org

Alternative treatment for cancer and other chronic degenerative diseases; also, the Gerson Clinic in Mexico

• • •

Herb Research Foundation
5589 Arapahoe Ave, Suite 205
Boulder, CO 80303
303-449-2265
303-449-7849 (fax)
www.herbs.org

• • •

Hypnobirthing® Institute
110-2 Sheep Davis Rd.
Pembroke, NH 03275
603-856-8792 / 603-856-8341
603-856-8745 (fax)
www.hypnobirthing.com

The Mongan Method philosophy and technique aids birthing mothers in comfortable, stress-free, natural birthing.

• • •

ISMP: Institute for Safe Medication Practices
200 Lakeside Drive; Suite 200
Horsham, PA 19044-2321
215-947-7797
215-914-1492 (fax)
www.ismp.org

A nonprofit organization educating the Healthcare community and consumers about safe medication practices.

• • •

International Academy of Medical Acupuncture
John A. Amaro, D.C., L.Ac., FIAMA, Dipl. Ac.
P.O. Box 1003
Carefree, AZ 85377
800-327-1113
480-595-9881 (fax)
www.IAMA.edu

Academic programs and training seminars for professionals who wish to become certified in acupuncture.

• • •

International Association for Colon Hydrotherapy
P.O. Box 461285
San Antonio, TX 78246
210-366-2888
210-366-2999 (fax)
www.i-act.org

National referral of therapists, seminars, training and information

• • •

International Chiropractors Association
6400 Arlington Blvd, Suite 800
Falls Church, VA 22042
800-423-4690
703-528-5023 (fax)
www.Chiropractic.org

National database of Chiropractors, seminars, training and information

• • •

International Chiropractic Pediatric Association
610-565-2360
www.ICPA4kids.org

Member directory, wellness articles, pre- and post-natal care information

• • •

International College of Applied Kinesiology (ICAK)-U.S.A.
ICAK-USA Central Office
6405 Metcalf Ave., Suite 503
Shawnee Mission, KS 66202
913-384-5336
913-384-5112 (fax)
icak@dci-kansascity.com
www.icakusa.com

National referral for applied Kinesiologists, certification courses

• • •

International Institute for Building Biology® & Ecology (IBE)
P.O. Box 8520
Santa Fe, NM 87504
866-960-0333
www.BuildingBiology.net

Non-profit organization that informs and educates the general public about environmental concerns adversely impacting personal health. Seminars, lectures, professional certification classes, and information addressing toxic chemicals and EMF pollution.

• • •

International Institute of Reflexology Inc.
5650 First Avenue North
P.O. Box 12642
Saint Petersburg, FL 33733
727-343-4811
727-381-2807 (fax)
www.reflexology-usa.net

Information, worldwide certification training, publications, referrals

• • •

International Kinesiology College
+61 0478 244-744
www.ikc-info.org

• • •

Microwave News
Louis Slesin
155 East 77th Street, Suite 3D
New York, NY 10075
212-517-2800
212-734-0316 (fax)
www.MicrowaveNews.com

Online newsletter informing the public about the risks of EMFs

• • •

Nambudripad's Allergy Elimination Techniques
Devi S. Nambudripad, M.D. (WI), D.C., L.Ac., Ph.D. (Acu.)
6714 Beach Blvd
Buena Park, CA 90621
714-523-8900
www.NAET.com

Appointments or referrals for doctors using Nambudripad Allergy Elimination Technique, pain clinic, newsletter and books

• • •

National Center for Homeopathy
1760 Old Meadow Road, Suite 500
McLean VA, 22102
703-506-7667
703-506-3266 (fax)
www.homeopathic.org

Referrals of homeopathic health professionals

• • •

National Vaccine Information Center
21525 Ridgetop Circle, Suite 100
Sterling, VA 20166
703-938-0342
571-313-1268 (fax)
www.nvic.org

National non-profit educational center devoted to preventing vaccine injury and death. Information, and advocate line.

• • •

Simonton Cancer Center
PO Box 6607
Malibu, CA 90264
800-459-3424
818-879-7904
simontoncancercenter@msn.com
www.simontoncenter.com

Center for guided imagery healing, information and referrals

• • •

Suicide Prevention Lifeline
1-800-273-TALK (8255)
www.suicidepreventionlifeline.org

Staff is trained to listen and offer support to people in emotional crisis. if you are in immediate medical crisis, please call 911(U.S. only) or your country's emergency line.

• • •

Sweet Beginnings
5661 S. Curtice Street
Littleton, CO 80120
303-317-5795
720-283-6575
michelle@oursweetbeginnings.com
www.oursweetbeginnings.com

Premier pregnancy, breastfeeding support, parenting resource center and retail boutique catering to natural family living.

• • •

Touch for Health Kinesiology Association (TFHKA)
4917 Waters Edge Drive, Suite 125
Raleigh, NC 27606
919-637-4938
517-321-0495 (fax)
www.TouchForHealth.us

• • •

The Weston A. Price Foundation
PMB 106-380
4200 Wisconsin Avenue, NW
Washington, DC 20016
202-363-4394
202-363-4396 (fax)
info@westonaprice.org
www.westonaprice.org

A nonprofit organization founded in 1999 to disseminate the research of nutrition pioneer Dr. Weston Price, whose studies of isolated nonindustrialized peoples established the parameters of human health and determined the optimum characteristics of human diets.

• • •

The Yeast Connection
www.YeastConnection.com

Dr. William Crook was the author of 14 books and numerous articles on Candida Albicans. Refer to this website for more information.

PRODUCT RESOURCE GUIDE

<u>Amino Acids</u>
Jo-Mar Laboratories
583 Division Street Suite B
Campbell, CA 95008
800-538-4545
408-374-5922
www.JoMarLabs.com

Mail order distributor of amino acids to both professionals and the public

• • •

<u>Bach Original Flower Remedies</u>
Nelson's Natural World
21 High Street, Suite 302
North Andover, MA 01845
800-319-9151
978-988-0233 (fax)
www.BachRemedies.com
Main Website: *www.NelsonsNaturalWorld.net*
U.S. Bach International Education Program
– 800-334-0843

Supplier of Bach Flower Remedies, certification courses

• • •

Pegasus Products, Inc.
P.O. Box 228
Boulder, CO 80306
800-527-6104
www.PegasusProducts.com

Over 700 flower essences, gem elixirs, and information

• • •

Caprylic Acid
Nutri-West®
P.O. Box 950
2132 East Richard Street
Douglas, WY 82633
800-443-3333
www.nutriwest.com

Distributor of many high-quality professional nutrients including Exspore™, and Total Yeast Redux™, both containing caprilic acid

• • •

Citricidal
Nutribiotic
P.O. Box 238
Lakeport, CA 95453
800-225-4345
www.nutribiotic.com

Information, referrals, and high-quality products

• • •

Core-Level and Total Nutritional Supplements
Nutri-West®
P.O. Box 950
2132 East Richard Street
Douglas, WY 82633
800-443-3333
www.nutriwest.com

Distributor of Dr. Alan Beardall's Core-Level nutrients including Core-Level Heart™, Core-Level Thyro™, Core-Level Thymus™, Core-Level Kidney™, Core-Level D-Tox™, Core-Level Prostate™, and other Core-Level™ formulas.

Also distributes the Total Nutrient Line including Total Brain™, Total Green™, Total Liver D –Tox™, Total Yeast Redux™, and many others. Information and professional referrals available.

• • •

EMF Detection and Clearing Devices
Advanced Living Comfort
Kenneth Lesser, CEO
98 Wadsworth Boulevard, Ste. 127-120
Lakewood, CO 80226
303-284-8461
ComfortClock@AdvancedLiving.com
www.advancedliving.com/

Environmental Kinesiologist, consultant, and global distributor for EMF detecting devices and EMF-clearing devices (the Comfort Clocks and other personal protection items) that protect against electromagnetic radiation. Full product lines.

• • •

Herbal Remedies
Herb Pharm
P.O. Box 116
Williams, OR 97544
541-846-6262 (information)
800-348-4372 (orders)
800-545-7392 (fax)
www.herb-pharm.com

Distributor of organic and wild crafted herbal tinctures to healthcare professionals.

Provides retail sales to the public.

• • •

Magnesium (topical)
Pure Magnesium Flakes
Life-flo®
800-258-8337
care@life-flo.com
www.life-flo.com

Magnesium oil
Swanson Health Products
P.O.Box 2803
Fargo, ND 58103-2803
1-800-451-9304
800-254-1885 (Español)
800-726-7691 (fax)
customercare@swansonvitamins.com
www.swansonvitamins.com

• • •

Professional Botanicals
1069 South Stewart Drive, #2
Ogden, UT 84404
877-745-0850
www.ProfessionalBotanicals.com

Distributor of vitamins, herbs, and combinations to healthcare professionals. A select group of items are also available to the public.

• • •

Standard Process Inc.
1200 W. Royal Lee Drive
Palmyra, WI 53156
800-558-8740
800-438-3799 (fax)
www.StandardProcess.com

Medi-Herb is a comprehensive herbal division. Distributor of quality nutrients, formulations, and herbal remedies to professional health care providers for their patients.

∙∙∙

Homeopathic Remedies
Mountain States Health Products (MHP)
P.O. Box 1129
Lyons, CO 80540
800-647-0074
303-823-9359 (fax)
www.MHPvitamins.com

Distributor of quality nutrients and formulations to professional health care providers for their patients. Information and referrals, product sales exclusive to health care providers

∙∙∙

Natural Progesterone and Other Hormonal Support Items
Klabin Marketing
2067 Broadway, Suite 700
New York, NY 10023
800-933-9440
212-877-2513 (fax)
www.longevity-science.net

Distributors of natural progesterone, as well as a combination of pregnenolone, DHE, and progesterone.

∙∙∙

Mountain States Health Products (MHP)
P.O. Box 1129
Lyons, CO 80540
800-647-0074
303-823-9359 (fax)
www.MHPvitamins.com

Distributor of quality nutrients and formulations to professional health care providers for their patients. Topical progesterone is available, as well as homeopathic versions of progesterone, estrogen, testosterone, DHEA, cortisol, thyroid, and others. Information and referrals, product sales exclusive to health care providers for their patients.

∙∙∙

Nutri-West®
P.O. Box 950
2132 East Richard Street
Douglas, WY 82633
800-443-3333
www.nutriwest.com

Distributor of quality nutrients and formulations to professional health care providers.

Distributor of Dr. Alan Beardall's Core-Level nutrients including Core-Level Ovary™, Core-Level Uterus™, Core-Level Prostate™, and other Core-Level™ formulas. Also distributes many hormone and gland supporting products including Total Female™, Total Fem-Bal™, Total Tri-Estro™, Total Male™, Total Andro-Bal™, Total DHEA™, and Total Pregnenolone™. Information and professional referrals available.

∙∙∙

Neuro Emotional Remedies
Dr. Theresa Dale's Wellness Center
1237 S. Victoria Avenue #169
Oxnard, CA 93035
800-219-1261
www.WellnessCenter.net

Distributor of Dr. Theresa Dale's Neuro Emotional

∙∙∙

Professional Grade Nutritional Supplements
Mountain States Health Products (MHP)
P.O. Box 1129
Lyons, CO 80540
800-647-0074
303-823-9359 (fax)
www.MHPvitamins.com

Distributor of quality nutrients and formulations to professional health care providers for their patients. Information and referrals, product sales exclusive to health care providers.

∙∙∙

Nutri-West®
P.O. Box 950
2132 East Richard Street
Douglas, WY 82633
800-443-3333
www.nutriwest.com

Distributor of quality nutrients and formulations to professional health care providers for their patients. Product examples include Dr. Alan Beardall's Core-Level nutrients including Core-Level Thyro™, Core-Level Thymus™, Core-Level Kidney™, Core-Level D-Tox™, Core-Level Prostate™, and other Core-Level™ formulas Also distributes Nutri-West's Total Nutrient Line including Total Brain™, Total Green™, Total Liver D-Tox™, Total Yeast Redux™, and many others.

Information and professional referrals available.

∙∙∙

Standard Process Inc.
1200 W. Royal Lee Drive
Palmyra, WI 53156
800-558-8740
800-438-3799 (fax)
www.StandardProcess.com

Distributor of quality nutrients and formulations to professional health care providers for their patients.

• • •

OXY-OXC, OXY-MAG
Teamwork Concepts, Inc.
4460 Redwood Hwy #16C
San Rafael, CA 94903
www.oxyoxc.com

Distributor of OXY-OXC and OXY-MAG

• • •

High Vibe™
138 East 3rd Street
New York, NY 10009
888-554 6645
www.HighVibe.com

Distributor of OXY-OXC and OXY-MAG, Raw Foods, Supplements, Books and DVDs

• • •

XanGo (Mangosteen Juice)
XANGO, LLC
www.DrSusan.mymangosteen.com
FeelBetterAndBetter@yahoo.com

Dr. Levy is an authorized distributor of XanGo products including Juice and Skin Products.

• • •

<u>Salt</u>
Redmond Real Salt
475 West 910 South
Heber City, UT 84032
800-367-7258
realsalt.com

• • •

SaltWorks®
Himalayan Pink Salt
16240 Wood-Red Road NE
Woodinville, WA 98072
800-353-7258
www.saltworks.us

• • •

Selina Naturally
4 Celtic Drive
Arden, NC 28704
800-867-7258
www.CelticSeaSalt.com

Endnotes

CHAPTER 1
1. Beardall, Alan G., D.C. "Differentiating The Muscles of the Low Back and Abdomen," *Selected Papers of the International College of Applied Kinesiology.*" Lawrence, Kansas: International College of Applied Kinesiology, 1980.
2. Beardall, Alan G., D.C. *Clinical Kinesiology, Vols. I, II, III, IV, V.* Lake Oswego, Ore.: A.G. Beardall, D.C, Inc., 1980, 1981, 1982, 1983, 1985.
3. Bond, Jack, ed. "Clinical Kinesiology—A Personal Focus." *Clinical Kinesiology Organization for Research and Education.* Portland, Ore.: Human Bio-dynamics, Inc., 1993.

CHAPTER 2
1. Diamond, John, M.D. *Your Body Doesn't Lie.* New York: Warner Books, 1979, 27.
2. Matsumoto, Kiiko and Stephen Birch. *Five Elements & Ten Stems: Nan-Ching theory, diagnosis, and practice.* Brookline, Mass.: Paradigm Publications, 1989.

CHAPTER 3
1. Needham, Joseph. *Science and Civilisation in China. Volume 5: Chemistry and Chemical Technology, Part 3: Spagyrical Discovery and Invention: Historical Survey, from Cinnabar Elixirs to Synthetic Insulin.* New York: Cambridge University Press, 1976, 5.
2. Wang Shu He. *Commentary on the Nan Ching.* (Nan Ching, Classic of Difficulties.) Anon., circa 100 B.C-100 A.D., Second edition, 1970.
3. Matsumoto, Kiiko and Stephen Birch. Five *Elements & Ten Stems: Nan-Ching theory, diagnosis, and practice.* Brookline, Mass.: Paradigm Publications, 1989.
4. Dale, Theresa, N.D. *NERs* (Neuro Emotional Remedies). Douglas, Wyo.: Nutri-West® Publishers, 1992, 2.
5. King Solomon. Proverbs 18:21. *The Holy Bible: Old and New Testaments.* Wichita, Kansas: Heirloom Bible Publishers, Inc. 1964, 410.
6. Dale, 2.
7. Borysenko, Joan, Ph.D. *Fire in the Soul: A New Psychology of Spiritual Optimism.* New York: Warner Books, 1993.
8. Beardall, Alan G., D.C. *Clinical Kinesiology, Vols. I, II, III, IV, V.* Lake Oswego, Ore.: A.G. Beardall, D.C, Inc., 1980, 1981, 1982, 1983, 1985.
9. Justice, Blair, Ph.D. *Who Gets Sick.* Los Angeles, Calif.: Jeremy Tarcher, Inc., 1988.
10. Ibid., 30.
11. Cousins, Norman. *Anatomy of an Illness as Perceived by the Patient.* New York: Norton, 1979.
12. Cousins, Norman. *The Healing Heart.* New York: Norton, 1983.
13. Justice, 39.
14. Ornstein, Robert. *The Amazing Brain.* Boston: Houghton-Mifflin, 1984.

CHAPTER 4
1. Mann, John and Lar Short. *The Body of Light.* Boston: Charles E. Turtle Company, Inc., 1990, 31.
2. Leadbeater, C.W. *The Chakras.* Adyar, Madras, India: Theosophical Publishing House, 1927, 4.
3. Ibid., 5.
4. Idem.
5. Ibid., 12.
6. Mann and Short, 27, 28.
7. Leadbeater, 15.
8. Idem.

9. Bach, Edward. *Heal Thyself.* London: C.W Daniel Co. Ltd., 1931.
10. Bates, William H. *The Bates Method for Better Eyesight Without Glasses.* New York: H. Holt Co., 1943.
11. Leadbeater, 15.

CHAPTER 5

1. Murphy, Anne S. et al. "Kindergarten students' food preferences are not consistent with their knowledge of the dietary Guidelines." *Journal of the American Dietetic Association.* 95: no. 2, 1995, 219-223.
2. Bland, Jeffrey, Ph.D. "Managing Arthritis" Audiotape lecture of the KEEPING HEALTHY SERIES. Side 1, Gig Harbor, Wash.: HealthComm, Inc. 1986.
3. Null, Gary, Ph.D. *Gary Nulls Complete Guide to Healing Your Body Naturally.* New York: McGraw-Hill Book Company, 1988, p. 183.
4. Bowen, R. Colorado State University, "Lactose Intolerance (Lactase Non-Persistence)." Last modified April 25, 2009. Accessed February 6, 2014. *http://www.vivo.colostate.edu/hbooks/pathphys/digestion/smallgut/lactose_intol.html.*)
5. Sanchez, Albert, et al. "Role of sugars in human neutrophilic phagocytosis." *The American Journal of Clinical Nutrition*, 26: no. 11, 1180-1184.
6. Nambudripad, Devi S. *Say Goodbye To Illness.* Buena Park, CA: Delta Publishing, 1993.

CHAPTER 6

1. Justice, Blair, Ph.D. *Who Gets Sick.* Los Angeles, CA: Jeremy Tarcher, Inc., 1988, p. 154.
2. Geison, Gerald L. *The Private Science of Louis Pasteur.* Princeton, N.J.: Princeton University Press, 1995, 163; and from Pasteur, Louis. *Oeuvres VI,* 290-291. (Refer to the "Table chronique.")
3. Lanctot, Guylaine, M.D. *The Medical Mafia: How to Get Out of it Alive and Take Back our Health and Wealth.* Miami: Here's The Key, Inc., 1995, 123-130; and *What you NEED to know about immunizations (to protect your health and your rights!)* World Chiropractic Alliance pamphlet, 1995.
4. Moskowitz, Richard, M.D. "The Case Against Immunizations." *Journal of the American Institute of Homeopathy,* American Institute of Homeopathy, Washington, D.C: 1983, 15.
5. Ibid., 7.
6. Ibid., 7-25.
7. Coulter, Harris, M.D. *Vaccination, Social Violence and Criminality—The Medical Assault on the American Brain.* Berkeley, Calif.: North Atlantic Books, 1990.
8. Moskowitz, 7-25.
9. Lanctot.
10. Mendelsohn, Robert S., M.D. *Male Practice: How Doctors Manipulate Women.* Chicago: Contemporary Books, Inc., 1981, 84.
11. Rogers, Sherry A., M.D. *Tired or Toxic? A Blueprint for Health.* Syracuse, New York: Prestige Publishing, 1990, 359.
12. Geison.
13. Ibid., 128.

CHAPTER 7

1. Rasic, Jeremija Lj and Joseph A. Kurmenn. *Bifidobacteria and Their Role.* Boston, Mass.: Birkhauser Verlag, 1983, 22.
2. Hentges, D.J. "Does diet influence human fecal microflora composition?" *Nutrition Review* 38: 329-337; and Jawetz, E., J.L. Melnick and E.A. Adelberg. *Review of Medical Microbiology* 13th edition, Los Altos, Calif.: LANGE Medical Publications, 1978.
3. Mintz, Morton. *The Therapeutic Nightmare.* Boston: Houghton-Mifflin, 1965.
4. Bland, Jeffrey, Ph.D. *New Clinical Breakthroughs in the Management of Chronic Fatigue Syndrome, Intestinal Dysbiosis, Immune Dysregulation and Cellular Toxicity.* Gig Harbor, Washington: Health Comm, Inc., 1992, 33.
5. International Dairy Food Association, "Pasteurization: Definition and Methods." Last modified June 2009. Accessed February 4, 2014. *http://www.idfa.org/files/249_Pasteurization Definition and Methods.pdf.*

CHAPTER 8

1. Sampaolo, Marco, ed. Encyclopædia Britannica. Encyclopædia Britannica Inc., 2014. s.v. "Human Digestive System." *http://www.britannica.com/EBchecked/topic/1081754/human-digestive-system/242920/Absorption* (accessed February 6, 2014).
2. Yamaguchi, Eri. *The Well Flavored Vegetable: Novel and Traditional Vegetable Recipes from Japan.* New York: Kodansha International, 1988.
3. Kapil, Vikas, Syed M.A. Haydar, Vanessa Pearl, Jon O. Lundberg, Eddie Weitzberg, and Amrita Ahluwalia. "Physiological role for nitrate-reducing oral bacteria in blood pressure control." *Free Radical Biology and Medicine.* no. February (2013): 93-100. *http://www.sciencedirect.com/science/article/pii/S0891584912018229* (accessed March 2, 2014).

CHAPTER 9

1. Becker, Robert O., M.D. *Cross Currents: The Perils of Electropollution, The Promise of Electromedicine.* Los Angeles: Jeremy P. Tarcher, Inc., 1990, 69.
2. Havas, Magda. *Biological Effects of Low Frequency Electric and Magnetic Fields.* Derek Clements-Croome (Ed.). Electromagnetism and Health, London: Taylor & Francis Books, Ltd., 2004, 207-231.
3. Ibid., 216.
4. Pelletier, Kenneth. *Longevity: Fulfilling Our Biological Potential.* New York: Delacorte Press, 1981, 161.
5. Gittleman, Ann Louise. *Zapped: Why Your Cell Phone Shouldn't Be Your Alarm Clock and 1,268 Ways to Outsmart the Hazards of Electronic Pollution.* New York: HarperCollins, 2010, 29.
6. Becker, 92.
7. Ibid., 108.
8. "Can Technology make Us Ill?" *Natural Life* (Jan, 2008): 7-9. http://search.proquest.com/docview/212913981?accountid=39001
9. Becker, 187.
10. Ibid.
11. Brodeur, Paul. *The Great Power-Line Cover-Up: How the Utilities and the Government Are Trying to Hide the Cancer Hazards Posed by Electromagnetic Fields.* New York: Little, Brown and Company, 1993.
12. Pinsky, Mark A. *The EMF Book.* New York: Warner Books, 1995, 121.
13. Slesin, Louis, "Ed. Draft NCRP Report Seeks Strong Action to Curb EMFs." *Microwave News*, Vol. XV, No. 4, July/August, 1995, 1.
14. The National Council on Radiation Protection and Measurements (NCRP). Section 8 of the "Report of NCRP Scientific Committee 89-3 on Extremely Low Frequency Electric and Magnetic Fields." United States Congress. Reprinted in *Microwave News*, Vol. XV, No. 4, July/August, 1995, 12-15.
15. NV Energy, a subsidiary of MidAmerican Energy Holdings Company, "Understanding EMF." Last modified 2014. Accessed March 26, 2014. https://www.nvenergy.com/home/safety/understandingEMF.cfm.
16. Wertheimer, Nancy and Edward Leeper. "Electric Wiring Configurations and Childhood Cancer." *American Journal of Epidemiology*, 109: 273-284.
17. Savitz, D.A., H. Wachtel, F. A. Barnes, et al. "Case Control Study of Childhood Cancer and Exposure to 60-Hz Magnetic Fields." *American Journal of Epidemiology*, 128: 21-38.
18. Ahlbom, Anders and Maria Feychting. "Magnetic Fields and Cancer in Children Residing Near Swedish High Voltage Power Lines." *American Journal of Epidemiology*, 138: no. 7: 467-481.
19. Wertheimer, Nancy and Edward Leeper. "Possible Effects of Electric Blankets and Heated Waterbeds on Fetal Development." *Bioelectromagnetics*, 7: 13-22.
20. Associated Press wire report, June 15, 1994, and National Institute of Environmental Health Sciences and U.S. Dept. of Energy (DOE/EE-0040), "Questions and Answers About E.M.F. Electric and Magnetic Fields Associated With the Use of Electric Power." January, 1995, 20.
21. Sobel, Eugene, Zoreh Davanipour and Lee Pey-Jiuan. "Occupations with Exposure to Electromagnetic Fields: A Possible Risk Factor for Alzheimer's Disease." *American Journal of Epidemiology*, 142: no 5, 515.
22. M. Riversong, personal communications, 1992-2014.
23. Ibid.
24. Becker, Robert O., M.D. and Gary Seldon. *The Body Electric: Electromagnetism and the Foundation of Life.* New York: William Morrow and Company, Inc., 1985, 316.
25. Ibid.
26. National Institute of Environmental Health Sciences and U.S. Dept. of Energy (DOE/EE-0400), "Questions and Answers About Electric and Magnetic Fields Associated With the Use of Electric Power." January, 1995.
27. Wertheimer and Leeper.
28. National Institute of Environmental Health Sciences.
29. Becker, *Cross Currents*, 249.
30. Ibid, 248-266.
31. K. Lesser, personal communications, 1992-2014.

CHAPTER 10

1. Gazella, Karolyn A., Ed., *Health Counselor.* Green Bay: IMPART Communications, Inc. 7: No. 6, December/January, 1996, 7.
2. Lark, Susan, M.D., *PMS: Self-Help Book: A Woman's Guide.* Berkeley, Calif.: Celestial Arts, 1984.
3. Wigmore, Ann. *The Wheatgrass Book.* Garden City Park, N.Y.: Avery Publishing, 1985.
4. Fuhrman, Joel, M.D. *Fasting and Eating for Health: A Medical Doctor's Program for Conquering Disease.* New York: St. Martin's Press, 1995, 1.

CHAPTER 11

1. Rodale, J.I. *The Healthy Hunzas.* Emmaus, Penn.: Rodale Press, 1948.

CHAPTER 12

1. Airola, Paavo, M.D. *Stop Hair Loss.* (Revised Edition) Sherwood, Ore.: Health Plus Publishers, 1994.
2. Covey, Stephen R. *The 7 Habits of Highly Effective People.* New York: Fireside, 1989.
3. Quillin, Patrick, Ph.D., R.D. *The Wisdom of Amish Folk Medicine.* North Canton, Ohio: The Leader Co, Inc., 1993.
4. Kulvinskas, Viktoras. *Survival into the 21st Century.* Fairfield, Iowa: Omangod Press, 1975.
5. Aesoph, Lauri M., N.D. "Coping With Male Infertility." *Delicious!*, September, 1995, 50.
6. Green, James. *The Male Herbal.* Freedom, Calif.: The Crossing Press, 1991.
7. Gerson, Max, M.D. *A Cancer Therapy: Results of Fifty Cases.* 5th edition. Bonita, Calif.: Gerson Institute, 1990.
8. Green, 15.
9. Available at: *http://www.cdc.gov/uscs*
10. Fink, John M. *Third Opinion.* Garden City Park, N.Y.: Avery Publishing, 1992.

CHAPTER 13

1. Waddington, C.H. *An Introduction to Modern Genetics.* New York: Macmillan, 1939.
2. Aamodt, Sandra and Sam Wang. *Welcome to Your Child's Brain: How the Mind Grows from Conception to College.* New York: Bloomsbury, 2011, 268.
3. Heller, H. Craig. Orians, Gordon H., Purves, William K. & Sadava, David. *Life: The Science of Biology, 6th Ed.* Sinauer & Freeman, 2000, 171.
4. Asprey, David and Lana Asprey. *The Better Baby Book: How to Have a Healthier, Smarter, Happier Baby.* Hoboken, New Jersey: John Wiley & Sons, 2013, 181-182.
5. Krapp, Kristine & Wilson, Jeffrey (Eds.). *The Gale Encyclopedia of Children's Health Vol. 1.* New York: Gale, 2005, 92-94.
6. Levine, Peter A., Ph.D and Maggie Kline. *Trauma Through a Child's Eyes: Awakening the Ordinary Miracle of Healing.* Berkeley, Calif.: North Atlantic and ERGOS, 2007, 298.
7. Berman, Jessica. (September 20, 2013). *Voice of America.* "Study: Pregnant Women Who Smoke Predispose Great-Grandchildren to Asthma." *http://www.voanews.comlcontentlstudy-shows-pregnant-women-who-smoke-predispose-grandchildren-to-asthma* H 754238.html
8. *Voice of America* (May 6, 2005). "Grandmothers' Smoking Linked to Grandchildren's Asthma Decades Later." Science Daily. *http://www.sciencedaily.conl/releases/2005/05/050505224059.htm*
9. Ibid.
10. h*ttp://www.usda.gov/factbook/chapter2.pdf*
11. Jensen, Robert G. *Handbook of Milk Composition.* San Diego, Calif.: Academic, 1995.
12. Robert D. Bremel's course notes and information from *The Handbook of Milk Composition*, (see note above) edited by Robert G. Jensen, were relied upon to produce a comprehensive chart depicting numerous constituents of mammalian milks. This work addressed 31 species. For the purposes of this book, I have modified Mr. Bremel's and Mr. Jensen's work. This abbreviated and modified version of Robert Bremel's chart is based on data from the handbook on milk consumption. His original chart addresses the first six columns. The remaining columns were added to promote though and discussion about appropriate duration of nursing in relationship to growth and maturation patterns.
13. Adams, Case, Ph.D. *Increased Intestinal Permeability aka Leaky Gut Syndrome: The Science of Achieving Digestive Health.* Wilmington, Delaware: Logical Books, 2012.
14. Kemsley, Jyllian. "Breast Milk Science: Toward Preemie Probiotics." *Chemical & Engineering News.* no. 27 (2013): 28-29. *http://cen.acs.org/articles/91/i27/Breast-Milk-Science-Toward-* Preemie.html (accessed February 15, 2014).
15. Siggers, Jayda, Mette V. Ostergaard, Richard H. Siggers, Kerstin Skovgaard, Lars Molbak, Thomas Thymann, Mette Schmidt, Hanne K. Moller, Stig Purup, Lisbeth N. Fink, Hanne Fokiaer, Mette Boye, Per T. Sangild, and Stine B. Bering. "Postnatal amniotic fluid intake reduces gut inflammatory responses and necrotizing enterocolitis in preterm neonates." *American Journal of Physiology Gastrointestinal and Liver Physiology.* no. G864-G875 (2013). *http://ajpgi.physiology.org/content/304/10/G864* (accessed February 15, 2014).

16. Thomas, Jenny, M.D., M.P.H., IBCLC, FAAP, FABM. *Dr. Jen 4 Kids*, "The Normal Newborn and Why Breastmilk is Not Just Food." Accessed March 2, 2014. *http://www.drjen4kids.com/*.

17. Cabrera-Rubio, Raul, M. Carmen Collado, Kirsi Laitenen, Seppo Salminen, Erika Isolauri, and Alex Mira. "The Human Milk Microbiome Changes Over Lactation and is Shaped by Maternal Weight and Mode of Delivery." *The American Journal of Clinical Nutrition.* no. 3 (2012): 544-551. *http://ajcn.nutrition.org/content/96/3/544.full.pdf html* (accessed February 15, 2014).

18. Nordqvist, Joseph. "Bacteria In Breast Milk Identified." *Medical News Today*. MediLexicon, Intl., (2013). <*http://www.medicalnewstoday.com/articles/254758*> (accessed February 15, 2014).

19. Queen Mary University of London. "Magic Ingredient In Breast Milk Protects Babies' Intestines." *ScienceDaily*. www.sciencedaily.com/releases/2009/06/090629200754.htm (accessed February 15, 2014).

20. Abrams, Barbra, et al. *Nutrition During Lactation*. Washington, D.C.: National Academy, 1991, 244-278.

21. Arms, Suzanne and Chloe Fisher. *Bestfeeding: How to Breastfeed Your Baby*. New York: Random House, 2004. 45.

22. Ibid.

23. Joshi, J.V., S.D. Bhandarkar, M. Chadha, D. Balaiah, and R. Shah. "Menstrual irregularities and lactation failure may precede thyroid dysfunction or goiter." *J Postgrad Med* [serial online] 1993 [cited 2013 Nov 5]; 39:137. Available from: *http://www.jpgmonline.com/text.asp?1993/39/3/137/614*

24. Huggins, Kathleen, R.N. M.S. *The Nursing Mothers Companion 5th Edition*. Boston: Harvard Common Press: 2005, 78-79.

25. Smith, Ed. *Therapeutic Herb Manual: A guide to the Safe and Effective Use of Liquid Herbal Extracts*. Oregon: Ed Smith, 2008, 114.

26. Weston A. Price Foundation. *Formula-Homemade Baby Formula*. December 31, 2001. *http://www.westonaprice.org/childrens-health/recipes-for-homemade-baby-formula*

27. Original source: *Nourishing Traditions The Cookbook that Challenges Politically Correct Nutrition and the Diet Dictocrats;* by Sally Fallon with Mary G. Enig, Ph.D. *Revised Second Ed.* Washington, DC: New Trends Publishing Inc., 2000. This recipe was posted at: *http://www.westonaprice.org/childrens-health/recipes-for-homemade-baby-formula*

28. Ibid.

29. Huggins.

30. Pitman, Teresa, Diana West and Diane Wiessinger. *The Womanly Art of Breastfeeding*. New York: Ballantine Books: 2010.

31. Carruth, B.R., P.J. Ziegler, A. Gordon, and S.I. Barr, (2004). "Prevalence of picky eaters among infants and toddlers and their caregivers' decisions about offering a new food. *Journal of the Academy of Nutrition and Dietetics,* 104, S57-S64.

32. Pero R. "Medical Researcher Excited by CBS=RF Project Results." *The Chiropractic Journal*, August 1989, 32.

33. Brennan, P., M. Graham, J. Triano, and M. Hondras. "Enhanced phagocytic cell respiratory bursts induced by spinal manipulation: Potential Role of Substance P." *J Manip Physiolog Ther* 1991; (14)7:399-400.

34. Elenkov, I.J., R.L. Wilder, G.P. Chrousos, and E.S. Vizi: "The sympathetic nerve—an integrative interface between the two supersystems: the brain and the immune system." *Pharmacol Rev* 2000;5 2:295-63.

35. Levine and Kline, 4.

36. Ullman, Dana, M.P.H. *Homeopathic Medicine for Children and Infants*. New York: Tarcher, 1992, 105.

CHAPTER 14

1. Gold, Robert Steven. *Are Your Meds Making You Sick?: A Pharmacist's Guide to Avoiding Dangerous Drug Interactions, Reactions and Side-Effects*. Alameda, Calif.: Hunter House, 2011, 126.

2. American Pharmacists Association | Improving medication use. Advancing patient care. Accessed March 24, 2014. *http://www.pharmacist.com/sites/default/files/Great_Moments_in_Pharmacy_Article.pdf.*

3. Angell, Marcia. *The Truth About the Drug Companies: How They Deceive Us and What to Do About It.* New York: Random House, 2004, 17.

4. Elliot, Carl. *White Coat Black Hat: Adventures on the Dark Side of Medicine*. Boston: Beacon, 2010, 3.

5. Angell, 16-17.

6. Bartholow, Michael. "Top 200 Drugs of 2011." *Pharmacology Times*. July 10, 2012. Acessed April 4, 2013. *http://www.pharmacytimes.com/publications/issue/2012/July2012/Top-200-Drugs-of-2011.*

7. Haley, Boyd. "The Relationship of Toxic Effects of Mercury to Exacerbation of the Medical Condition Classified as Alzheimer's Disease." *Medical Veritas* 4, (2007): 1484-1498.

8. Schmidt, Michael A., Lendon H. Smith, and Keith W. Sehnert. *Beyond Antibiotics: Healthier Options for Families.* Berkeley, Calif.: North Atlantic, 1993. 47.
9. Perdomo, Daniela. "100,000 Americans Die Each Year from Prescription Drugs, While Pharma Companies Get Rich." *Alter.net*. June 24, 2010. Accessed June 30, 2013. *http://www.alternet.org/story/147318/100,000_americans_die_each_year_from_prescription_drugs,_while_pharma_companies_get_rich.*
10. Roberts, Barbara. *The Truth about Statins: Risks and Alternatives to Cholesterol-Lowering Drugs.* New York: Pocket Books, 2012. 195.
11. Enig, Mary and Sally Fallon. *Eat Fat, Lose Fat: The Healthy Alternative to Trans Fats.* New York: Hudson Street, 2005.
12. Price, Weston A. *Nutrition and Physical Degeneration: A Comparison of Primitive and Modern Diets and Their Effects, 8th Ed.* Washington, DC: Price Pottenger Nutrition, January, 31, 2008.
13. Cholesterol Treatment: A Review of the Clinical Trials Evidence. *U.S. Government Accountability Office.* 1996.
14. Price, Weston A. *Nutrition and Physical Degeneration: A Comparison of Primitive and Modern Diets and Their Effects, 8th Ed.* Washington, DC: Price Pottenger Nutrition, January, 31 2008.
15. Breggin, Peter. *The Antidepressant Fact Book.* Cambridge, Mass: Da Capo, 2001, 25-26.
16. Lambert, Kelly. *Lifting Depression.* Philadelphia, Penn.: Basic, 2008, 7.
17. Tracy, Ann Blake. *Prozac: Panacea or Pandora 2nd Ed.* West Jordan, Utah: Cassia, 1994. Back cover.
18. Breggin, 181.
19. Penckofer, Sue, Kouba, Joanne, Byrne, Mary, Estwing Ferrans, Carol. "Vitamin D and Depression: where is all the Sunshine". *Mental Health Nursing.* 31 (2010):385-393.
20. Cohen, Suzy. *Diabetes Without Drugs: The 5-Step Program to Control Blood Sugar Naturally and Prevent Diabetes Complications.* Emmaus, Penn : Rodale Books, 70.
21. Balch, James F., Mark Stengler, and Robin Young-Balch. *Prescription for Drug Alternatives: All-Natural Options for Better Health without the Side Effects.* Hoboken, New Jersey: Wiley & Sons, 2008, 46.
22. Cohen, 70.
23. Ibid., 2-3.

Index

A
Abrasions, 259
Acidophilus, 125, 128, 150
Acid Reflux (*See* Indigestion)
Acne, 127, 138, 146, 193, 228, 259
Acupressure, 46-47, 52, 53, 46, 231
Acupuncture, 4, 17, 24, 27, 45-48, 165, 207, 212
    and Alarm point, 48-52
    and Allergies, 108
    and Ch'i, 24-26
    and Bedwetting, 218
    and Hemorrhoids, 223
    and Kinesiology, 4-6, 10, 18, 24-25, 45
    and Lupus, 140
    and Meridians, 208 (Also see individual meridians)
    and Ryodoraku, 26-27
    and Scars, 42-44, 226
Addiction, 94 (*Also see* Food; Alcohol)
Additives (*See* Diet)
AIDS, 113, 129, 150, 174
Alcohol, 106, 131, 138, 150-153, 192, 222, 229-230
Allergies, 35, 95, 99, 108, 170, 174, 218 (*Also see* Food allergies)
    and Children, 255-257, 266
Aloe vera, 157, 222-223
Alzheimer's disease, 168-169, 174, 284
Amalgam, 284 (*Also see* Mercury amalgams)
Amaro, John, 26-27, 49
American Academy of Pediatrics, 256
Amino acids, 9, 66-67, 188, 192, 209-210, 218, 222, 224
Amniocentesis, 241
Amniotic fluid, 241, 248-249
Anger, 59-62, 70, 78, 174
Anorexia, 94
Antibiotics, 104, 116-117, 229, 284-285, 294-297
    and Candida, 125-128, 136, 138
    and Culture and susceptibility test, 160
    and Leaky gut syndrome, 149, 151, 159
Anxiety, 67-67, 82, 127, 146
    and EMF, 174
    and Men, 221, 227
    and PMS, 187-188, 192, 196
APGAR score, 236
Appendicitis, 37
Applied Kinesiology, 4-5, 233
Arms, Suzanne, 257-258
Arteriosclerosis, 41-42, 298-301 (*Also see* Heart)
Arthritis, 45, 99-100, 284, 322-326 (*Also see* Inflammation; Rheumatoid arthritis)
Asthma, 20, 30, 61, 128, 146, 151, 255, 266
    and Smoking, 243-244
Attention Deficit Hyperactivity Disorder (ADHD), 216-217
Autoimmune diseases, 61, 113, 118, 129, 137, 146, 151 (*Also see* AIDS; Chronic fatigue syndrome; Lupus; Multiple sclerosis; Rheumatoid arthritis; Scleroderma)

B
B Vitamins, 21-22, 121, 125, 135, 188, 307
    B_3 (Niacin), 66, 218
    B_5 (Pantothenic acid), 135, 158
    B_6, 66, 188, 191
    B_9 (Folic acid), 66, 158
    B_{12}, 256
    B-complex, 67, 188, 210, 218, 223, 230, 306
Bach flower remedies, 81-82, 86-88
Bacteria, 105, 113-115, 118, 122, 125, 159, 222, 229
Bacterial flora, 146, 159, 223 (*Also see* Probiotics)
Bates method, 84
Beardall, Alan, 4, 14, 115, 165, 210
    and Acupuncture, 24
    and Chakras, 81
    and Clinical kinesiology, 5-6
    and Five element theory, 54
    and Handmodes, 12, 64, 86
Beardall, Christopher, 10
Bedwetting, 99-100, 215, 218
Bile, 145, 149
Biofeedback, 65
Biotin, 221
Birth control 202, 204 (*Also see* Vasectomy)
Birth plan, 236-237
Bladder, 21, 62, 206, 218, 228, 231
    and Alarm point test, 50
    and Emotions, 62, 70
    and Energy, 38
    and Imbalance, 38
    and Infections, 38, 127
    and Meridian, 37-38, 218
Bland, Jeffrey, 100, 125, 129, 137
Bloating, 99, 127, 138, 146, 187, 196, 223
Block Buster drug, 281, 299
Blood, 34, 50, 61, 65, 94, 100, 102, 114-116, 184, 189-190, 204 (*Also see* Red blood cells; White blood cells)
Blood clots, 327-331
Blood sugar, 133, 185, 188-189, 304-307, 310-314, 310-314 (*Also see* Red blood cells; Sugar; White blood cells)
Blood pressure, 315-321
Bovine growth formula, 187
Brain, 5-6, 66, 116, 146, 169, 183, 188, 211
    and Amino acids, 66
    and Brain waves, 65
    and Cancer, 168
    and Circulation/ sex meridian, 41
    and Emotions, 65-66
    and Hypothalamus, 41
    and Imbalances, 17, 41, 188, 217
    and Injury, 119
    and Tumors, 164
Breast cancer, 164, 168, 204, 250
Breast milk, 59, 102, 187, 245-273
Breast feeding, 246, 248-252, 256-259, 262, 268
Brow chakra, 78-79, 81, 87
Brown rice water, 270
Brush border, 149

C
Caffeine, 104-105, 190-191, 218, 223, 229-230
Calcium, 150, 189, 209, 218, 230, 248
Cancer, 98, 103, 113, 128, 137, 150, 167, 202, 205 (*Also see* Breast cancer; Prostate cancer)
    and Children, 168, 255
    and Clinical kinesiology, 4
    and EMF, 163-164, 167, 172, 174
    and Men, 215, 221, 226, 229-230
    and the Simonton Cancer Center, 65
    and Women, 168, 203-204
Candida, 124-141, 146, 150-151
    and Handmode test, 139-140
    and Questionnaire, 135
Carpal tunnel syndrome, 8, 35
Cardio pulmonary resuscitation (CPR), 8
Cardiovascular disease, 204, 215, 221
Cells, 165, 169, 191 (*Also see* Red blood cells; T-cells; White blood cells)
    and Superoxide dismutase, 43
    and Spleen, 61
    and the Triple warmer meridian, 42
Central nervous system (*See* Nervous system)
Chakras, 73-74, 76, 77-79 (*Also see individual chakras*)
    and Bach Remedies, 82, 87
    and Colors, 84
    and Divine energy, 73, 76
    and Imbalances, 73-74, 81, 85-86
    and Kundalini energy, 76
Chemotherapy, 128, 149
Ch'i, 24-26, 45-46, 56
Chicken pox, 259-260, 267
Children, 236-274
    and ADHD, 216-217
    and Bedwetting, 218-219
    and Cancer, 164, 166
    and Diet, 94, 96-98, 106
    and EMF, 164, 166, 170, 176
    and Fetal alcohol syndrome, 106
    and Immune system, 113, 117, 121
    and Immunizations, 117-120
Chinese Five Element Theory, 54-57, 63, 74, 225
Chlorophyll, 158, 189-190, 223
Cholesterol, 255, 298-299

Choline, 67, 192
Chromium, 188-189
Chronic fatigue syndrome, 42, 141, 146
Circulation/sex or pericardium meridian, 40-42, 223, 225
Circumcision, 216, 258
Clinical Kinesiology, 3-6, 9-11, 19, 22, 32, 67, 86 (*Also see* Alan Beardall; Muscle testing)
    and Acupuncture, 24-25, 27, 45, 47-49, 165
    and Bach flower remedies, 82-83
    and Candida, 130-131, 140
    and Chakras, 74, 81-84,
    and EMF, 165, 170, 176-177
    and Emotions, 54, 56, 59, 64, 68, 71
    and Food sensitivities, 88
    and Homeopathy, 56
    and Hypothalamus, 232
    and Leaky gut syndrome, 152-153
    and Menopause, 211-213
    and PMS, 192, 195, 197
    and Prostate, 231
    and Psychological kinesiology, 10
Colds and flu, 35, 42, 61, 81, 116, 146, 259, 267-268
Cold sores, 259
Colic, 268
Colitis, 30, 129, 146, 151
Colon, 99, 137, 147
Colostrum, 158, 249-250, 254, 258-259
Concussion, 264
Conjunctivitis, 259, 269, 271
Constipation, 30-31, 35, 99, 127, 138, 146, 223, 228
Copper, 115, 121-122, 135, 150, 230
Corn, 97-98, 103
Coronary artery disease, 255, 327-331
Cough, 259
Crohn's disease, 36, 129, 146, 151, 255
Crook, William G., 127, 132, 137
Croup, 269
Crown chakra, 79
Cystic fibrosis, 146

D

Dairy, 101, 128, 132-133, 187, 190, 218
Dale, Theresa, 54, 56, 64, 68
Deep vein thrombosis (DVT), 327
Deoxyribonucleic acid (DNA), 118, 238-240, 243-244
Depression, 115, 303-309, 332, 337-339
    and Amino acids, 66
    and Candida, 127, 130, 138
    and Circulation/sex meridian, 41, 47
    and EMF, 174
    and Leaky gut syndrome, 143, 146
    and Men, 221, 227, 232
    and PMS, 185, 187, 191-192, 195-196, 203, 211
Dermatitis, 45, 146, 193 (*Also see* Eczema)
Desmosomes, 148-149
Detoxification, 3, 193-194, 210, 226-227
Diabetes, 22, 64, 146, 151, 174, 215, 218, 227, 255, 310-314
Diaper rash, 259
Diarrhea, 30, 35, 105, 195, 223, 255, 270
Diet, 9, 66, 88, 148 (*Also see* Food sensitivities)
    and Additives, 102, 104-105, 114, 116, 217-218
    and Candida, 124-125, 127, 131-133
    and Energetic compatibility, 93, 95-96
    and Energetic incompatibility, 93-111
    and Fats, 209
    and Food addiction, 105-106
    and Gallbladder, 44
    and Leaky gut syndrome, 153-157
    and Liver, 21
    and Milk based foods, 154
    and Microwave use, 109
    and Pancreas, 22
    and Prebiotics, 156-157
    and Preservatives, 102, 105, 114, 116, 217-218
    and Red meat, 106
    and Small intestine, 37
    and Sugar, 127, 131-133, 138, 141, 152, 284, 298, 306 (*Also see* Blood sugar)
Digestion, 42, 99-101, 132-133, 135, 151, 209, 217, 221-223, 233 (*Also see* Indigestion)
Digestive enzymes, 97, 100-101, 132-133, 147, 149-150, 154, 158, 165, 223, 233
Digestive system, 35, 40, 144-149, 153
Diphtheria-pertussis (DPT), 119
Diuretics, 191
Divine energy (*See* Chakras)
Dizziness, 59

E

Ear ache, 271
Ear infection, 99, 102, 127, 255, 259
Earth element, 60
Eczema, 45, 146, 255, 259
Eggs, 97, 104, 128, 133, 187
Electromagnetic body, 163-165, 169
Electromagnetic clearing device, 162-163, 176-177
Electromagnetic frequency (EMF), 85, 162-175, 242
Electromagnetic imbalance, 14, 22, 24, 47-48
Electromagnetic pollution, 85, 95
Electromagnetics, 9-10, 13-14, 17, 25, 56
    and Laser therapy, 47
    and Ryodoraku, 26-27
Enemas, 137
Emotions, 10, 14, 54-57, 63-67, 74, 80-81, 94-96, 104, 115 (*Also see* Neuro-emotional remedies)
    and Amino acids, 66
    and Chinese five element theory, 57, 63
    and Depression, 41-42, 66, 115
    and Disease, 56
    and Imbalances, 54, 57, 63, 68, 71, 73, 81, 86
    and Meditation, 58, 79
    and Organs, 56, 68
Energy, 3-17, 22, 25-29, 47, 49-52, 54-58, 67, 71, 83-84 (*Also see* Ch'i)
Environmental pollution, 21, 98, 116
Environmental toxins, 143, 145, 150
Enzymes (*See* Digestive enzymes)
Epigenetics, 98, 238-239
Espy, Burt, 7, 33, 39, 61, 115, 119, 122, 130, 140, 242
Essential fatty acids, 135-136, 157-158, 191, 209, 230
Estrogen, 128, 183, 185-186, 191, 202, 204-205, 210-211 (*Also see* Hormones)
Eye disorders, 95, 99
Eyes, 42, 45 (*Also see* Third eye)

F

False negative, 241
False positive, 241
Fasting, 79, 94, 193-194
Fats, 21, 44, 209
Fatigue, 138, 141, 151 (*Also see* Chronic fatigue syndrome)
Fear, 57, 62, 66, 70, 77-78, 80-82, 188, 191, 234
Fermented foods, 132, 153, 156
Fetal alcohol syndrome, 106
Fever blisters, 259
Fiber, 157-158
Fibromyalgia, 146
Finger mode, 130, 140, 152
Fire element, 56, 59-60, 74, 78, 225
Flatulence, 146
Flower remedies (*See* Bach flower remedies)
Folic acid (B9) (*See* B vitamins)
Food, 32 (*Also see* Diet)
Food allergies, 95, 98-110, 127-128, 132, 136, 141, 145-146, 149-151, 218
    and children, 255-257, 266
Food and Drug Administration (FDA), 280-281, 305-306
Food sensitivity, 96, 101, 104, 106-107, 109, 190, 217, 218
    and Candida, 127-128, 131-132
    and Leaky gut syndrome, 146, 149-151, 154
Formula, 245-246, 249-251, 253-255
Fungus, 124-125, 131, 134-136, 138

G

Galactogogue, 252
Gallbladder, 20, 42-44, 58, 70, 100, 145-147, 193
    and Emotions, 58, 70
    and Meridian, 42-44
Gastroenteritis, 97
Gastrointestinal disorders, 99
Genetically modified organisms (GMOs), 96-98, 103, 244-245, 250, 326
Genetics, 205, 238-241
Genetic testing, 240-241
Genitourinary system, 215, 226
Geopathic imbalances, 162
GERD (*See* Indigestion)
Germs, 119
Gerson cancer therapy program, 226
Glandulars, 198, 203, 209-210, 213, 217, 221, 230
Gluten intolerance, 146, 151
GMOs (*See* Genetically modified organisms)
Goodheart, George, 4-5, 233
Grain, 67, 97, 101-103, 189, 192, 194, 209, 218, 220, 223
Growing pains, 272
Gut, 144-145, 159 (*Also see* Leaky gut syndrome)

H

Hair loss, 146, 215, 220-221
Handmodes, 4-5, 12, 64, 86
Hashimoto's disease, 151
Hashimoto's thyroiditis, 146
Hay fever, 95, 99
Headaches, 8, 32, 35, 42, 95, 105, 127, 139, 141, 146
    and EMF, 170, 174
    and PMS, 188, 195
Head injuries, 264-265
Heart, 7-9, 19, 40, 42, 44, 51, 59-60, 146, 159, 174, 210
    and Bach flower remedies, 87
    and Chakras, 78, 81, 85
    and Disease, 205, 223, 298-301
    and Emotions, 59, 69
    and Imbalance, 141, 162, 205
    and Menopause, 205
    and Meridians, 34-35, 50, 141, 205, 223, 225
    and PMS, 196
Heart attacks, 327-331
Heart burn (*See* Indigestion)
Heavy metal toxicity, 174, 217, 227
Heel stick (*See* PKU test)
Hemorrhoids, 39, 99, 223
Herbology, 280,
Herbs, 135, 157, 280, 289, 291,
    and Clinical kinesiology, 109-110
    and Immune system, 121
Hernia, 32, 39, 215, 219, 222, 223
Hip pain (*See* Pain)
Histamine, 157
Hives, 146
Homeopathy, 56-58
Hormones, 128, 135, 145
Hormone replacement therapy, 128, 149
Hormones, 184-185
    and EMF, 174
    and Men, 228
    and Menopause, 200, 202-204, 208, 210-211
    and PMS, 183, 185-187, 191
Hot flashes, 42, 194, 203, 212
Hydrochloric acid (HCL), 32, 100, 211, 222-223, 232-233
Hyperactivity, 127, 146, 215-218, 221, 232
Hypertension (*See* Blood pressure)
Hypotension (*See* Blood pressure)
Hypno-birthing, 238
Hypoglycemia, 22,
Hypothalamus, 41, 69, 79, 183-184, 195-204, 211-213, 217-218, 221, 228, 232
Hypothyroidism, 146, 251-252

I

Immune system, 51, 61, 115, 122, 93-106, 111-122, 294-297
    and Candida, 127-129
    and Children, 248-250, 256, 258
    and EMF, 174-175
    and Herbs, 135
    and Leaky gut syndrome, 149-150
    and Men, 226, 229-230
    and Menopause, 210
    and Supplements, 135
Immunizations, 111-112, 117-121
Impetigo, 272
Impotence, 226-227, 232
Incontinence, 38-39, 62, 206, 228
Increased intestinal permeability (*See* Leaky gut syndrome)
Influenza (*See* Colds and flu)
Indicator muscle, 12-14, 18, 27, 49, 61, 86
Indigestion, 8, 35, 99, 332-335
Inflammation, 45-46, 127, 145-150, 187, 190-191, 209-210, 223, 229, 322-326 (*Also see* Arthritis; Colitis; Crohn's disease; Rheumatoid arthritis)
Inflammatory bowel disease, 146
Insect bites, 259
Institute for Sane Medication Practices (ISMP), 280
Insomnia, 146, 191, 196, 203, 221, 336-341
Insulin, 188, 310, 314 (*Also see* Diabetes; Blood sugar)
International College of Applied Kinesiology, 4
Intestinal flora, 153, 156 (*Also see* Probiotics)
Intestinal mucosal lining, 145
Iodine, 252, 254
Iron, 189-190, 230, 255-256
Irritable bowel syndrome, 3, 99, 146
Irritability, 255, 273

J

Joints, 99-101, 113 (*Also see* Arthritis; Pain)
Juicing, 193

K

Kefir, 132, 154, 156
Kegel exercises, 206, 230-231
Kidney, 110, 206, 218, 220, 223
    and Bach flower remedies, 81
    and Chakras, 77
    and Emotions, 62, 70
    and Meridians, 17, 38-39, 218-219, 223, 227
Kundalini energy (*See* Chakras)

L

Lactose, 246-249, 253
Lactose intolerance (*See* Probiotics)
Large intestine, 49, 61, 125, 127, 1129, 147
    and Chakras, 77
    and Emotions, 62, 70
    and Meridians, 30-31
Laser therapy, 36, 44-47
Leaky gut questionnaire, 151
Leaky gut syndrome, 100, 127, 137, 141, 143-160, 255-256, 285
Lesser, Ken, 162, 171, 176
Liver, 19-20, 43-44, 51, 57-58, 145, 147, 184-185, 192-193, 227
    and Dysfunction, 146
    and Emotions, 57, 70
    and Imbalance, 182, 215, 220
    and Meridians, 44-45, 228, 227-228, 230-231
    and Statin drugs, 298-299
    and Toxicity, 93, 97, 100-101, 285-286, 290
Liver flush, 193-194
Lung, 19-20, 49, 61
    and Emotions, 61, 69
    and Imbalance, 215
    and Meridians, 27, 29-30
Lupus, 113, 129, 137, 140-141, 146, 151, 202
Lymphatic system, 114

M

Magnesium, 133, 150, 158, 189-192, 209, 218, 230
Magnet therapy, 47-48
Magnetic resonance imaging (MRI), 163, 173-174
Malabsorption of nutrients, 146
Malnutrition, 146
Manganese, 98, 121, 135, 150, 252
Massage, 46
Measles, 117, 119
Meat, 97, 101, 104
Meditation, 22, 58, 65, 76-77, 82
Memory loss, 130, 138, 143, 146, 151
Mendel, Gregor, 238-239
Menopause, 194, 200-214
Menstrual cycle, 42, 174, 181, 185, 193-198, 203-208, 212
Mercury amalgams, 95, 226 (*Also see* Amalgam)
Meridians (*See* Acupuncture; *and individual meridians*)
Metal element, 61
Microbes, 134, 147, 156, 250, 262
Microbiome, 250
Microwaves (*See* EMF)
Migraines, 127, 146, 151
Milk, 97-100, 128, 132, 135, 154, 156, 187, 218 (*Also see* Breast milk)
Mold, 126-127, 131, 138
Monsanto, 97-98, 187
Mother's lactation tonic, 252, 268
Mucosal membrane, 144-145, 148-150
Multiple sclerosis, 113, 129-130, 137, 146, 151, 174, 227, 284, 298
Mumps, 117
Muscle testing, 7-11, 13-18, 86, 109, 165, 210
Myocardial infarction, 327-331

N

Nambudripad's allergy elimination techniques (NAET), 108
Nasal congestion, 139, 146, 259
Nausea, 34-35, 99, 170, 174, 194, 204, 211, 253, 268
Naval chakra, 77-78
Necrotizing enterocolitis (NEC), 248-249, 255
Nervous system, 25, 66, 74, 118-119, 127, 129, 134, 144, 146, 168
    and EMF, 164, 168, 170
    and PMS, 188,
    and Men, 218
Neuro-emotional remedies, 56-57
Neuro-linguistic programming, 10
Neurotransmitters, 66-67, 195, 209
Niacin (*See* B vitamins)
Nightshades, 101
Nutrition (*See* Diet)

O

Okra, 157-158

Omega 3 fatty acids, 304, 307
Organ-emotion questionnaire, 68
Organic food, 104-105, 187, 193
Osteoporosis, 186, 203
Ovary, 45, 184, 198, 204, 208-209, 213
Oxytocin, 251
Oxygen, 114, 121

P

Pain, 4, 7-11, 18, 42, 58, 64, 176, 206, 216, 223, 229, 290-293 (*Also see* Headaches)
    and Arm, 30-31, 35, 42, 205
    and Back, 35, 38, 45, 206-207
    and Chest, 222
    and Foot, 183
    and Hip, 38, 42, 183, 206-207, 210
    and Joint, 99, 130, 138-139, 146, 151
    and Leg, 32, 34, 38-39, 183
    and Stomach, 31, 34-35, 99, 221-222
Pancreas, 19, 22, 60-61, 69, 78, 145, 147
    and Dysfunction, 146
    and Emotions, 60-61, 69
Pantothenic acid (B5) (*See* B vitamins)
Parasites, 124, 131, 136, 145, 149-151
Parkinson's disease, 174, 227
Pasteur, Louis, 116-117
Pasteurization, 101
Pathogenic bacteria, 145, 150, 159
Peristalsis, 147
Pharmaceutical drugs, 104, 110, 117, 125-126 (*Also see* Antibiotics)
Pharmacology, 280
Physician's Desk Reference (PDR), 280, 287-288
Phytonutrients, 156-157
Pink eye (*See* Conjunctivitis)
Pituitary gland, 40, 79, 183-185, 194, 198, 204, 213, 228
PKU test, 237
PMS questionnaire, 196
Poison ivy, 259-260
Polio, 117, 119-120
Potassium, 191, 210, 230
Prebiotics, 153, 156-157
Premenstrual syndrome (PMS), 139, 181-199
Prescription Drug Chart, 281-283
Preservatives (*See* Diet)
Probiotics, 124, 132, 134, 141, 147, 149, 248-249, 253
Progesterone, 128, 185-186, 191, 195, 201-204, 210-211 (*Also see* Hormones)
Prostate, 45, 60, 226, 228-232
Prostatitis, 229
Proton pump inhibitors (PPIs), 330 (*Also see* Indigestion)
Prozac, 305-306
Psoriasis, 130, 146
Psychoneuroimmunology, 64, 115-116

Q
Quercetin, 157-158

R
Radiation therapy, 149
Rashes, 127, 139, 146, 151
Rectum, 147
Red blood cells, 114

Reiter's syndrome, 146
Respiratory system, 42
Reticular activating system, 6
Rheumatoid arthritis, 113, 137, 146
Root chakra, 77
Rosacea, 146
Round Up®, 97-98
Ryodoraku (*See* Acupuncture)

S

Sadness, 57, 59, 61, 63, 69
Schizophrenia, 146
Scleroderma, 113
Seasonal affective disorder, 78
Selective serotonin reuptake inhibitor (SSRI), 305, 337
Selenium, 135, 210, 230, 256
Serotonin, 66, 248, 255
Shingles, 259
Sinus infections, 143, 146
Sinus, 31-32, 78, 95, 99
Sitz bath, 193, 195, 202, 209, 228
Skin cancer, 229
Sleep Disorders, 42, 336-341 (*Also see* Insomnia)
Small intestine, 144-148
    and Emotions, 59
    and Meridian, 35-36
Smith, Ed, 252-253
Smoking, 28, 191, 202, 243-244
Sore throat, 30, 32, 35, 42-45, 78, 139, 146
Spine, 38, 74, 76-77
Spleen, 60, 113-114
    and Bach flower remedies, 87
    and Chakras, 77, 81, 86
    and Emotions, 60-61, 69, 81
    and Meridians, 33-34, 50
Statins, 298-301, 311
Steroids, 128, 149, 151
Stomach, 32, 34, 60, 78, 97-99, 115, 145-146, 222 (*Also see* Pain)
    and Acid, 211, 222, 233
    and Emotions, 60, 69
    and Meridians, 31-32, 50, 223
Streptococcus, 126, 159
Stress, 10, 63, 67, 115-116, 210, 218
    and EMF, 176
    and Men, 215, 219-223
    and Menopause, 200, 202
    and PMS, 184, 187-188, 198
Stroke, 42, 223, 327-331
Suicide, 304-306
Sunburn, 259
Surgery, 11, 38, 42-43, 183, 206-209, 219, 226
Surrogate muscle testing, 250-251
Swelling, 138-139, 146
Symptom log, 28

T

T-cells, 113-115, 121
Tea, 190, 192, 194, 210
Teething, 273
Teishein, 46-47
Therapy localization, 18-20
Third eye, 79 (*Also see* Chakras)
Throat chakra, 78
Throat, 190 (*Also see* Sore throat)
Thymus, 78, 113-115

Thyroid, 42, 51, 60, 69, 78, 93, 114-117, 248, 251-252
    and EMF, 174
    and Imbalance, 100-101
    and Men, 228
    and Menopause, 203-205, 207-208, 210, 212-213
    and PMS, 183-185, 190, 194, 197
Tight junctions, 148-150
Tissues, 127, 146-148
Tonsillectomy, 284
Trace minerals, 22, 135
Triple warmer meridian, 41-42
Tryptophan, 248, 255
Tubal ligation, 183, 201, 208
Turmeric, 157

U

Ulcerative colitis, 146, 151, 255
Ulcers, 32, 99, 221-222
Ultrasound, 241
Upper respiratory infection, 256, 259
Uterus, 182-185, 194-197, 201, 205-213, 228

V

Vaccinations, 117-121, 258 (*Also see* Immunizations)
Vaginal infections, 127, 134-135, 139
Vasectomy, 225-226
Viruses, 113, 117-118, 120
Vitamins, 109-110, 192, 209-210 (*Also see* B vitamins)
    Vitamin A, 102, 121, 189, 221, 223
    Vitamin C, 66, 121, 158, 210, 218, 221, 223-224, 229-230
    and Children, 256
    Vitamin D_3, 102, 230, 254, 256, 298, 307
    Vitamin E, 121, 158, 191-192, 205, 221, 224, 226, 230, 314
    Vitamin K_2, 299
    Vitamin U, 155, 158
Vomiting, 99, 194, 204, 223

W

Warts, 259
Water element, 62, 74, 77
Weight gain, 146
Weston A. Price Foundation, 253
White blood cells, 105, 113-116, 149, 172, 284, 322-323, 327
Whole grains, 67, 133, 156, 311-314 (*Also see* Grains)
Wood element, 57

X

Xango® juice, 144, 158, 290, 333
Xanthones, 144, 158

Y

Yeast infections, 127
Yoga, 76, 88
Yogurt, 132, 154, 156

Z

Zinc, 121, 135, 188-189, 192, 218, 223-224, 228-230
    and Children, 248

Contact Information

ABOUT THE AUTHOR

SUSAN L. LEVY, D.C. has extensive training in massage, polarity therapy, nutrition, herbology, is a registered nurse, a Chiropractor, and is certified in acupuncture by the International Academy of Medical Acupuncture. Dr. Levy's positive, gentle, healing presence promotes an alternative method for restoring and maintaining your health. She approaches the broad topics of human body function and dysfunction from several vantage points, including multiple health care disciplines, traditions, and philosophies. Her popular seminars, newsletters and articles emphasize natural health care through balance, harmony, expertise and love. She continues to research pathways to assist her patients as expediently as possible, and is eager to share this remarkable approach with her colleagues. She lives in Colorado where she was named Chiropractor of the Year in 1985.

Contact:
Advanced Health Systems / Natural Solutions: 800-770-6704
YourBodyCanTalk@gmail.com; *www.yourbodycantalk.com*

ABOUT KALINDI PRESS

KALINDI PRESS, an affiliate of HOHM PRESS, proudly offers books in natural health and nutrition, as well as the acclaimed *Family and World Health Series* for children and parents, covering such themes as nutrition, dental health, reading, and environmental education.

Contact:
hppublisher@cableone.net; www.kalindipress.com